CLINICAL SYMPOSIA
ANTHOLOGY

Dedicated to

THE NEW PHYSICIAN

CLINICAL SYMPOSIA ANTHOLOGY

J. HAROLD WALTON, M.D., *Editor*

FRANK H. NETTER, M.D., *Illustrator*

CIBA PHARMACEUTICAL COMPANY

SUMMIT, NEW JERSEY

C I B A

CIBA PHARMACEUTICAL COMPANY

SUMMIT, NEW JERSEY

DIVISION OF CIBA CORPORATION

PRINTED IN U.S.A.   B/00/6294

FOREWORD

This volume contains seven of the most popular issues of *Clinical Symposia* published during the last decade. *Clinical Symposia* is published four times a year by CIBA for the medical profession. Each issue contains one or more articles of clinical significance in medicine and surgery. The text is supplied by leading authorities. The illustrations — most of them in full color — are by the renowned medical illustrator, Frank H. Netter, M.D.

Some of the accompanying illustrations appear in *The CIBA Collection of Medical Illustrations.* This is a continuing series of atlases portraying normal and pathologic anatomy — including surgical and manipulative techniques — involving all systems of the human organism. Volume 4 in the series will be issued October, 1965.

CONTENTS

SECTION A

CIBA

SURGICAL ANATOMY OF THE HAND
Ernest W. Lampe, M.D.

SURGICAL ANATOMY OF THE HAND

With Special Reference to Infections and Trauma

ERNEST W. LAMPE, M.D.

Assistant Professor of Surgery, Assistant Professor of Clinical Anatomy
Cornell University Medical College, New York City

EDITOR'S NOTE: Dr. Lampe's monograph, *Surgical Anatomy of the Hand,* was originally published in our December 1951 edition. Scarcely a day has passed in the interim without requests for additional copies, and hence our supply became exhausted long ago. Thus, for all who have found "The Hand" so invaluable in the past and for the many who have never been able to acquire it, we are happy to republish this masterpiece of concise exposition.

Chemotherapy and better early care have decreased the incidence of serious infections of the hand. Still, a considerable number become sufficiently severe to warrant surgery. Add to these the vastly increased number of traumatized hands that demand repair, and it becomes quite evident that surgery of the hand is still an important part of surgical therapeutics. Other qualifications being equal, the surgeon with the sounder knowledge of the surgical anatomy of the hand should achieve the better end-results.

While nothing especially new is presented in this monograph, we have attempted to emphasize, by figures, diagrams, and text, certain anatomical structures and relationships, which may be found helpful to the surgeon called upon to treat a serious tendon-sheath-space infection or a badly lacerated hand.

SKIN AND SUBCUTANEOUS FASCIA OF THE HAND

Figures 1, 2, 3, and 25 demonstrate the important structural differences between the subcutaneous tissue of the palm and that of the dorsum of the hand.

In the palm, innumerable minute, but strong, fibrous fasciculi extend from the palmar aponeurosis to the skin. These hold the skin close to the underlying palmar aponeurosis, permitting comparatively little sliding movement of one upon the other. Also, these thread-like fibrous strands divide the subcutaneous fat into small, irregular masses. Numerous, minute blood vessels pass through this subcutaneous tissue to the derma.

Clinically, it is important to remember the relationship of the fibrous fasciculi to the skin, fat, and blood vessels. In *Dupuytren's contracture,* hypertrophy and hyperplasia of this fibrous tissue result in ultimate displacement of the fat masses and partial obliteration of the blood vessels, thereby interfering markedly with the nutrition of the skin. Obviously, this points to the wisdom of early surgical excision of the palmar aponeurosis in Dupuytren's contracture.

Contrast the tight relationship of the palmar aponeurosis, subcutaneous tissue, and skin of the palm with the looseness of these structures on the dorsum of the hand! Figures 3 and 25 show the looseness of areolar tissue which creates the so-called *dorsal subcutaneous space.*

This tissue is so lax that a fold of the skin grasped between one's thumb and index finger can be elevated several centimeters off the underlying deep fascia. In fact, it is so loose that the skin can be separated readily from the deep fascia by blunt dissection — quite different from the palm where this must be done by very sharp dissection. The course of the sensory nerves, veins, and lymphatics through this loose areolar layer is clearly shown in Figure 3.

It is important to emphasize that most of the lymph from the palmar aspects of the fingers, web-areas, hypothenar and thenar eminences flows into myriads of lymph channels and lacunae located in the loose areolar layer on the dorsum of the hand (see pages 12 and 16).

This anatomic fact accounts for the marked lymphedematous swelling frequently seen on the back of the hand even when the focus of infection is on the palmar aspect of the finger, web-space, hypothenar or thenar area. Occasionally, the unwitting one mistakenly incises the back of such a swollen hand and to his dismay finds lymphedema instead of pus.

Dorsal Deep Fascia

On the dorsum of the hand, the deep fascia and extensor tendons fuse to form the roof for the *dorsal subaponeurotic space* (Figures 3, 17, 25). Because of the barrier formed by the metacarpal bones and interosseous muscles and the manner of flow and location of the lymphatics, this space is not very frequently involved in hand infections. Metacarpal osteomyelitis and direct penetration of the space by a sharp, contaminated instrument are causes for those rare accumulations of pus found in this space.

Palmar Deep Fascia

Figures 1 and 2 show the intimate contact of the deep fascia to the thenar and hypothenar groups of muscles. This relationship prevents formation of a space over these muscles within which pus may accumulate.

The central, triangular-shaped part of the palmar aponeurosis has several anatomical features worthy of mention. In *Dupuytren's contracture,* the clinical significance of its attachment to the derma and its relationship to the subcutaneous fat and blood vessels have already been mentioned. Figures on page 9 show that the proximal end is continuous with the tendon of the palmaris longus muscle. It is this attachment that enables the palmaris longus muscle to assist in flexion of the hand.

Figures 1, 2, 4, and 25 demonstrate the protective thickness of the central triangular part and also the manner of its fusion medially and laterally with the deep fascia covering the hypothenar and thenar muscles, respectively. An understanding of this relationship helps one realize why the great majority of hand infections, excluding fingers, are found in the hollow of the palm between or distal to the hypothenar and thenar eminences.

At the base of the aponeurotic triangle, the interlacing fasciculi of the superficial transverse metacarpal ligament add protection to the underlying digital vessels and nerves (Figure 2). Fasciculi extend to the proximal phalanges to fuse with the fibrous annular tendon sheath on its palmar, medial, and lateral aspects. These insertions enable the palmaris longus muscle to help in flexing the proximal phalanges.

In the distal part of the palm, septa

extend from the deep aspect of the palmar aponeurosis to the deep transverse palmar ligament forming the sides of annular fibrous canals for the passage of the ensheathed flexor tendons and lumbrical muscles as well as blood vessels and nerves (Figures 4, 5, 25).

The semidiagrammatic cross section on page 25 shows a septum extending from the palmar aponeurosis to the third metacarpal. Frequently, but not always, this septum separates the thenar space or bursa from the midpalmar space or bursa. The beginnings of the other less well-developed septa are also shown in this figure. Since this section is proximal to the deep transverse metacarpal ligament, located at the distal ends of the metacarpal bones, these septa appear unattached on their deep aspect. However, just distal to the ends of the midpalmar and thenar spaces, they are actually attached to the deep transverse metacarpal ligament.

BLOOD AND LYMPH VESSELS

Figures 4, 6, and 7 show how the *radial* and *ulnar arteries* terminate by dividing into superficial and deep branches. The former anastomose in the palm to form the *superficial palmar arterial arch*, the latter to form the *deep arch*.

A line drawn across the palm at the level of the distal border of the fully abducted thumb marks the approximate location of the superficial arterial arch. This is shown as a broken line in Figure 6. The deep arch is a finger's breadth proximal.

The pulsation of the *ulnar artery* can usually be felt just lateral to the pisiform bone. Immediately distal to this point the artery divides into its larger branch which forms most of the superficial arch and the smaller branch which forms

the lesser part of the deep palmar arch.

Just proximal to the pisiform bone the ulnar artery gives off volar and dorsal carpal branches which unite with the volar and dorsal branches of the radial artery to form the arterial wristlet about the carpal bones. Perforating branches passing between the proximal ends of the middle metacarpal bones connect the deep palmar arch with the dorsal carpal arch, as shown in Figure 17. The latter sends small branches to the phalanges.

The pulsation of the *radial artery* is usually palpated near the proximal volar carpal skin crease. Here the superficial branch arises to continue distally over or through the thenar eminence to the palm to complete the formation of the superficial palmar arterial arch (Figures on page 14).

The much larger, deep radial branch, whose pulsations can be felt in the anatomical snuffbox, Figures 17 and 20, passes under the "snuffbox" tendons and plunges between the two heads of the first dorsal interosseous muscle to reach the palm where it forms the greater part of the deep palmar arch, Figure 6.

It is to be remembered that the superficial arterial arch is much larger and more important than the deep arch.

The superficial arch gives off *digital branches* which bifurcate into *phalangeal branches* about a finger's breadth proximal to the web-border of the hand, Figures 6 and 7. The superficial arch and its digital branches are immediately deep to the tough central part of the palmar aponeurosis and are superficial to the branches of the median and ulnar nerves. This relationship to the nerves is reversed in the fingers (Figures 6, 7, 16).

As shown in Figure 6, the *metacarpal branches* of the *deep arch* empty into the *digital branches* of the *superficial arch* just proximal to their bifurcation into the phalangeal arteries.

CLINICAL IMPORTANCE OF OSSEOUS
BLOOD SUPPLY

The *lunate bone* (semilunar) is the most frequently *dislocated* of all the carpal bones. Therefore, it is important to remember a few points about its blood supply. As shown in Figure 10, branches from the dorsal and volar carpal arteries reach the bone via its dorsal and volar ligaments from the radius. The bone can survive only if one ligament is torn, and good results can be expected if early reduction is effected. On the other hand, atrophic necrosis is the rule if both ligaments have been ruptured (Figure 12).

Since the *navicular* (scaphoid) is the most frequently *fractured* of the carpal bones, it is important to remember that in about two-thirds of the cases the blood vessels are evenly enough distributed to expect survival of both fragments with some chance for union. In the remaining third, however, so many of the blood vessels are located nearer one end than the other that necrosis is apt to occur in the meagerly supplied fragment (Figure 13).

A *felon* may cause necrosis of the distal end of the terminal phalanx. Unless antibiotics and supportive therapy are administered very early, edema and toxins will cause thrombosis of some of the terminal branches of the digital arteries and thus interfere sufficiently with the blood supply of the bony tuft (Figures 14, 16) to eventuate in its necrosis. Figure 15 schematically shows the numerous fibrous septa in the palmar part of the terminal phalanx — especially its distal half. The terminal vessels are found in these irregu-

larly formed expansionless compartments. It does not require much edema and toxin to cause early thrombosis with subsequent necrosis of the tuft of the phalanx.

VEINS

The hand, like the remainder of the upper extremity, is drained by two sets of veins: a superficial group located on the superficial fascia and a deep set associated with the arteries. These are illustrated in Figures 3, 4, 8, and 9.

The *superficial venous system* is the more important of the two sets because it is the larger, and most of the finger and hand lymphatics accompany its tributaries (Figures 3, 8, 9). A few small veins are found in the tight superficial or subcutaneous fascia of the palm and palmar aspects of the fingers. However, they compare neither in size nor number with those located in the loose areolar subcutaneous tissue of the dorsum of the hand and fingers. While Figure 3 offers an idea of the venous arrangement on the dorsum of the hand, one needs but hang the hand at the side for a moment to demonstrate quite clearly the dorsal venous arch. This arch receives digital veins from the fingers and frequently becomes continuous with the *cephalic* and *basilic* veins on the radial and ulnar borders of the wrist. A glance at the volar aspect not uncommonly reveals the distal end of the *median antebrachial* vein near the carpal creases, where it receives the few, small and usually invisible, superficial palmar veins.

The above-mentioned veins — *cephalic*, *basilic*, and *median antebrachial* — continue proximad; and they, with their tributaries, make up the superficial venous drainage of the upper extremity.

The *deep venous* return is not difficult

to review if one recalls that the very small digital veins, helping to drain the fingers, empty into small superficial and deep venous arches associated respectively with the superficial and deep arterial arches, Figures 4 and 6. These two venous arches help form the venae comites which accompany the radial and ulnar arteries; and they, with their tributaries, make up the deep venous drainage of the forearm. At the elbow the radial and ulnar venae comites unite to form the venae comites of the brachial artery, and they in turn unite with the basilic vein at the pectoral fold to form the axillary vein.

In the hand, forearm, and arm the superficial and deep sets of veins anastomose with each other by means of a variable number of communicating or perforating veins.

If one knows the venous drainage of the hand, one can easily visualize the lymph drainage because, generally speaking, the lymph vessels follow the veins, having originated from the same mesenchymal tissue. This implies the presence of a *superficial* and *deep* set of lymph vessels corresponding to the superficial and deep sets of veins.

Superficial Lymph Vessels

While some of the proximal phalangeal and web-area lymph vessels proceed palmward, most of them head for the dorsum of the fingers and hand (Figure 9).

Most of the lymph from the thenar and hypothenar areas flows toward the vessels and lacunae in the subcutaneous loose areolar tissue — the so-called dorsal subcutaneous space. This should remind one again of the reason for the frequent swelling (lymphedema) of the dorsum of the hand in the presence of an infection on the palmar aspect of a finger, web-area, or edge of the thenar or hypothenar eminence.

Most of the lymph from the dorsum leaves via lymph vessels accompanying the cephalic and basilic veins. This is shown by the black arrows in Figure 3. In theory at least, bacteria or tumor cells from a focus on the thumb or index finger have easier access to the thoracic ducts, since they tend to follow the cephalic vein. The lymph gland in the deltopectoral triangle is the first sizable node encountered by the lymph channels following this vein. Contrast this relatively gland-free pathway with the gland-studded route along the basilic and axillary veins (Figure 8).

Deep Lymph Vessels

Figure 9 shows schematically how most of the central palmar lymph vessels proceed deeply to join the lymph vessels associated with the superficial and deep venous arches. From here lymph channels follow the venae comites of the radial and ulnar arteries.

The median, ulnar, and radial nerves furnish most of the motor and sensory control of the hand. The dorsal antebrachial cutaneous and lateral antebrachial cutaneous nerves assist variably in supplying sensory nerves.

Motor Nerves

The intrinsic muscles of the hand are controlled by the ulnar and median nerves (Figures 5, 6, 7, 28). Since these muscles are not the sole manipulators of the hand, the radial nerve, which assists in supplying the extrinsic muscles, must also be considered.

Ordinarily, the muscles on the anterior or volar-medial aspect of the forearm are referred to as the volar forearm group, and those on the posterior or dorsolateral side as the dorsal group — names which tell nothing more than their location.

It might be even more helpful if broad functional names were applied to them because they would always remind one of what these important muscle groups do. For example: It is known that the flexors of the hand (flexors carpi radialis and ulnaris), Figures 21 and 23; flexors of the fingers (flexors digitorum sublimis and profundus), Figure 24; and the pronators (pronators radii teres and quadratus) are located in this so-called volar group of muscles. Would it not be a bit more practical to think of the group as the *flexor-pronator group*—a name which would tell in a general way what these muscles do?

The same applies to the dorsal group of muscles consisting of the extensors of the hand (extensors carpi radialis longus and brevis and extensor carpi ulnaris), Figure 26; the extensors of the proximal phalanges and assistant extensors of the middle phalanges (extensors digitorum communis, indicis proprius, and digiti quinti proprius); the extensors and abductor of thumb (extensors pollicis brevis and longus and abductor pollicis longus), Figures 20 and 26; and finally, the assistant supinator of the forearm or supinator muscle (the supinator muscle is referred to as the assistant supinator because the biceps muscle, supplied by the musculocutaneous nerve, is the much more important supinator). Therefore, why not call the whole dorsal forearm group of muscles the *extensor-assistant supinator* group

— supplied by the *extensor-assistant supinator nerve* — the functional name for the *radial nerve?*

In his first course in surgical diagnosis, the junior medical student learns that the usual test for *ulnar nerve* palsy is to spread and approximate the fingers; and the more common test for *median nerve* palsy is to approximate successively the tip of the thumb to the tips of the fingers.

The ulnar nerve controls certain muscles which flex the hand and fingers (flexor carpi ulnaris and the ulnar half of the flexor digitorum profundus) as well as the intrinsic muscles of the hand except those in the thenar eminence and two adjacent lumbrical muscles.

Since the interosseous muscles which spread and approximate the fingers are exclusively controlled by the ulnar nerve, this action of the interossei can serve as a test of ulnar nerve function. If the nerve is damaged, one will have difficulty in holding a piece of paper between adjacent fingers which are fully extended. Thus, the action of these muscles gives to the ulnar nerve a logical functional name: the *finger-spreader-approximator nerve.*

The median nerve controls the whole flexor-pronator group except one and one-half muscles (the ulnar nerve controls only the flexor carpi ulnaris and ulnar half of the flexor digitorum profundus), and because the median nerve innervates the lateral two lumbrical muscles and the thenar eminence muscles whose opponens muscle is *the* important muscle in approximating the thumb-tip successively to the finger tips, it seems reasonable to give the *median nerve* a functional name: the *flexor - pronator - thumb - finger - approximator nerve* — a rather long name, but it summarizes the chief motor rôle of the median nerve.

8

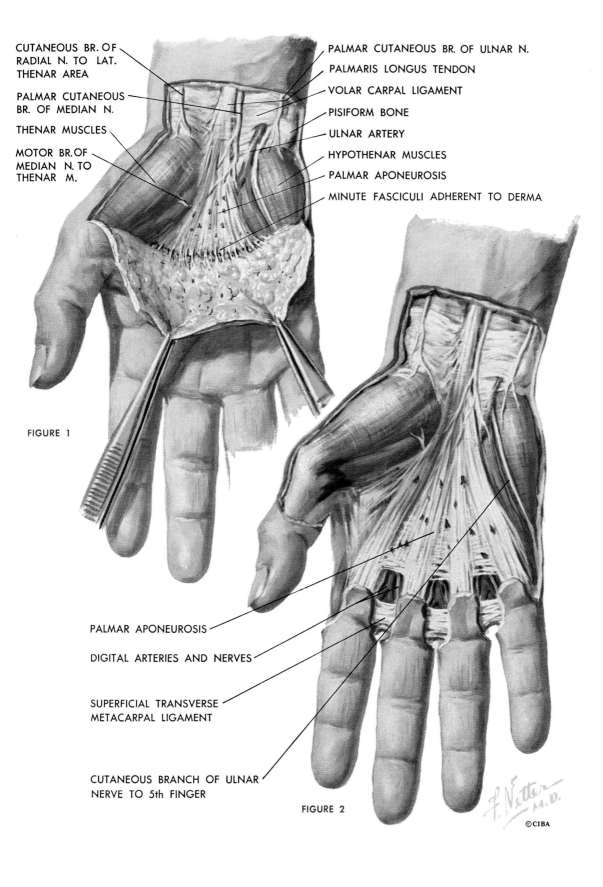

CUTANEOUS BR. OF
RADIAL N. TO LAT.
THENAR AREA

PALMAR CUTANEOUS
BR. OF MEDIAN N.

THENAR MUSCLES

MOTOR BR. OF
MEDIAN N. TO
THENAR M.

PALMAR CUTANEOUS BR. OF ULNAR N.

PALMARIS LONGUS TENDON

VOLAR CARPAL LIGAMENT

PISIFORM BONE

ULNAR ARTERY

HYPOTHENAR MUSCLES

PALMAR APONEUROSIS

MINUTE FASCICULI ADHERENT TO DERMA

FIGURE 1

PALMAR APONEUROSIS

DIGITAL ARTERIES AND NERVES

SUPERFICIAL TRANSVERSE
METACARPAL LIGAMENT

CUTANEOUS BRANCH OF ULNAR
NERVE TO 5th FINGER

FIGURE 2

F. Netter
M. D.

©CIBA

Sensory Nerves

Figure 18 shows diagrammatically a palmar view of the hand with the *median nerve* supplying the median or central palmar area and the palmar surfaces of the lateral three and one-half fingers; Figure 19, a dorsal view, charts the median nerve distribution to the dorsum of the distal two phalanges of the lateral three and one-half fingers.

Note how the *ulnar nerve* supplies sensory nerves to the volar and dorsal aspects of the medial third of the hand and the volar and dorsal aspects of the medial one and one-half fingers, Figures 3, 7, 17, 18, and 19.

The *radial nerve* conveys sensation from the lateral two-thirds of the dorsum of the hand and a portion of the thenar eminence area, as well as from the dorsum of the proximal phalanges of the lateral three and one-half fingers.

Variations of the sensory distribution of the above three nerves are quite common. For example, on the palmar surface, the median nerve may supply only the central third of the palm and the skin of two and one-half fingers, with the ulnar nerve innervating the *medial* half of the palm and two and one-half fingers. Furthermore, the lateral antebrachial cutaneous (volar branch of musculocutaneous) occasionally extends its control as far as the web-area of the thumb, index, and middle fingers. On the dorsum, the ulnar nerve may give sensory nerves to the medial half of the dorsum of the hand as well as to the dorsum of two and one-half fingers. This leaves the radial nerve offering sensory nerves to only the lateral half of the dorsum of the hand and proximal phalanges of two and one-half fingers. Occasionally, the dorsal branch of the medial antebrachial cutaneous nerve may extend distally almost to the web-area between the fifth, fourth, and third fingers; and sometimes the dorsal antebrachial cutaneous nerve may reach the web-areas between the second, third, and fourth fingers.

Figures 1 and 7 show the median and ulnar nerves in the distal forearm giving off their palmar cutaneous branches which are destined to supply the skin of the proximal palm. The median nerve passes under the tough transverse carpal ligament and divides into (a) three lateral branches — two supplying either side of the thumb and the third to the lateral aspect of the index finger, and (b) two medial branches — one dividing to innervate adjacent surfaces of the index and middle finger and the other to the adjacent aspects of the third and fourth fingers.

It is of considerable clinical importance to remember that the main muscular branch of the median nerve arises from the lateral cutaneous branch to the thumb just distal to the transverse carpal ligament, Figure 7. Observe that en route to the thenar eminence and its muscles (the flexor pollicis brevis, abductor pollicis brevis, and opponens pollicis) this small but important nerve passes over the flexor pollicis longus tendon and its sheath, Figures 4, 5, and 7. **Every surgeon opening this sheath in a case of suppurative tenosynovitis must make certain that the proximal end of his thumb incision extends no farther than the midpoint of the first metacarpal bone, thereby avoiding section of the motor nerve to the thenar eminence muscles (Figure 54).**

From the nerves supplying the lateral aspect of the index finger and adjacent sides of the second and third fingers arise small branches respectively to the first and second lumbrical muscles.

The *ulnar nerve,* shown in Figures 4, 6, 7, and 28, passes lateral to the pisiform bone, and just distally it bifurcates into superficial and deep rami. The former, after giving a filament to the unimportant palmaris brevis muscle, promptly divides into a branch to the medial aspect of the fifth finger, a branch supplying contiguous surfaces of the fifth and fourth fingers, and finally a fine twig which unites with the most medial branch of the median nerve (Figure 7). The deep ramus of the ulnar nerve furnishes muscular branches to the hypothenar eminence muscles (the abductor dig. quinti, flexor dig. quinti, opponens dig. quinti) and to the three volar and dorsal interosseous muscles, and the adductor pollicis muscle (Figure 28). The tiny branches to the third and fourth lumbrical muscles and the deep head of the flexor pollicis brevis muscle can be seen.

Lesions of the radial, median, and ulnar nerves will be discussed after the muscles have been reviewed.

MUSCLES OF THE HAND

Muscles of the hand can be grouped as *extrinsic* and *intrinsic.* While the muscle bellies of the former are in the forearm, their tendons, nevertheless, are in the hand and play a very important part in its movements.

Supination of the hand, be it recalled, is controlled chiefly by the biceps located in the arm and inserted into the radial tuberosity, assisted by the supinator muscle originating from the proximal dorsolateral aspect of the ulna, wrapping itself laterally around the proximal fourth of the radius to insert on its volar aspect. As previously mentioned, supination is controlled mainly by the musculocutaneous nerve supplying the powerful biceps and assisted by the radial nerve supplying the supinator muscle.

Pronation is controlled by the median nerve which supplies branches to the *pronator radii teres* and *pronator quadratus muscles* found respectively in the proximal half and distal one-fourth of the forearm.

Adduction of the hand at the wrist is produced by the combined action of the *flexor carpi ulnaris* and the *extensor carpi ulnaris muscles* — the former innervated by the *ulnar* nerve and the latter by the *radial* nerve. Figure 21 shows the *ulnar flexor* tendon on its way to insert into the pisiform, hamate, and fifth metacarpal bones. In Figures 17 and 26, the *ulnar extensor* tendon is seen proceeding to the dorsum of the fifth metacarpal bone.

Abduction, like adduction, is effected by the combined action of two or more muscles. To produce abduction, the *flexor carpi radialis* contracts synergistically with the *extensors carpi radialis longus* and *brevis.* Figure 21 shows the *radial flexor* tendon en route to the volar aspect of the base of the second and third metacarpal bones. In Figures 17 and 20, the terminal ends of the two *radial extensors* are seen just before they insert into the proximal dorsal parts of the second and third metacarpal bones.

In addition to producing abduction, these three muscles have another important rôle. Recall that the second and third metacarpal bones are fixed *proximally* by ligaments to each other and to the *capitate* and *lesser multangular* bones of the *transverse carpal arch.* Distally, they are firmly anchored to each other by the *deep transverse metacarpal ligament.* These strong proximal and distal attachments of the second and third metacarpal bones

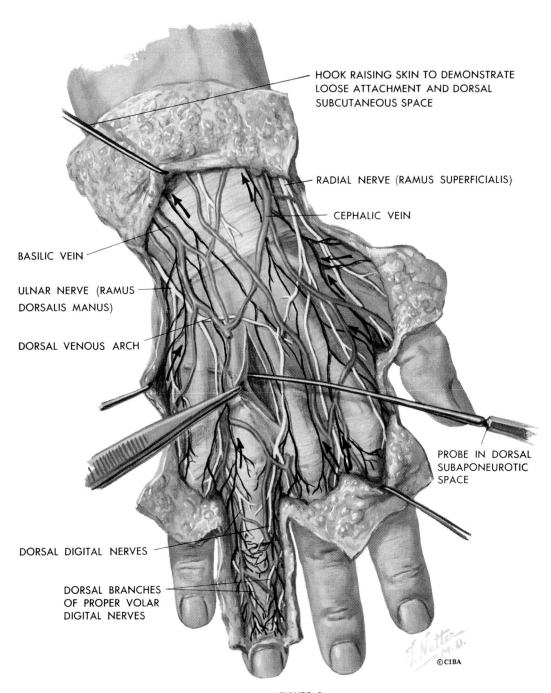

HOOK RAISING SKIN TO DEMONSTRATE LOOSE ATTACHMENT AND DORSAL SUBCUTANEOUS SPACE

RADIAL NERVE (RAMUS SUPERFICIALIS)

CEPHALIC VEIN

BASILIC VEIN

ULNAR NERVE (RAMUS DORSALIS MANUS)

DORSAL VENOUS ARCH

PROBE IN DORSAL SUBAPONEUROTIC SPACE

DORSAL DIGITAL NERVES

DORSAL BRANCHES OF PROPER VOLAR DIGITAL NERVES

FIGURE 3

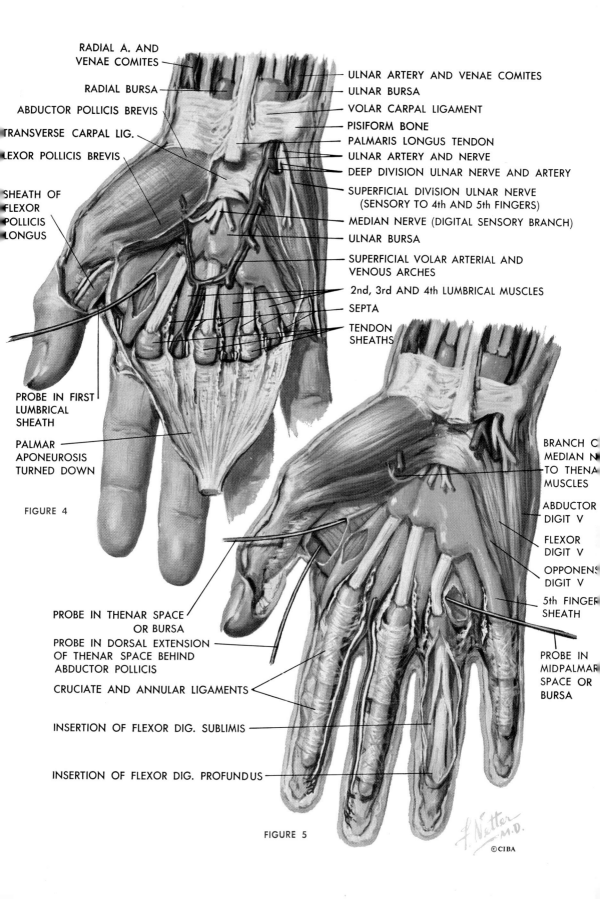

RADIAL A. AND VENAE COMITES

RADIAL BURSA

ABDUCTOR POLLICIS BREVIS

TRANSVERSE CARPAL LIG.

FLEXOR POLLICIS BREVIS

SHEATH OF FLEXOR POLLICIS LONGUS

PROBE IN FIRST LUMBRICAL SHEATH

PALMAR APONEUROSIS TURNED DOWN

FIGURE 4

ULNAR ARTERY AND VENAE COMITES

ULNAR BURSA

VOLAR CARPAL LIGAMENT

PISIFORM BONE

PALMARIS LONGUS TENDON

ULNAR ARTERY AND NERVE

DEEP DIVISION ULNAR NERVE AND ARTERY

SUPERFICIAL DIVISION ULNAR NERVE
(SENSORY TO 4th AND 5th FINGERS)

MEDIAN NERVE (DIGITAL SENSORY BRANCH)

ULNAR BURSA

SUPERFICIAL VOLAR ARTERIAL AND VENOUS ARCHES

2nd, 3rd AND 4th LUMBRICAL MUSCLES

SEPTA

TENDON SHEATHS

BRANCH C MEDIAN N TO THENA MUSCLES

ABDUCTOR DIGIT V

FLEXOR DIGIT V

OPPONENS DIGIT V

5th FINGER SHEATH

PROBE IN MIDPALMAR SPACE OR BURSA

PROBE IN THENAR SPACE OR BURSA

PROBE IN DORSAL EXTENSION OF THENAR SPACE BEHIND ABDUCTOR POLLICIS

CRUCIATE AND ANNULAR LIGAMENTS

INSERTION OF FLEXOR DIG. SUBLIMIS

INSERTION OF FLEXOR DIG. PROFUNDUS

FIGURE 5

f. Netter M.D.

©CIBA

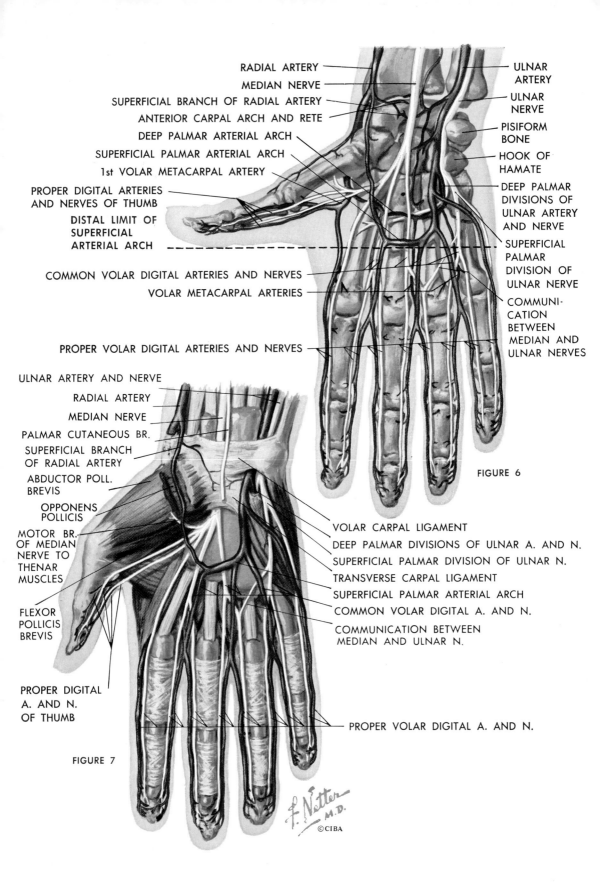

RADIAL ARTERY

MEDIAN NERVE

SUPERFICIAL BRANCH OF RADIAL ARTERY

ANTERIOR CARPAL ARCH AND RETE

DEEP PALMAR ARTERIAL ARCH

SUPERFICIAL PALMAR ARTERIAL ARCH

1st VOLAR METACARPAL ARTERY

PROPER DIGITAL ARTERIES AND NERVES OF THUMB

DISTAL LIMIT OF SUPERFICIAL ARTERIAL ARCH

COMMON VOLAR DIGITAL ARTERIES AND NERVES

VOLAR METACARPAL ARTERIES

PROPER VOLAR DIGITAL ARTERIES AND NERVES

ULNAR ARTERY

ULNAR NERVE

PISIFORM BONE

HOOK OF HAMATE

DEEP PALMAR DIVISIONS OF ULNAR ARTERY AND NERVE

SUPERFICIAL PALMAR DIVISION OF ULNAR NERVE

COMMUNICATION BETWEEN MEDIAN AND ULNAR NERVES

FIGURE 6

ULNAR ARTERY AND NERVE

RADIAL ARTERY

MEDIAN NERVE

PALMAR CUTANEOUS BR.

SUPERFICIAL BRANCH OF RADIAL ARTERY

ABDUCTOR POLL. BREVIS

OPPONENS POLLICIS

MOTOR BR. OF MEDIAN NERVE TO THENAR MUSCLES

FLEXOR POLLICIS BREVIS

PROPER DIGITAL A. AND N. OF THUMB

VOLAR CARPAL LIGAMENT

DEEP PALMAR DIVISIONS OF ULNAR A. AND N.

SUPERFICIAL PALMAR DIVISION OF ULNAR N.

TRANSVERSE CARPAL LIGAMENT

SUPERFICIAL PALMAR ARTERIAL ARCH

COMMON VOLAR DIGITAL A. AND N.

COMMUNICATION BETWEEN MEDIAN AND ULNAR N.

PROPER VOLAR DIGITAL A. AND N.

FIGURE 7

F. Netter M.D.

©CIBA

make them the most *stable* or *fixed* part of the hand.

The *extensors carpi radialis longus* and *brevis* insert into the dorsum of the proximal end of the second and third metacarpals; and, while there is only one *flexor carpi radialis,* it is very powerful and gains insertion into the volar aspects of the proximal ends of the second and third metacarpal bones. With this arrangement, it is easy to see how these three strong muscles, along with the above-mentioned ligaments, aid in stabilizing the most fixed part of the hand, especially in flexion and extension movements of the fingers.

In many reconstructive procedures of the badly mutilated hand, it is imperative for the surgeon to remember this important muscle-tendon-bone-ligament combination. *Flexion of the hand* at the wrist is effected by the *flexors carpi radialis* and *ulnaris* supplied respectively by the median and ulnar nerves. The former originates from the medial humeral epicondyle, the latter from the same epicondyle plus the proximal three-fifths of the ulna.

Extension of the hand at the wrist is produced by the *extensors carpi radialis longus* and *brevis* and the *extensor carpi ulnaris.* The *radial extensors* originate from the lateral epicondyle and distal part of the lateral epicondylar ridge, the *ulnar extensor* from the medial epicondyle and middle half of the ulna.

While the chief functions of these three muscles are extension of the hand, and abduction and adduction by working together with their fellow carpal flexors, they are also synergic muscles for flexion of the fingers because they counteract the flexor effect which the digital flexors would otherwise produce at the wrist.

Flexion of the fingers on the hand is produced mainly by the *flexors digitorum*

sublimis and *profundus.* The assistant flexor rôle of the lumbrical and interosseous muscles (flexion of proximal phalanges) will be discussed in the paragraphs dealing with the intrinsic hand muscles.

The *flexor digitorum sublimis* originates from the medial humeral epicondyle, the coronoid process of ulna, and the proximal two-thirds of the volar margin of the radius. Proximal to the volar carpal ligament, the muscle gives rise to four tendons inserting into the proximal thirds of the middle phalanges of the medial four digits. The vincula longa and breva give additional insertion into the proximal and middle phalanges.

For *clinical reasons,* the following points regarding the tendons of this muscle deserve to be remembered:

1. As is shown on pages 24 and 25, just proximal and deep to the volar carpal ligament, the third and fourth sublimis tendons lie superficial to the second and fifth tendons. This is a quite constant arrangement. However, in some cases the third, fourth, and fifth sublimis tendons will be in the superficial plane with the second or index finger tendon deep to the third sublimis tendon. Seldom are all four in one plane in this region as are the flexor digitorum profundus tendons.

2. Next, note the manner of insertion of a sublimis tendon, Figures 5, 24, and 32. The sublimis tendon first splits at the proximal end of the first phalanx to permit passage of the profundus tendon and then reunites, only to split a second time to gain insertion on each side of the proximal third of the second phalanx.

The *flexor digitorum profundus* originates from the proximal two-thirds of the ulna and the adjacent interosseous mem-

LYMPHATIC DRAINAGE

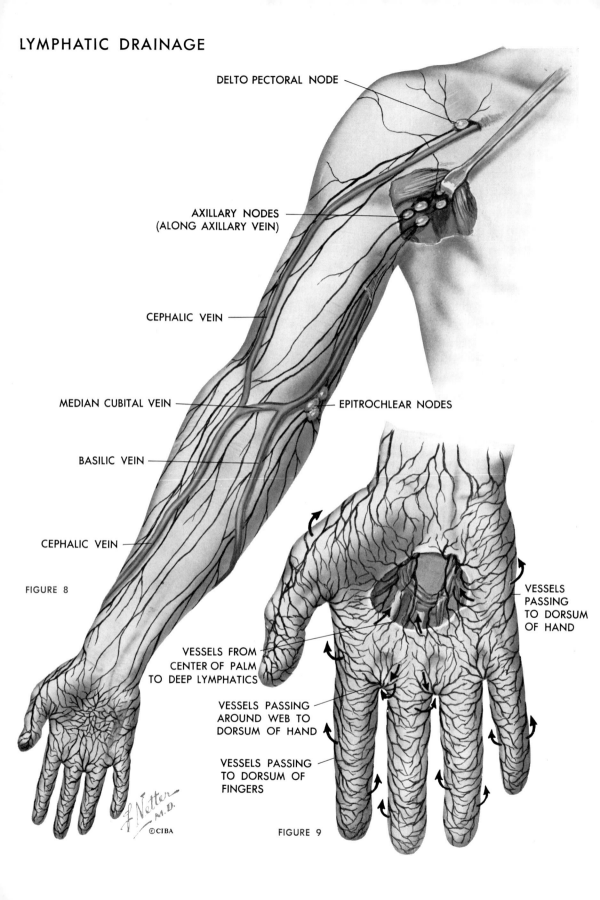

DELTO PECTORAL NODE

AXILLARY NODES
(ALONG AXILLARY VEIN)

CEPHALIC VEIN

MEDIAN CUBITAL VEIN

EPITROCHLEAR NODES

BASILIC VEIN

CEPHALIC VEIN

FIGURE 8

VESSELS
PASSING
TO DORSUM
OF HAND

VESSELS FROM
CENTER OF PALM
TO DEEP LYMPHATICS

VESSELS PASSING
AROUND WEB TO
DORSUM OF HAND

VESSELS PASSING
TO DORSUM OF
FINGERS

FIGURE 9

F. Netter
M.D.
©CIBA

brane. It inserts into the proximal half of the palmar aspect of the terminal phalanx of the medial four digits. The vincula offer additional insertion.

Figure 24 shows the flexor digitorum profundus as already having given rise to its four tendons. Actually, however, at this point it is not uncommon to see only the profundus tendon to the index finger and the large, distal fibromuscular part of the remainder of the profundus muscle, which then divides about two centimeters distad into the tendons going to the third, fourth, and fifth fingers.

Extension of the fingers and thumb is produced by the combined action of the *extrinsic* and *intrinsic muscles.*

The extensor muscles, their tendons, and the compartment through which they pass at the wrist are shown on page 28. The chief extrinsic extensor of the fingers is the *extensor digitorum communis.* The *extensor indicis proprius* and *digiti quinti proprius* assist in extending respectively the index and fifth fingers.

The *extensor digitorum communis* originates from the lateral humeral epicondyle, intermuscular septa, and antebrachial fascia. It divides into four tendons which pass through the fourth dorsal compartment. In this connection, it is worthy of mention that not uncommonly the extensor digitorum communis has only three tendons passing through the fourth dorsal compartment. The fourth tendon arises on the dorsum of the hand from the fourth finger extensor and goes from there to the fifth finger. The *extensor indicis proprius* also passes through this compartment.

The manner of the *insertion* of the *extensor digitorum communis* tendons deserves special mention. Figure 33 shows the deep part of the extensor digitorum communis tendon inserting into the dor-

sum of the proximal phalanx. This insertion gives purchase to the muscle for the performance of its chief functions: (1) to extend the proximal phalanx to extension and hyperextension and (2) to stabilize the proximal finger joints so that the intrinsic muscles (lumbricals and interossei) not only can extend the middle and distal phalanges but are also able to give lateral movement to the fingers.

As the extensor communis tendon continues distally, it divides into three parts (shown on page 30). A central slip inserts into the dorsum of the proximal end of the middle phalanx. Two lateral tendinous slips unite with the tendons of the lumbrical and interosseous muscles and continue distally to the proximal end of the dorsum of the terminal phalanx for insertion. Despite the insertions of the extensor digitorum communis into the middle and terminal phalanges, this muscle can extend these two phalanges only very slightly, if at all, when the proximal phalanges are in extension. This occurs because so much of each of the extensor digitorum communis tendons is inserted into the dorsum of the proximal phalanges that when the muscle contracts, most of its power is concentrated in extending the proximal phalanges.

Furthermore, this firm anchoring of the tendons to the proximal phalanges permits but little extension of the middle and terminal phalanges by the extensor communis when the proximal phalanges are in the extended position. The arrows on page 30 show how the tendons of the lumbrical muscles and interosseous muscles, especially the volar interossei, inserted into the lateral slips of the extensor digitorum communis, are able to do most of the extending of the middle and terminal phalanges *when the proximal*

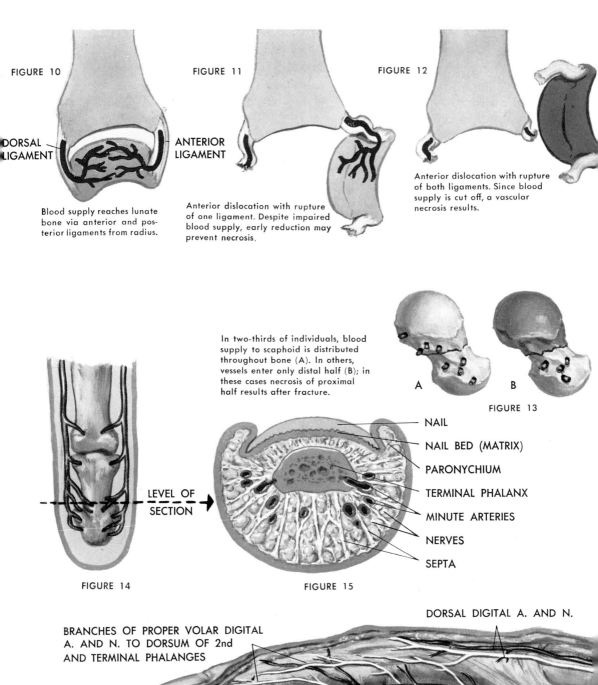

FIGURE 10

DORSAL
LIGAMENT

ANTERIOR
LIGAMENT

Blood supply reaches lunate
bone via anterior and posterior ligaments from radius.

FIGURE 11

Anterior dislocation with rupture
of one ligament. Despite impaired
blood supply, early reduction may
prevent necrosis.

FIGURE 12

Anterior dislocation with rupture
of both ligaments. Since blood
supply is cut off, a vascular
necrosis results.

In two-thirds of individuals, blood
supply to scaphoid is distributed
throughout bone (A). In others,
vessels enter only distal half (B); in
these cases necrosis of proximal
half results after fracture.

A   B

FIGURE 13

LEVEL OF
SECTION

NAIL

NAIL BED (MATRIX)

PARONYCHIUM

TERMINAL PHALANX

MINUTE ARTERIES

NERVES

SEPTA

FIGURE 14

FIGURE 15

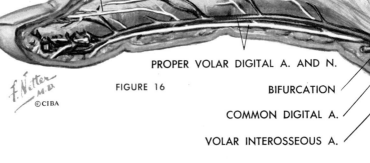

DORSAL DIGITAL A. AND N.

BRANCHES OF PROPER VOLAR DIGITAL
A. AND N. TO DORSUM OF 2nd
AND TERMINAL PHALANGES

PROPER VOLAR DIGITAL A. AND N.

FIGURE 16

F. Netter M.D.
©CIBA

BIFURCATION

COMMON DIGITAL A.

VOLAR INTEROSSEOUS A.

phalanges are extended. The situation changes, however, as soon as the extensor digitorum communis relaxes sufficiently to permit the flexors digitorum sublimis and profundus to begin flexing the middle and terminal phalanges. Simultaneously, this causes the extensor communis "hood" to be pulled distal to the metacarpophalangeal joint just enough, so that when the lumbricals and interossei contract, they then flex the proximal phalanges. In fact, *the* important flexors of the proximal phalanges are the lumbricals and interosseous muscles.

It seems almost paradoxical to have these intrinsic muscles flex the proximal phalanges and extend the middle and terminal phalanges. But a study of the figures on page 30 will show that if the dorsal expansion or "hood" is pulled proximally to the metacarpophalangeal joint (this occurs when the extensor digitorum communis has extended the proximal phalanges), contraction of the lumbricals and interossei extends the middle and terminal phalanges. On the other hand, when the "hood" is pulled distal to the metacarpophalangeal joint (this occurs with the synergistic relaxation of the extensor digitorum communis and flexion of the digitorum sublimis and profundus), contraction of the lumbricals and interossei results in flexion of the proximal phalanges. Now when the fingers are flexed (for example, 45 degrees), the extensor digitorum communis via its lateral slips takes over about half the control of the extension of the middle and terminal phalanges; and when the fingers are three-fourths flexed, the extensor digitorum communis assumes full control in the extension of these phalanges.

The interosseous muscles gain partial insertion into not only the lateral aspects of the proximal ends of the proximal phalanges but also into the lateral aspects of the capsules of the metacarpophalangeal joints (Figures 31, 32, and 33). It is these insertions which enable the ulnar-nerve-controlled interossei to spread and approximate the fingers. More will be said of this in the discussion on the intrinsic muscles of the hand.

Needless to say, it is important to understand the synergistic play of extrinsic and intrinsic muscles in the production of hand and finger movements; and it is equally obvious that it can be understood only if one has a clear picture of the detailed origins, insertions, and nerve supply of these muscles.

The tendon of the fifth finger proprius muscle *(extensor digiti quinti)* passes through the fifth compartment under the dorsal carpal ligament, Figures 26 and 27. It arises by a thin, tendinous slip from the common extensor in the forearm, and it inserts into the dorsal aponeurotic expansion hood on the dorsum of the proximal phalanx of the fifth finger. It aids in extending this phalanx and the hand at the wrist.

The tendon of the *extensor indicis proprius* passes through the fourth dorsal compartment with the three or four extensor communis tendons, as the case may be, Figures 26 and 27. The muscle arises from the dorsum of the ulna, near the junction of its proximal three-fourths and distal one-fourth. It assists in extending the proximal phalanx of the index finger and the hand at the wrist.

Whenever a tendon transplant is needed for repair of the very important extensor pollicis longus tendon, the tendon of the palmaris longus muscle is used. If the latter is absent, the tendon of the extensor indicis proprius muscle serves the purpose.

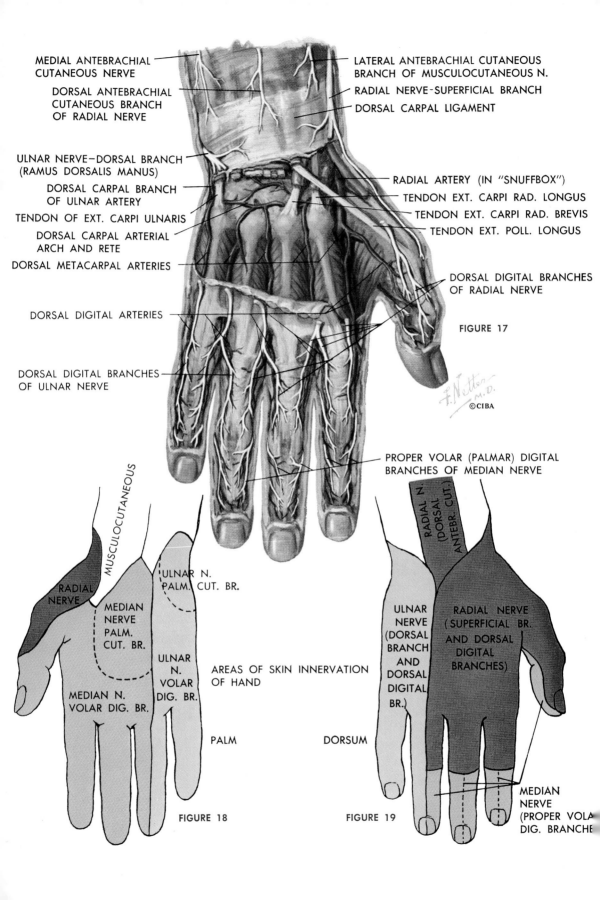

MEDIAL ANTEBRACHIAL CUTANEOUS NERVE

DORSAL ANTEBRACHIAL CUTANEOUS BRANCH OF RADIAL NERVE

ULNAR NERVE—DORSAL BRANCH (RAMUS DORSALIS MANUS)

DORSAL CARPAL BRANCH OF ULNAR ARTERY

TENDON OF EXT. CARPI ULNARIS

DORSAL CARPAL ARTERIAL ARCH AND RETE

DORSAL METACARPAL ARTERIES

DORSAL DIGITAL ARTERIES

DORSAL DIGITAL BRANCHES OF ULNAR NERVE

LATERAL ANTEBRACHIAL CUTANEOUS BRANCH OF MUSCULOCUTANEOUS N.

RADIAL NERVE-SUPERFICIAL BRANCH

DORSAL CARPAL LIGAMENT

RADIAL ARTERY (IN "SNUFFBOX")

TENDON EXT. CARPI RAD. LONGUS

TENDON EXT. CARPI RAD. BREVIS

TENDON EXT. POLL. LONGUS

DORSAL DIGITAL BRANCHES OF RADIAL NERVE

FIGURE 17

PROPER VOLAR (PALMAR) DIGITAL BRANCHES OF MEDIAN NERVE

F. Netter
M.D.
©CIBA

MUSCULOCUTANEOUS

ULNAR N. PALM. CUT. BR.

RADIAL NERVE

MEDIAN NERVE PALM. CUT. BR.

ULNAR N. VOLAR DIG. BR.

AREAS OF SKIN INNERVATION OF HAND

MEDIAN N. VOLAR DIG. BR.

PALM

FIGURE 18

RADIAL N. (DORSAL ANTEBR. CUT.)

ULNAR NERVE (DORSAL BRANCH AND DORSAL DIGITAL BR.)

RADIAL NERVE (SUPERFICIAL BR. AND DORSAL DIGITAL BRANCHES)

DORSUM

FIGURE 19

MEDIAN NERVE (PROPER VOLA DIG. BRANCHE

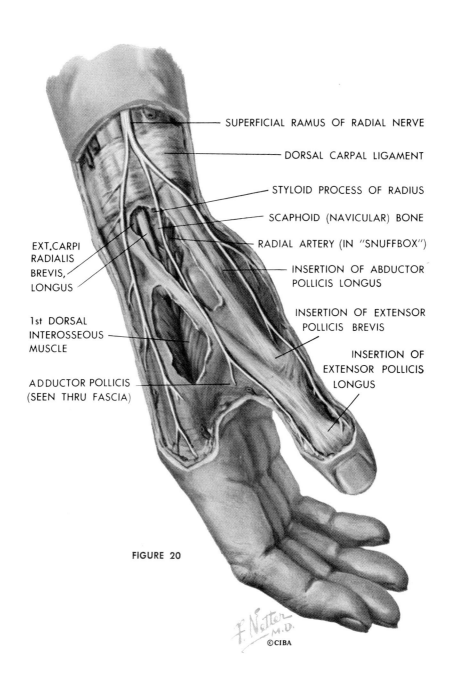

SUPERFICIAL RAMUS OF RADIAL NERVE

DORSAL CARPAL LIGAMENT

STYLOID PROCESS OF RADIUS

SCAPHOID (NAVICULAR) BONE

RADIAL ARTERY (IN "SNUFFBOX")

INSERTION OF ABDUCTOR POLLICIS LONGUS

INSERTION OF EXTENSOR POLLICIS BREVIS

INSERTION OF EXTENSOR POLLICIS LONGUS

EXT.CARPI RADIALIS BREVIS, LONGUS

1st DORSAL INTEROSSEOUS MUSCLE

ADDUCTOR POLLICIS (SEEN THRU FASCIA)

FIGURE 20

F. Netter M.D.
©CIBA

The *thumb* is an extremely important part of the hand. Its metacarpal bone, Figure 6, is the most mobile of all the metacarpal bones. Attached to the dorsum of its proximal end is the surprisingly stout *abductor pollicis longus* tendon, which may insert by one, two or even three tendinous slips, Figures 20 and 26. Just as this strong muscle can give rise to as many as three tendinous slips for insertion, it may have as many as three heads of origin: the proximal part of the ulna, the interosseous membrane, and middle third of the radius. This muscle abducts or extends the first metacarpal and stabilizes the first metacarpocarpal joint. The thumb could not function without this muscle. A stenosing tenosynovitis occasionally besets this tendon at the point where it passes through the first compartment on the radius, Figures 20, 26, and 27. This condition is also known as *de Quervain's disease*. Surgical removal of the roof of the compartment usually effects a cure.

The *extensor pollicis brevis*, Figure 20, arises from the interosseous membrane and dorsum of the radius just distal to the above-mentioned abductor pollicis longus and inserts into the dorsum of the proximal end of the first phalanx of the thumb. It extends this phalanx and also assists in extending and abducting the hand at the wrist.

The *extensor pollicis longus*, Figure 20, larger and more powerful than the preceding muscle, originates from the middle *third* of the dorsum of the ulna and interosseous membrane and is inserted into the dorsum of the proximal end of the terminal phalanx of the thumb. It extends the terminal phalanx, and like the extensor pollicis brevis, on continued action, it assists in extending the hand at the wrist. The tendon is quite frequently ruptured in a severe Colles' fracture; if not at the time of fracture, it may occur five to six weeks after the accident.

It should be observed that each of the three bones associated with the thumb (first metacarpal bone, and proximal and distal phalanges) has a tendon of one of the above-mentioned muscles inserted into the dorsum of its proximal end, Figures 7 and 20. The saddle-shaped surface of the greater multangular bone, articulating with the concavo-convex surface of the first metacarpal bone, permits a very wide range of movement of the thumb when acted upon by the above muscles, as well as the flexor pollicis longus and related intrinsic muscles of the hand, Figure 30.

Because lacerations involving tendons, vessels, and nerves about the wrist are quite common, it is important to review the anatomic relationships of these structures.

ARRANGEMENT OF
TENDONS, VESSELS, AND NERVES
AT THE WRIST

Figures 21 and 23 show schematically the general arrangement of the tendons, vessels, and nerves under the volar carpal ligament. By clenching the fist tightly and flexing the wrist as though against resistance, one can usually palpate the palmaris longus tendon (absent in 10 per cent of hands), the flexors carpi radialis and ulnaris tendons, and the superficial tendons of the flexor digitorum sublimis.

Next palpate the **median duo**, consisting of the *palmaris longus tendon* (superficial to the volar carpal ligament) and *median nerve*, the latter being deep and slightly lateral to the tendon.

Palpation of the radial pulse reminds

one of the **radial trio,** consisting of the *radial artery,* and ulnarward from it, the *radial flexor* (flexor carpi radialis), and deep and ulnarward of this stout tendon, the *flexor pollicis longus tendon.* With the fist tightly clenched and the wrist flexed, one has little difficulty in palpating accurately with one's thumbnail the sharp-bordered *ulnar flexor* tendon (flexor carpi ulnaris). If the ball of the thumb is used for palpation, it not only presses upon the ulnar flexor but also upon the superficial tendons of the flexor digitorum sublimis.

Palpation of the sharp-bordered ulnar flexor tendon brings to mind the **ulnar trio** which consists of the *ulnar flexor tendon,* the laterally placed *ulnar nerve,* and the adjacent *ulnar artery.* Again, with fist clenched and wrist flexed, one is reminded that the two **digital flexor tendon quartets** are medial to the centrally located palmaris longus tendon. Figure 23 shows schematically the relationship of the sublimis tendons. Those acting on the third and fourth fingers are superficial to those of the second and fifth fingers. This is most easily remembered by placing one's second and fifth fingers behind the third and fourth fingers as in Figure 22 and having in mind that 34 is a higher number than 25. Not uncommonly, sublimis tendons to the third, fourth, and fifth fingers are in the superficial plane, and the index finger sublimis tendon is deep to the third sublimis tendon.

Figure 23 shows the four *flexor digitorum profundus tendons* lying in one plane which is deep to the sublimis tendons. As previously mentioned, it is not uncommon to find at this point only the profundus tendon to the index finger separated from the distal fibromuscular end of the flexor digitorum profundus — the other three tendons arising one to two

centimeters distad. A *subtendinous space (Parona)* exists between all the above structures and the square pronator muscle *(pronator quadratus).* In discussing hand infections, this space will again be mentioned.

By insular attachments on the *dorsal and lateral aspects* of the radius and ulna, the dorsal carpal ligament creates six compartments for the passage of extensor and abductor tendons to the hand and fingers. Figure 26 shows the three thumb tendons bounding the *anatomical snuffbox:* the *abductor pollicis longus* and *extensor pollicis brevis* on the volar boundary, and the *extensor pollicis longus* on the dorsal boundary.

The first two tendons of the *snuffbox (abductor pollicis longus* and *extensor pollicis brevis)* are in the **first compartment,** and the *third* tendon of the *snuffbox (extensor pollicis longus)* is in the **third compartment.** The *two radial extensor tendons (extensors carpi radialis longus* and *brevis)* are in the **second compartment.**

One can associate the *four communis tendons* with the **fourth compartment;** and, as one wag expressed it, the *extensor indicis proprius tendon* is a "fellow-traveler" accompanying these four tendons. As previously mentioned, the *extensor digitorum communis* may give rise directly to only three tendons, in which case the *extensor indicis proprius tendon* will be the fourth tendon. The tendinous slip to the fifth finger from the *extensor digitorum communis* will then branch off from the tendon going to the fourth finger.

The *extensor digiti quinti proprius* fits well into the **fifth compartment.** The *ulnar extensor tendon (extensor carpi ulnaris)* falls easily into the *ulnar,* or **sixth compartment.**

Figures 20 and 26 show the *anatomical*

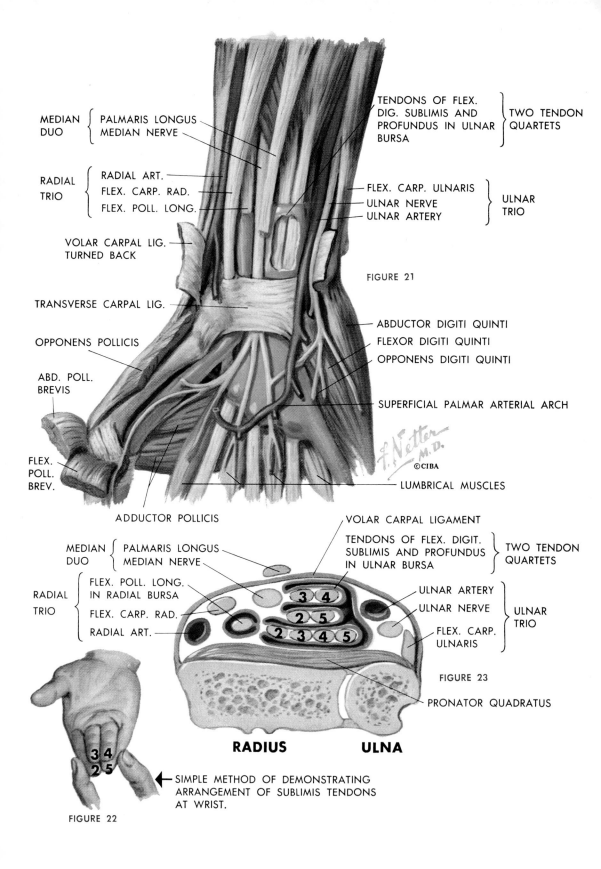

MEDIAN { PALMARIS LONGUS
DUO { MEDIAN NERVE

RADIAL { RADIAL ART.
TRIO { FLEX. CARP. RAD.
{ FLEX. POLL. LONG.

VOLAR CARPAL LIG.
TURNED BACK

TRANSVERSE CARPAL LIG.

OPPONENS POLLICIS

ABD. POLL.
BREVIS

FLEX.
POLL.
BREV.

ADDUCTOR POLLICIS

TENDONS OF FLEX.
DIG. SUBLIMIS AND } TWO TENDON
PROFUNDUS IN ULNAR } QUARTETS
BURSA

FLEX. CARP. ULNARIS
ULNAR NERVE } ULNAR
ULNAR ARTERY } TRIO

FIGURE 21

ABDUCTOR DIGITI QUINTI
FLEXOR DIGITI QUINTI
OPPONENS DIGITI QUINTI

SUPERFICIAL PALMAR ARTERIAL ARCH

LUMBRICAL MUSCLES

VOLAR CARPAL LIGAMENT

MEDIAN { PALMARIS LONGUS
DUO { MEDIAN NERVE

RADIAL { FLEX. POLL. LONG.
TRIO { IN RADIAL BURSA
{ FLEX. CARP. RAD.
{ RADIAL ART.

TENDONS OF FLEX. DIGIT.
SUBLIMIS AND PROFUNDUS } TWO TENDON
IN ULNAR BURSA } QUARTETS

3 4
2 5
2 3 4 5

ULNAR ARTERY
ULNAR NERVE } ULNAR
FLEX. CARP. } TRIO
ULNARIS

FIGURE 23

PRONATOR QUADRATUS

RADIUS   ULNA

3 4
2 5

SIMPLE METHOD OF DEMONSTRATING
ARRANGEMENT OF SUBLIMIS TENDONS
AT WRIST.

FIGURE 22

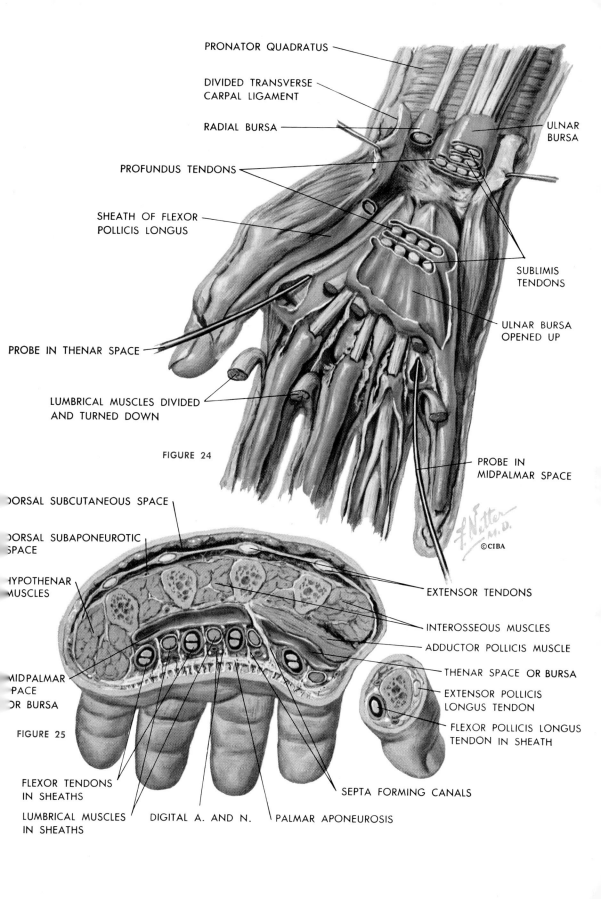

PRONATOR QUADRATUS

DIVIDED TRANSVERSE CARPAL LIGAMENT

RADIAL BURSA

PROFUNDUS TENDONS

SHEATH OF FLEXOR POLLICIS LONGUS

PROBE IN THENAR SPACE

LUMBRICAL MUSCLES DIVIDED AND TURNED DOWN

ULNAR BURSA

SUBLIMIS TENDONS

ULNAR BURSA OPENED UP

PROBE IN MIDPALMAR SPACE

FIGURE 24

DORSAL SUBCUTANEOUS SPACE

DORSAL SUBAPONEUROTIC SPACE

HYPOTHENAR MUSCLES

MIDPALMAR SPACE OR BURSA

FIGURE 25

EXTENSOR TENDONS

INTEROSSEOUS MUSCLES

ADDUCTOR POLLICIS MUSCLE

THENAR SPACE OR BURSA

EXTENSOR POLLICIS LONGUS TENDON

FLEXOR POLLICIS LONGUS TENDON IN SHEATH

FLEXOR TENDONS IN SHEATHS

LUMBRICAL MUSCLES IN SHEATHS

DIGITAL A. AND N.

PALMAR APONEUROSIS

SEPTA FORMING CANALS

snuffbox and its important contents. The tip of the styloid process of the radius can be felt at its proximal end. A small part of the extensors carpi radialis longus and brevis tendons can be seen, as well as the radial artery. Deep to the radial artery is the capsule of the wrist joint and navicular (scaphoid) bone. Because the navicular bone (Figure 13) is the most frequently fractured carpal bone, it is clinically more important than the greater multangular bone — a small part of which also lies in the *snuffbox.* Figure 3 shows sensory branches of the *radial nerve,* which are found in the *snuffbox.* Awareness of their presence prompts the surgeon to preserve them in surgical procedures in this area.

INTRINSIC MUSCLES OF THE HAND

These may be grouped into those forming the *hypothenar eminence,* the *thenar eminence,* and a third group — the muscles between these two eminences, Figures 2, 5, 28, 29, and 30.

Muscles of Hypothenar Eminence

The *abductor digiti quinti,* the *flexor digiti quinti brevis* and the *opponens digiti quinti* comprise this group, Figures 1, 5, and 21. The *abductor digiti quinti* originates chiefly from the pisiform bone and pisohamate ligament and inserts into the joint capsule of the fifth metacarpophalangeal joint, the ulnar side of the base of the proximal phalanx of the fifth finger, and the ulnar border of the aponeurosis of the *extensor digiti quinti proprius.* It is supplied by the ulnar nerve, abducts the fifth finger when its proximal phalanx is extended, and flexes the proximal phalanx when the long extensor is relaxed.

The *flexor digiti quinti brevis* arises from the hamate bone and transverse carpal ligament and is inserted into the ulnar side of the base of the first phalanx. It is innervated by the ulnar nerve and assists in abducting the fifth finger and in flexing the proximal phalanx.

The *opponens digiti quinti* originates from the hamate bone and transverse metacarpal ligament. It is inserted into the ulnar border of the fifth metacarpal bone and innervated by the ulnar nerve. It lies deep to the other two muscles, next to the fifth metacarpal bone.

The fifth is the second most mobile of all the metacarpal bones, being movable about 15 degrees palmarward and dorsalward, Figure 30. Because of this mobility, the *opponens digiti quinti* is able to draw the fifth metacarpal forward, thereby helping to deepen the hollow of the palm. The unimportant palmaris brevis merely corrugates the skin on the ulnar side of the palm.

Muscles of Thenar Eminence

This group consists of the *abductor pollicis brevis,* the *flexor pollicis brevis,* and *opponens pollicis* muscles, Figures 1, 4, 7, 21, and 28. These muscles, which are functionally much more important than those of the hypothenar eminence, are supplied almost entirely by the median nerve.

The *abductor pollicis brevis* muscle originates from the transverse carpal ligament and from the navicular and greater multangular bones. It inserts into the radial side of the proximal phalanx of the thumb and into the capsule of the metacarpophalangeal joint. It aids in abducting the thumb away from the palm.

The *opponens pollicis* muscle originates from the transverse carpal ligament and greater multangular bone. It inserts into the whole radial side of the first metacarpal bone and because of this is largely responsible for the movement which enables the thumb to be approximated successively to the tips of each of the fingers. This is recognized as the *thumb-finger-approximator test*, frequently used to test the motor function of the median nerve.

The *flexor pollicis brevis* muscle consists of two parts: (1) a *superficial* portion, innervated by the median nerve, originating from the transverse carpal ligament and greater multangular bone and inserting into the radial side of the proximal phalanx and (2) a *deep* and very small portion, innervated by the ulnar nerve, arising from the ulnar side of the first metacarpal and inserting into the ulnar side of the proximal end of the first phalanx.

All the hypothenar and thenar eminence muscles, except the abductor digiti quinti, get part of their origin from the transverse carpal ligament — a purchase which enables them (abductor excepted) to help preserve the carpal arch.

INTEROSSEOUS MUSCLES

There are seven interosseous muscles: four interossei in the dorsal group and three interossei in the volar group, Figures 29 and 30.

The *four dorsal interosseous* muscles are bipennate with their muscular heads of origin from adjacent sides of the metacarpal bones. From the figures on pages 28 and 29, one can see how the tendon of one head of the muscle inserts into the tubercle on the lateral aspect of the proximal phalanx or the capsule of the metacarpophalangeal joint, or into both tubercle and joint capsule. The other head inserts into the dorsal expansion and

its volar border — the lateral band which continues distally to the dorsum of the proximal end of the terminal phalanx. It is not uncommon for the tendinous slip to the capsule to arise from the tendon joining the lateral band instead of the one going to the tubercle.

Because the tendon of one of these two-headed or bipennate dorsal interosseous muscles has a stout insertion into the lateral aspect of the proximal end of the proximal phalanx (and this insertion is slightly more volar than dorsal) and because it fuses with the transverse fibers of the hood, contraction of the muscle belly associated with this tendon will cause lateral motion of the proximal phalanx. When the *extensor digitorum communis* relaxes, flexion of this same phalanx occurs.

Because the tendon of the other belly blends with the lateral band of the dorsal expansion (hood) which continues distally to the dorsum of the middle and terminal phalanges, contraction of its associated muscle fibers will aid in extending the middle and terminal phalanges (Figures 31, 32).

It is to be noted, however, that the *first* dorsal interosseous is *different* from the second, third, and fourth in that it has its second metacarpal head inserting into the lateral tubercle of the proximal phalanx and its first metacarpal head inserting into the dorsal expansion hood with no contribution to the lateral band slip of the first lumbrical muscle.

This different mode of insertion enables the second metacarpal component of the first dorsal interosseous to be more effective in flexing the proximal phalanx, and the first metacarpal belly to be the more important in lateral motion, especially so in the pinching gesture with the thumb.

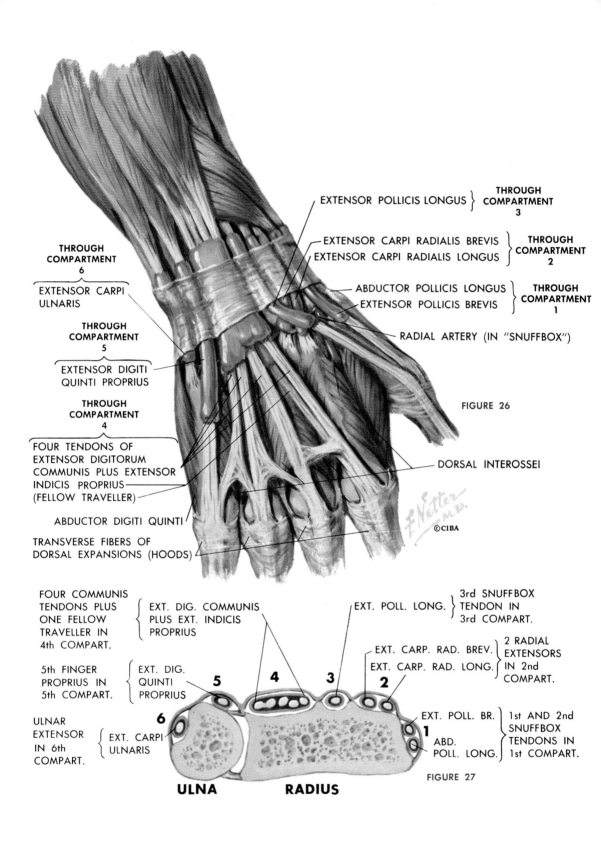

EXTENSOR POLLICIS LONGUS } THROUGH COMPARTMENT 3

EXTENSOR CARPI RADIALIS BREVIS } THROUGH COMPARTMENT 2
EXTENSOR CARPI RADIALIS LONGUS

THROUGH COMPARTMENT 6

EXTENSOR CARPI ULNARIS

ABDUCTOR POLLICIS LONGUS } THROUGH COMPARTMENT 1
EXTENSOR POLLICIS BREVIS

THROUGH COMPARTMENT 5

RADIAL ARTERY (IN "SNUFFBOX")

EXTENSOR DIGITI QUINTI PROPRIUS

THROUGH COMPARTMENT 4

FIGURE 26

FOUR TENDONS OF EXTENSOR DIGITORUM COMMUNIS PLUS EXTENSOR INDICIS PROPRIUS (FELLOW TRAVELLER)

DORSAL INTEROSSEI

ABDUCTOR DIGITI QUINTI

TRANSVERSE FIBERS OF DORSAL EXPANSIONS (HOODS)

F. Netter M.D.
©CIBA

FOUR COMMUNIS TENDONS PLUS ONE FELLOW TRAVELLER IN 4th COMPART.
{ EXT. DIG. COMMUNIS PLUS EXT. INDICIS PROPRIUS

EXT. POLL. LONG. } 3rd SNUFFBOX TENDON IN 3rd COMPART.

5th FINGER PROPRIUS IN 5th COMPART.
{ EXT. DIG. QUINTI PROPRIUS

EXT. CARP. RAD. BREV. } 2 RADIAL EXTENSORS IN 2nd COMPART.
EXT. CARP. RAD. LONG.

ULNAR EXTENSOR IN 6th COMPART.
{ EXT. CARPI ULNARIS

EXT. POLL. BR. } 1st AND 2nd SNUFFBOX TENDONS IN 1st COMPART.
ABD. POLL. LONG.

5   4   3   2

6   1

FIGURE 27

ULNA   RADIUS

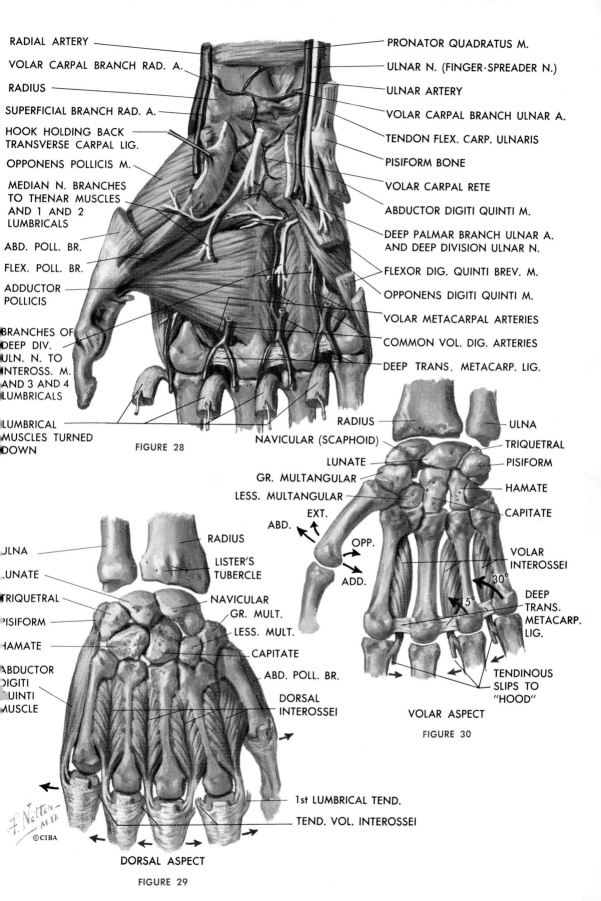

RADIAL ARTERY

VOLAR CARPAL BRANCH RAD. A.

RADIUS

SUPERFICIAL BRANCH RAD. A.

HOOK HOLDING BACK
TRANSVERSE CARPAL LIG.

OPPONENS POLLICIS M.

MEDIAN N. BRANCHES
TO THENAR MUSCLES
AND 1 AND 2
LUMBRICALS

ABD. POLL. BR.

FLEX. POLL. BR.

ADDUCTOR
POLLICIS

BRANCHES OF
DEEP DIV.
ULN. N. TO
INTEROSS. M.
AND 3 AND 4
LUMBRICALS

LUMBRICAL
MUSCLES TURNED
DOWN

PRONATOR QUADRATUS M.

ULNAR N. (FINGER-SPREADER N.)

ULNAR ARTERY

VOLAR CARPAL BRANCH ULNAR A.

TENDON FLEX. CARP. ULNARIS

PISIFORM BONE

VOLAR CARPAL RETE

ABDUCTOR DIGITI QUINTI M.

DEEP PALMAR BRANCH ULNAR A.
AND DEEP DIVISION ULNAR N.

FLEXOR DIG. QUINTI BREV. M.

OPPONENS DIGITI QUINTI M.

VOLAR METACARPAL ARTERIES

COMMON VOL. DIG. ARTERIES

DEEP TRANS. METACARP. LIG.

FIGURE 28

RADIUS

NAVICULAR (SCAPHOID)

LUNATE

GR. MULTANGULAR

LESS. MULTANGULAR

EXT.

ABD.

OPP.

ADD.

ULNA

TRIQUETRAL

PISIFORM

HAMATE

CAPITATE

VOLAR
INTEROSSEI

30°

5°

DEEP
TRANS.
METACARP.
LIG.

TENDINOUS
SLIPS TO
"HOOD"

VOLAR ASPECT

FIGURE 30

ULNA

LUNATE

TRIQUETRAL

PISIFORM

HAMATE

ABDUCTOR
DIGITI
QUINTI
MUSCLE

RADIUS

LISTER'S
TUBERCLE

NAVICULAR
GR. MULT.

LESS. MULT.

CAPITATE

ABD. POLL. BR.

DORSAL
INTEROSSEI

1st LUMBRICAL TEND.

TEND. VOL. INTEROSSEI

F. Netter
M.D.
©CIBA

DORSAL ASPECT

FIGURE 29

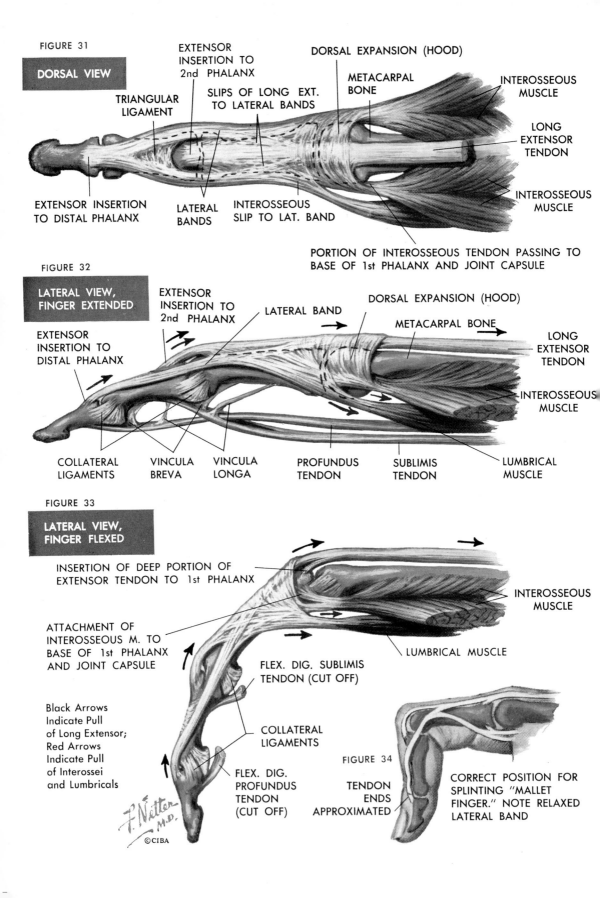

FIGURE 31

DORSAL VIEW

EXTENSOR INSERTION TO 2nd PHALANX

TRIANGULAR LIGAMENT

SLIPS OF LONG EXT. TO LATERAL BANDS

DORSAL EXPANSION (HOOD)

METACARPAL BONE

INTEROSSEOUS MUSCLE

LONG EXTENSOR TENDON

EXTENSOR INSERTION TO DISTAL PHALANX

LATERAL BANDS

INTEROSSEOUS SLIP TO LAT. BAND

INTEROSSEOUS MUSCLE

PORTION OF INTEROSSEOUS TENDON PASSING TO BASE OF 1st PHALANX AND JOINT CAPSULE

FIGURE 32

LATERAL VIEW, FINGER EXTENDED

EXTENSOR INSERTION TO 2nd PHALANX

LATERAL BAND

DORSAL EXPANSION (HOOD)

METACARPAL BONE

LONG EXTENSOR TENDON

EXTENSOR INSERTION TO DISTAL PHALANX

INTEROSSEOUS MUSCLE

COLLATERAL LIGAMENTS

VINCULA BREVA

VINCULA LONGA

PROFUNDUS TENDON

SUBLIMIS TENDON

LUMBRICAL MUSCLE

FIGURE 33

LATERAL VIEW, FINGER FLEXED

INSERTION OF DEEP PORTION OF EXTENSOR TENDON TO 1st PHALANX

INTEROSSEOUS MUSCLE

ATTACHMENT OF INTEROSSEOUS M. TO BASE OF 1st PHALANX AND JOINT CAPSULE

LUMBRICAL MUSCLE

FLEX. DIG. SUBLIMIS TENDON (CUT OFF)

Black Arrows Indicate Pull of Long Extensor; Red Arrows Indicate Pull of Interossei and Lumbricals

COLLATERAL LIGAMENTS

FLEX. DIG. PROFUNDUS TENDON (CUT OFF)

FIGURE 34

TENDON ENDS APPROXIMATED

CORRECT POSITION FOR SPLINTING "MALLET FINGER." NOTE RELAXED LATERAL BAND

F. Netter M.D.

©CIBA

Because the first dorsal interosseous muscle gives no notable tendinous contribution to the lateral tendinous slip of the first lumbrical muscle, it obviously gives practically no aid in the extension of the middle and terminal phalanges of the index finger. Their extension is effected by the first lumbrical muscle and first volar interosseous muscle whose tendinous slips insert into the dorsum of the middle and proximal phalanges.

The *second* and *third dorsal interosseous* muscles insert respectively into the tubercles on the radial and ulnar side of the proximal phalanx of the middle finger and into the lateral slips of the dorsal expansion hood which extend distally to the middle and terminal phalanges for insertion. When the tendon of the *extensor digitorum communis* extends the proximal phalanx of the third finger, the second and third dorsal interosseous muscles can extend the middle and terminal phalanges via the lateral slips and "wig-wag" the middle finger, *i.e.,* move it respectively radialward and ulnarward because of their insertion into the proximal phalanx. The arrows on pages 29 and 30 depict these movements. With the tendon of the *extensor digitorum communis* to the third finger relaxed, contraction of the second and third dorsal interosseous muscles causes flexion of the proximal phalanx.

The *fourth dorsal interosseous muscle* inserts into the ulnar side of the proximal phalanx of the fourth finger, the ulnar side of the joint capsule, and the ulnar side of the dorsal expansion. With the proximal phalanx extended, the fourth dorsal interosseous muscle will pull the fourth finger away from the third finger and aid in extending the middle and terminal phalanges via its attachment to the hood,

Figure 32. When the extensor tendon is relaxed, the fourth dorsal interosseous muscle flexes the proximal phalanx of the fourth finger, Figure 33.

Volar or *palmar* interosseous muscles are three in number. The *first* arises from the ulnar side of the volar aspect of the second metacarpal bone and is inserted into the same side of the proximal end of the first phalanx and lateral band of the dorsal expansion hood of the index finger. The *second* and *third* arise respectively from the radial side of the fourth and fifth metacarpal bones and are inserted into the same side of the proximal phalanx of the fourth and fifth fingers and lateral bands of their dorsal expansion.

The red arrows in Figure 30 show how contraction of these muscles results in approximating the second, fourth, and fifth fingers toward the middle finger. Red arrows on page 30 demonstrate how tendinous slips given to the lateral bands of the dorsal expansions enable these muscles to assist in extending the middle and terminal phalanges when the proximal phalanges are extended by the extensor digitorum communis muscle.

Some prefer including the two-headed *adductor pollicis* muscle, Figure 28, with the "median nerve-controlled" thenar eminence muscle group. However, because it is functionally under the control of the ulnar nerve as are the seven interossei and the two lumbrical muscles on the ulnar side of the hand, it seems more logical to include it with the latter group. The *oblique* head of the adductor pollicis muscle arises chiefly from the capitate bone and the bases of the second and third metacarpals. The *transverse* part arises from the distal two-thirds of the volar aspect of the third metacarpal bone. All of the transverse head and most of the

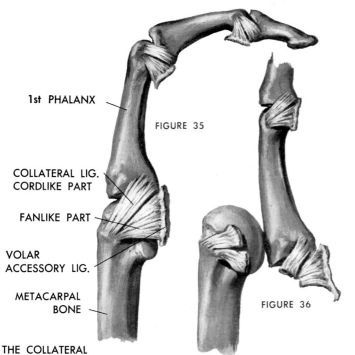

1st PHALANX

FIGURE 35

COLLATERAL LIG.
CORDLIKE PART

FANLIKE PART

VOLAR
ACCESSORY LIG.

METACARPAL
BONE

THE COLLATERAL
AND VOLAR ACCESSORY
LIGAMENTS IN A
TYPICAL DIGIT

FIGURE 36

ANTERIOR DISLOCATION OF
PROXIMAL PHALANX
DUE TO DIVISION OF
COLLATERAL LIGAMENTS

FIGURE 37

FRACTURE OF
METACARPAL
BONE. FLEXION
DEFORMITY
CAUSED BY
PULL OF
INTEROSSEOUS
MUSCLE

INTEROSSEOUS
MUSCLE

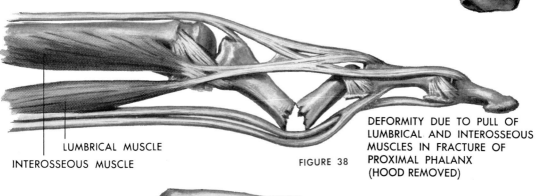

LUMBRICAL MUSCLE

INTEROSSEOUS MUSCLE

FIGURE 38

DEFORMITY DUE TO PULL OF
LUMBRICAL AND INTEROSSEOUS
MUSCLES IN FRACTURE OF
PROXIMAL PHALANX
(HOOD REMOVED)

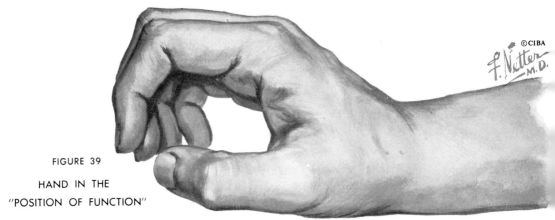

FIGURE 39

HAND IN THE
"POSITION OF FUNCTION"

©CIBA

F. Netter
M.D.

oblique head insert into the ulnar side of the base of the proximal phalanx of the thumb. A sesamoid bone is not uncommonly found in this tendon. Some of the fibers from the *oblique* head join the flexor pollicis brevis to insert into the radial side of the thumb's first phalanx. Here also is located a sesamoid bone. The tendon of the flexor pollicis longus is between these two points of insertion.

As the name implies, the *function* of the *adductor pollicis muscle* is adduction of the first metacarpal toward the third metacarpal bone. Note the difference between the action of the *opponens pollicis,* of the "median-nerve-supplied" thenar eminence group and the *adductor pollicis muscle* supplied by the ulnar nerve: The *opponens pollicis* swings the thumb in an arching manner toward the

tips of the fingers, whereas the *adductor pollicis* slides or scrapes the thumb across the palm and bases of the fingers toward the ulnar side of the hand.

With a functionless adductor pollicis, as in ulnar nerve paralysis, it is impossible to make a perfect "O" with the thumb and index finger or execute the pinch-movement between these digits.

In *ulnar nerve* paralysis, there is not only a "hollowing-out" due to atrophy of the interosseous muscle bulges on the dorsum of the hand, but there is a noticeable thinning of the thumb-index finger web-area due to atrophy of the adductor pollicis muscle. As stated previously, the *ulnar nerve* can be called the "*finger-spreader-approximator-nerve*" because spreading and approximating the fingers by the dorsal and volar interossei, respectively, tests

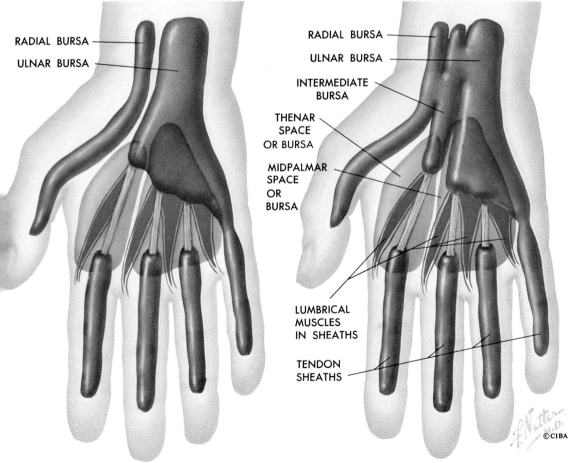

RADIAL BURSA

ULNAR BURSA

RADIAL BURSA

ULNAR BURSA

INTERMEDIATE BURSA

THENAR SPACE OR BURSA

MIDPALMAR SPACE OR BURSA

LUMBRICAL MUSCLES IN SHEATHS

TENDON SHEATHS

FIGURE 40

FIGURE 41

©CIBA

quite effectively the motor integrity of the ulnar nerve.

LUMBRICAL MUSCLES

On the radial side of the palmar portion of each flexor digitorum profundus tendon is a lumbricalis (worm-like) muscle, page 13. The *first* and *second* lumbricals originate respectively from the radial side of the first and second flexor profundus tendons, the third lumbrical originates from the adjacent sides of the second and third profundus tendons, and the fourth from adjacent sides of the third and fourth profundus tendons (Figure 21). Figures 32 and 33 show how these muscles send transverse fibrous elements to the dorsal expansion hood, and a substantial tendinous slip to fuse with a similar contribution from the interosseous muscles to form the lateral bands inserting into the middle and terminal phalanges.

This insertion enables these muscles to flex the proximal phalanges when the extensor digitorum longus muscle is relaxed; and the middle and terminal phalangeal insertions enable them to *extend* these phalanges when the extensor digitorum longus is extending the proximal phalanges.

The *first* and *second* or lateral two *lumbricals* arising from the first and second flexor profundus tendons are innervated by the *median nerve*, the *third* and *fourth* or medial two by the *ulnar nerve*. This is quite logical when one recalls that in the forearm the lateral half of the flexor digitorum profundus, from which arise the tendons to the first and second fingers, is innervated by the median nerve; the medial half, from which originate the tendons to the third and fourth fingers, is supplied by the ulnar nerve.

THE EFFECT ON THE HAND OF RADIAL, MEDIAN, AND ULNAR NERVE LESIONS

Severance of Radial Nerve

Because of the frequency of arm injuries such as shoulder dislocations and fractures of the surgical neck and middle third of the humerus, the radial is the most frequently injured of these three important nerves.

Sensory examination will reveal hypesthesia in an area along the dorsum of the forearm about half the width indicated in Figure 19 and also on the hand in most of the area diagrammed in Figures 18 and 19. There is usually anesthesia of the skin overlying the first dorsal interosseous muscle.

Motor examination reveals the typical "wrist drop" position of the hand. The adducted position of the thumb and the position of the already flexed hand makes flexion of the fingers somewhat difficult. The hand cannot be extended at the wrist, and the lateral movements of the hand are difficult because the ulnar and radial extensors are paralyzed. The proximal phalanges of the four fingers cannot be extended because of the involvement of the extensor digitorum communis; the thumb cannot be extended or abducted because of the paralysis of the abductor pollicis longus and of the extensors pollicis longus and brevis. The bulge of the dorsal forearm group of muscles (extensor-supinator group) is flattened or even hollowed. There is absence of the periosteal reflex on tapping the radius.

Severance of Median Nerve

While *sensory examination* will reveal varying degrees of hypesthesia and anesthesia as outlined in the medial nerve areas of Figures 18 and 19, complete anesthesia will usually be present only on the palmar and dorsal aspects of the terminal phalanges and parts of the middle phalanges of the index and middle fingers.

In a previous paragraph, it was suggested that the median nerve could also be known by its functional name: the flexor - pronator - thumb - finger - approximator nerve. In a general way, this name summarizes the motor control of the nerve and suggests what to expect in division of the nerve.

Motor examination in a case of severance of the median nerve just above the elbow reveals weakness in wrist-flexion because of paralysis of the powerful flexor carpi radialis muscle. The flexor carpi ulnaris (innervated by the ulnar nerve) has a tendency to flex the wrist ulnarward. There is inability to flex the thumb, index, and middle fingers. Pronation is very weak because the pronator radii teres (round pronator) and the pronator quadratus (square pronator) muscles are paralyzed. Because the thenar eminence muscles are paralyzed, there is considerable difficulty in trying to approximate the tip of the thumb successively to the tips of the fingers. In attempting to clasp the unaffected hand, the index and middle fingers will not flex as will the other fingers. With the hand flat on a desk, the index finger cannot scratch the desk.

Inspection reveals a hollowing-out of most of the normal forearm muscle bulge of the volar or flexor-pronator group of muscles and a hollowing-out of the thenar eminence or thumb-finger-approximator muscle group.

It is easy to appreciate the importance of the median nerve, since it has most of the motor and sensory control of the thumb, index, and middle fingers. It is no

wonder that causalgia, which seems to affect this nerve more than others, is such a painfully disabling affliction.

Severance of the Ulnar Nerve

Sensory examination reveals varying degrees of hypesthesia and anesthesia of the ulnar border of the hand and the volar and dorsal aspects of the fifth finger and ulnar half of the fourth finger, Figures 18 and 19. Total anesthesia is noted usually in the fifth finger.

Motor Examination: If the division of the nerve is above the elbow, there is loss of ulnar flexion due to paralysis of the flexor carpi ulnaris (ulnar flexor) and inability to flex the terminal phalanges of the fourth and fifth fingers because of paralysis of the ulnar half of the flexor digitorum profundus muscle.

Since the ulnar nerve supplies the hypothenar eminence muscles, the interosseous muscles, the two medial lumbrical muscles, the adductor pollicis muscle, and the deep head of the flexor pollicis brevis muscle, there is a marked weakness or loss of the so-called finger-spreading and approximating movements of the fingers. There is inability to scrape the thumb across the palm as well as the inability to form a perfect "O" with the thumb and index finger. It is also difficult to hold tightly a piece of paper between the thumb and index finger.

Inspection will reveal a hollowing-out of the hypothenar eminence and the muscle bulges of the interosseous muscles between the metacarpals. The normal bulge along the proximal ulnar border of the forearm will also be flattened due to atrophy of the flexor carpi ulnaris and the ulnar half of the flexor digitorum profundus muscles.

The so-called "claw-hand" is most

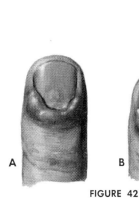
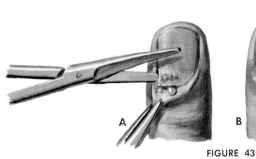
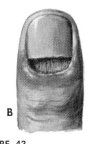

FIGURE 42

FIGURE 43

PARONYCHIA

TECHNIQUE IF LOCAL-
IZED TO ONE SIDE

PULLING DOWN NAIL FLAP
AND EXCISING NAIL ROOT.

AFTER REMOVAL
OF NAIL ROOT

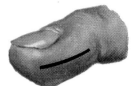
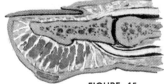
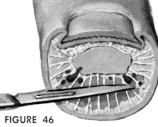

FIGURE 44

FELON
(SHOWING INCISION)

FIGURE 45

SAGITTAL SECTION
SHOWING PUS (GREEN)
BETWEEN SEPTA

FIGURE 46

SCHEMATIC CROSS SECTION
SHOWING HOW INCISION
DIVIDES SEPTA

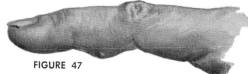

FIGURE 47

SUBCUTANEOUS ABSCESS
(NOTE *LOCALIZED* SWELLING)

TENOSYNOVITIS
(DEMONSTRATING KANAVEL'S
4 CARDINAL POINTS)

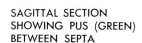
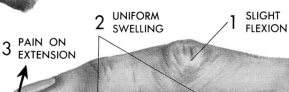

2 UNIFORM
SWELLING

1 SLIGHT
FLEXION

3 PAIN ON
EXTENSION

4 TENDERNESS ALONG SHEATH

FIGURE 48

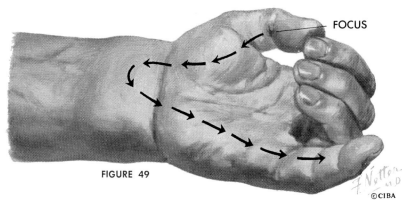

FOCUS

PATHOGENESIS OF
"HORSESHOE ABSCESS"
WITH RUPTURE
INTO PARONA'S
SUBTENDINOUS
SPACE

FIGURE 49

F. Netter
©CIBA

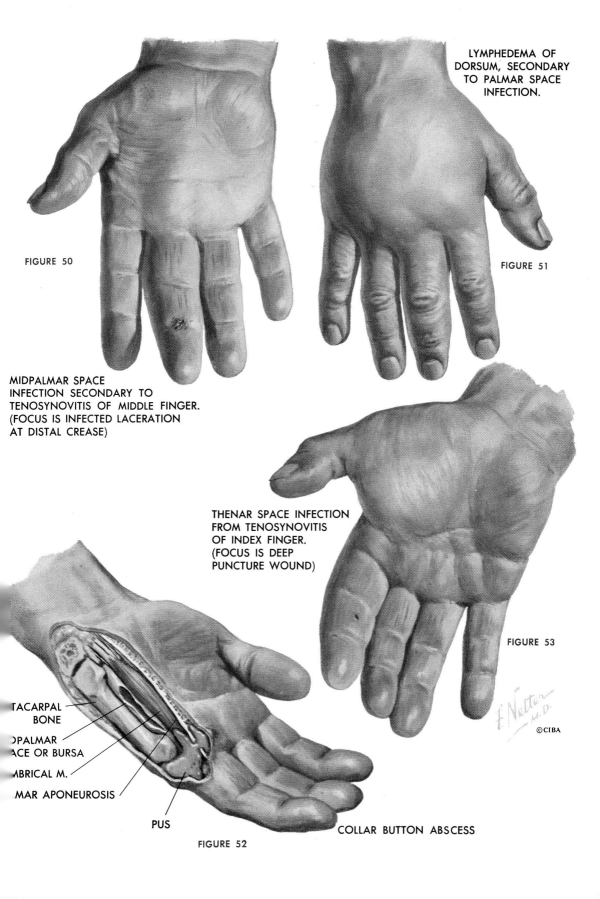

FIGURE 50

FIGURE 51

LYMPHEDEMA OF DORSUM, SECONDARY TO PALMAR SPACE INFECTION.

MIDPALMAR SPACE INFECTION SECONDARY TO TENOSYNOVITIS OF MIDDLE FINGER. (FOCUS IS INFECTED LACERATION AT DISTAL CREASE)

THENAR SPACE INFECTION FROM TENOSYNOVITIS OF INDEX FINGER. (FOCUS IS DEEP PUNCTURE WOUND)

FIGURE 53

TACARPAL BONE

DPALMAR ACE OR BURSA

MBRICAL M.

MAR APONEUROSIS

PUS

FIGURE 52

COLLAR BUTTON ABSCESS

noticeable when the ulnar nerve is severed in the distal half of the forearm; *i.e.*, after it has given motor branches to the flexor carpi ulnaris and especially to the ulnar half of the flexor digitorum profundus. The extensor digitorum communis (supplied by the radial nerve) will extend the proximal phalanges of the fourth and fifth fingers. The ulnar half of the flexor digitorum profundus (supplied by the ulnar nerve) will flex the terminal and middle phalanges, thus producing a claw-like position of the fourth and fifth fingers.

Severance of Median *and* Ulnar Nerves

Sensory examination reveals a variable amount of hypesthesia and anesthesia of the palm and of the volar and dorsal aspects of the fingers as outlined in Figures 18 and 19.

The findings in the *motor examination* depend upon the level at which the nerves are cut. If severed above the elbow, the entire flexor-pronator or volar forearm group of muscles, and all the intrinsic muscles of the hand will be paralyzed. With the flexors carpi radialis and ulnaris paralyzed, the extensors carpi radialis longus and brevis and extensor carpi ulnaris (supplied by radial nerve) will tend to extend and slightly supinate the hand at the wrist.

The extensor digitorum communis will hyperextend the proximal phalanges, and the thumb abductor and extensors will abduct the thumb and pull it in a plane slightly dorsal to that of the hand. The paralysis of the intrinsic muscles of the hand causes a flattening of the carpal and metacarpal arches, creating a flat "ape-like" hand. The subsequent contracture of the flexors digitorum profundus and of the sublimis and flexor pollicis longus produces a moderate "claw" position of the

fingers and thumb. If the nerves are severed in the distal part of the forearm, *i.e.*, after they have supplied motor branches to the flexors of the fingers, the "claw" position of the fingers will be very marked. This is understandable when one recalls that the extensor digitorum communis muscle (supplied by radial nerve) will hyperextend the proximal phalanges, and that the finger flexors, unopposed by the paralyzed intrinsic hand muscles, will sharply flex the middle and terminal phalanges, thus producing an extreme "claw" appearance of the fingers.

LIGAMENTS OF THE HAND

A thick but loose articular capsule holds together the saddle-shaped joint between the first metacarpal and greater multangular bone. Because of the configuration of these articular facets, the thumb enjoys a very wide range of movement, in fact, the widest range of movement of any of the metacarpal bones.

The bases of the second, third, fourth, and fifth metacarpal bones are held together by dorsal, volar, and interosseous ligaments.

The volar surfaces of the heads of the second, third, fourth, and fifth metacarpal bones are connected by a tough fibrous band — the *deep transverse metacarpal ligament*, Figures 28 and 30. This ligament and the dorsal, volar, and interosseous carpometacarpal ligaments give the hand stability. They permit the fifth metacarpal a thirty-degree range of movement, the fourth about fifteen degrees. They permit practically no mobility to the second and third metacarpal bones, thereby making this the most stable part of the hand. The *deep transverse metacarpal ligament* helps preserve the metacarpal arch, and its rupture weakens the hand to a marked degree. As shown in Figures 28 and 30, the lumbrical tendons lie on the palmar aspect and the interosseous tendons on the dorsal aspect of this ligament.

Mention should be made of the *accessory volar* ligament and the two *collateral* ligaments which strengthen the metacarpophalangeal joints. These are clinically important because, whether by rupture or capsulotomy, they may permit the base of the proximal phalanx to slide onto the palmar aspect of the head of the metacarpal bone, thereby creating a painfully disabling condition in the hand, Figures 35 and 36.

TENDON AND MUSCLE SHEATHS
OF THE HAND

Figure 54 shows the palmar creases. Figures 4, 5, 40, and 41 show the tendon sheaths of the *second, third,* and *fourth* fingers. In most hands these sheaths extend from the terminal phalanges approximately to a line drawn across the palm from the *medial* end of the distal palmar crease to the *lateral* end of the proximal crease. Note how the proximal ends of these sheaths overlie the distal ends of the thenar and midpalmar spaces or bursae, Figures 40 and 41. Any one of these sheaths occasionally may extend to the wrist.

If one remembers the extent of these sheaths, it is not difficult to realize how a suppurative tenosynovitis involving them can account for *Kanavel's four cardinal points* which are utilized in diagnosing pus in flexor tendon sheaths. Figure 48 illustrates *Kanavel's* four cardinal signs and symptoms:

1. The finger is held in slight flexion for comfort. In contrast it can be held straight without much pain in a localized inflammation (furuncle).
2. The finger is uniformly swollen in tendon sheath infections in contrast to localized swelling in local inflammation.
3. Intense pain accompanies any attempt to extend the partly flexed finger; this is absent in local involvement.
4. Tenderness is marked along the course of the inflamed sheath in contrast to its absence in a localized inflammation.

The *flexor sheath* of the thumb usually extends from the terminal phalanx to a point two or three centimeters proximal to the proximal volar crease of the wrist. The proximal half is commonly referred to as the *radial bursa*, Figures 4, 24, 40, and 41. Occasionally the proximal half of the flexor pollicis longus sheath is separated by a septum from the distal half of the sheath, making them entirely separate sheaths.

The *fifth-finger flexor sheath* commences at its terminal phalanx and, on reaching a point half way up the palm, expands laterally (Figures 4, 5, 24, 40, and 41) to envelop the tendons of the fourth, third, and second fingers. This expanded portion extends two or three centimeters proximal to the proximal volar crease of the wrist and is usually called the *ulnar bursa*. Occasionally the distal unexpanded part of the fifth-finger sheath is separated by a septum from the ulnar bursa.

In a much smaller number of hands, the sheath of the index finger may extend to and communicate with the *ulnar bursa.* The third-finger sheath or the fourth-finger sheath may occasionally do this. These are variations the surgeon should always keep in mind. In a large number of hands, a communication exists between the *radial* and *ulnar bursa.* This accounts

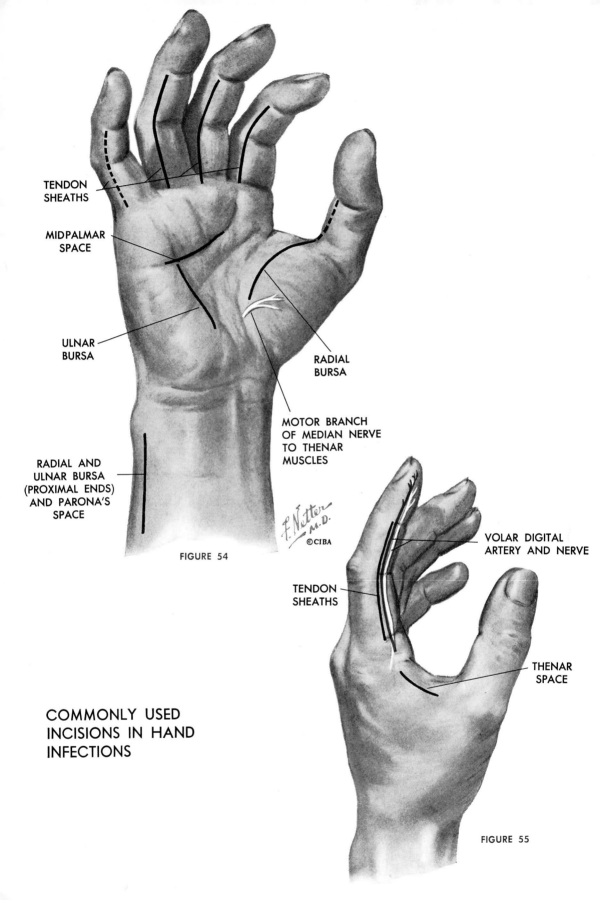

TENDON
SHEATHS

MIDPALMAR
SPACE

ULNAR
BURSA

RADIAL AND
ULNAR BURSA
(PROXIMAL ENDS)
AND PARONA'S
SPACE

RADIAL
BURSA

MOTOR BRANCH
OF MEDIAN NERVE
TO THENAR
MUSCLES

F. Netter
M.D.
©CIBA

FIGURE 54

VOLAR DIGITAL
ARTERY AND NERVE

TENDON
SHEATHS

THENAR
SPACE

FIGURE 55

COMMONLY USED
INCISIONS IN HAND
INFECTIONS

for the so-called "horseshoe abscess" (Figure 49) following a suppurative teno-synovitis of the thumb or fifth finger.

The potential space between the flexor pollicis longus tendon, the flexor digito-rum profundus tendons, and the pronator quadratus muscle is known as the *sub-tendinous space* of the wrist or *Parona's space*. It is easy to see how pus in a flexor pollicis longus sheath infection can ascend the radial bursa and eventually rupture into this space. The same can occur in a suppurative tenosynovitis involving the tendon sheath of the fifth finger and ulnar bursa. Figure 24 shows how it is possible for pus from a thenar abscess or midpal-mar abscess to rupture into Parona's space.

LUMBRICAL MUSCLE SHEATHS

Figures 4 and 5 show the ensheathed lumbrical muscles with a probe in the opened first lumbrical sheath. This sheath is adherent to the "roof" of the *thenar bursa* or *space* with no demonstrable opening into it. The second, third, and fourth lumbrical sheaths are not nearly so easily demonstrated, but when present, usually overlie the midpalmar bursa or space. Figures 25, 40, and 41 show sche-matically these relationships. These sheaths extend from the web-area to the center of the palm. They are demonstrated most easily in the hand of a heavy toiler and are surprisingly strong despite their being thin and semitransparent. It will be recalled that the ensheathed lumbrical muscles and flexor tendons lie in canals formed by septa from the palmar apo-neurosis, Figures 4, 5, and 25. From this description, it is not difficult to visualize how pus from a web-area infection can ascend the first lumbrical canal and sheath and rupture into the thenar bursa or space; the second, third, and fourth rupture into the midpalmar bursa or space. In the "pre-antibiotic" days when serious hand infec-tions were more common, cases were seen in which pus from a thenar or midpal-mar space abscess would erode into and descend a lumbrical sheath and canal finally to rupture through the skin in the dorsal web-area.

THENAR AND MIDPALMAR SPACES

There is some disagreement about the existence of these spaces. According to Kanavel, the *thenar* space extends medio-laterally from the third metacarpal bone to the thenar eminence and proximodis-tally from the transverse carpal ligament to a line about a thumb's breadth prox-imal to the webs of the fingers. The *mid-palmar space* extends lateromedially from the third metacarpal bone to the hypo-thenar eminence and proximodistally about a centimeter more proximally than the thenar space. Figures 24, 25, 40, and 41 show schematically the approximate extent of these spaces.

The use of the word "space" in the terms *thenar space* and *midpalmar space* is not entirely accurate. They are only potential spaces, demonstrable only when injected with a radiopaque fluid. Figures 4, 5, and 24 show rents in a thin, almost transparent, membranous layer colored green. In order to depict these so-called spaces in relation to surrounding structures, the artist had to make the membranes appear much thicker than they actually are. In fact, they are so thin that, unless extreme care is taken in palmar dissection, the membrane covering the thenar space is usually removed with the skin and superficial fascia. This no doubt accounts for the infrequency with which this membrane is seen. With careful dissection, a thin, semi-transparent membrane can be definitely demonstrated. In fact, the artist sketched these figures from a dissected palm with probes in the rents of the membranes covering the so-called thenar and midpalmar spaces. As stated previously, they are demonstrated best in hands which have done hard and rough work. For that reason, it seems logical to think of these membranes as parts of modified bursae which develop as a result of the extra friction to which laborers' palms are subjected. Therefore, why not call them the *thenar* and *midpalmar bursae* instead of purposeless spaces?

Recall that in the fingers proper and the proximal palmar and wrist regions, the flexor tendons have sheaths and bursae to make their sliding movement easier, Figure 24. Unlike the flexor tendons of the thumb and fifth finger, which have sheaths and bursae, the flexor tendons of the second, third, and fourth fingers have little or no sheath or bursal protection in their central palmar portions. Figures 4, 5, 24, and 25 show how the thenar bursa is interposed between the deep aspect of the index-finger flexor tendons, the ensheathed first lumbrical muscle, and the superficial aspect of the adductor pollicis muscle. Also, note in Figure 5 a probe within the dorsal extension of the thenar bursa or space interposed between the deep aspect of the adductor pollicis muscle and the palmar aspect of the first dorsal interosseous muscle, the second metacarpal bone, and the first palmar interosseous muscle. Figure 24 shows the end of the probe butting against the proximal end of the thenar bursa.

Figures 5 and 24 show a rent in the membrane covering the so-called *midpalmar* space. Actually, there is no space here; it is also a potential space in what can be more logically called the *midpalmar bursa*. This bursa is not nearly so easy to expose as the thenar bursa; and, similarly, it can be demonstrated only in a hand that has done hard, rough work. Figure 24 shows probes butting against the proximal ends of the thenar and palmar bursae.

The author has had an opportunity to dissect many hands, varying from those of delicate type to those which have obviously been exposed to hard, rough usage. In the former, the thenar bursa could usually be exposed, but the midpalmar bursa could not be demonstrated satisfactorily enough to be called a bursa. In the strong, tough hand, however, there was consistently a thenar bursa and usually a midpalmar bursa — or excellent imitations of bursae.

Considering the tremendous amount of friction to which the palm is subjected, it seems natural enough to have a *thenar bursa* present to enhance the sliding movements of the index-finger flexor tendons and ensheathed first lumbrical muscle over the underlying adductor pollicis muscle.

The *thenar bursa* also minimizes friction between the adductor pollicis and that part of the palmar skin between the index-finger tendons and thenar eminence. The dorsal extension of the thenar bursa makes smoother the movements between the adductor pollicis and the first dorsal interosseous muscle, the second metacarpal bone, and the first palmar interosseous muscle. Similarly, the *midpalmar bursa* when present minimizes friction between the flexor tendons of the third, fourth, and fifth fingers, the ensheathed lumbrical muscles, the underlying metacarpal bones, and interosseous muscles. As stated previously, in delicate hands both bursae seem to be absent or very difficult to demonstrate.

Figures 4, 5, and 24 show a sizable ulnar bursa. However, it fails to cover all of the palmar portions of the flexor tendons — especially that part of the palm where these tendons are subjected to considerable pressure and friction.

Figures 4, 5, 24, 25, 40, and 41 show somewhat schematically how the proximal end of the index-finger sheath and the sheath of the first lumbrical muscle are in contact with the thenar bursa. The proximal ends of the third, fourth, and fifth tendon sheaths, and associated lumbrical sheaths and canals are in contact with the midpalmar bursa. This enables one to understand how a suppurative tenosynovitis of the index-finger tendon sheath can rupture through its proximal end into the thenar bursa if present and cause the so-called thenar-space abscess, the clinical appearance of which is shown in Figure 53. On the same page is shown a midpalmar space abscess which can be produced by rupture of a suppurative tenosynovitis of the sheaths of the third, fourth, or fifth fingers into the so-called midpalmar bursa.

As previously mentioned, the loose areolar tissue of the *dorsal subcutaneous space* is loaded with minute lymph vessels which receive much of the lymph from the fingers, web-areas, and edges of the palm. Such lymphedema caused by a palmar space infection is shown in Figure 51. This occurs quite commonly and is on occasion mistakenly incised. The *dorsal subaponeurotic space* is an area not frequently involved in hand infections.

A clear picture of the muscle and ten-

don sheaths, the thenar and midpalmar spaces or bursae and their locations, and their extent and relation to each other should make it much easier to visualize the anatomic course which can be taken by acute pyogenic infections of the hand.

Figure 49 shows the uniform swelling when the tendon sheath of the second, third, or fourth finger is infected and depicts by arrows the spread of a suppurative tenosynovitis from the flexor pollicis longus sheath and radial bursa via the intermediate sheath to the ulnar bursa, fifth-finger sheath with eventual rupture into Parona's subtendinous space.

Figure 50 illustrates the appearance of a midpalmar abscess following a suppurative tenosynovitis of the third finger. The appearance of the palm is similar when abscess is due to infection of the fourth finger.

Figure 53 shows a thenar abscess with its swollen thenar area and abducted thumb resulting from an index finger suppurative tenosynovitis. In Figure 51 is shown the dorsal lymphedema which may develop with either thenar or midpalmar abscesses. Figure 52 illustrates how a subcutaneous abscess in the palmar web-area can erode through the palmar aponeurosis to reach the dorsum of the web-area to form a so-called *"collar button abscess."*

SURGICAL INCISIONS

Most surgeons prefer a general anesthetic for the patient and the use of a tourniquet (a blood pressure cuff inflated to 250 mm.) to obtain a bloodless field. It is axiomatic that the incision should be adequate and properly placed, and that utmost care be exercised in handling the small nerves, tendons, joints, and other pertinent structures. It goes without saying that chemotherapy, heat, rest, elevation, position of function (Figure 39), and physiotherapy be included in the plan of treatment.

Some of the more commonly used incisions are illustrated in Figures 42B, 43A, 44, 46, 54, and 55.

In treating *paronychia,* as a rule, it is *not* necessary to use an incision extending proximalward on the dorsum of the distal phalanx. Figure 42B shows the knife-point elevating the skin from the dorsum of the proximal end of the nail to release the drop or two of pus found in the early stage of a paronychia. This, with supportive therapy of heat, rest, and chemotherapy, usually cures the infection.

Should a paronychia be advanced to the stage of abscess formation under the root of the nail, gentle elevation of the edge of the skin, Figure 43, and excision of part or all of the loosened root of the nail, plus supportive therapy handles the situation adequately.

A *felon* is no longer drained by "fish mouth" or "hockey stick" incisions. These have been replaced by a simple lateral incision, Figures 44 and 46, which avoids the formation of a tender scar on the finger tip.

Figure 54 shows the placement of incisions for draining a *suppurative tenosynovitis of the second, third, or fourth finger.* Observe that the incisions are along lines placed at the dorsal limit of the finger-creases in order to avoid injuring the digital nerves and artery depicted in Figure 55.

The dotted line on the *fifth finger* in Figure 54 represents the position of the incision as it is on the *radial side* of the fifth finger. The reason for the incision on the radial side of the fifth finger and ulnar side of the second finger is obvious: to

have the scars where they will be subjected to the least friction and trauma.

The incision for draining a *thenar abscess* is placed on the dorsal aspect of the web between the thumb and index finger, Figure 55.

The incision for draining a *midpalmar abscess* is shown in Figure 54. This incision can be made along or slightly proximal to the *distal* palmar crease. Once through the palmar aponeurosis en route to the more deeply situated midpalmar abscess, it is important for the surgeon to avoid injuring the digital branches of the medial and ulnar nerve shown in Figure 7.

Pus from a suppurative tenosynovitis of the fifth-finger sheath may progress proximally to the ulnar bursa extending from the palm to a point four or five centimeters proximal to the crease of the wrist. Figure 54 depicts the three incisions which might be necessary to promote adequate drainage. Certainly the incision along the *radial* border of the fifth finger and radial border of the hypothenar eminence would be required. If swelling and tenderness are presented cephalad to the proximal wrist crease, a third incision extending five centimeters proximally from the crease and along the medial border of the ulna would be necessary. These three incisions usually allow efficient drainage.

Figures 24 and 40 demonstrate the pathway of pus from a thumb sheath infection to the proximal end of the radial bursa — four or five centimeters cephalad to the proximal crease of the wrist. In Figure 54 is seen an incision for opening the flexor pollicis longus sheath and the distal part of the radial bursa.

To avoid injuring branches of the median nerve that supply the thenar muscle, it is best *not to* extend the incision along the ulnar border of the thenar eminence proximally beyond the mid-point of the first metacarpal bone. To go farther jeopardizes the motor branches of the median nerve, Figure 54. If swelling and tenderness are noted over the proximal end of the radial bursa, it can be drained by using the same incision suggested for draining the proximal end of the ulnar bursa, Figure 54, or, as some surgeons prefer, a similarly placed incision on the radial side — making sure to hug the lateral border of the radius to avoid cutting the radial artery.

If pus from either the ulnar or radial bursa ruptures into *Parona's subtendinous space* (between the flexor tendons and pronator quadratus muscle, Figure 23), it can be drained by the same incision used for releasing pus from the proximal end of the ulnar bursa, Figure 54.

The so-called *"horseshoe abscess,"* Figure 49, has to be drained by a combination of fifth finger-ulnar bursa and flexor pollicis-radial bursa incisions as depicted in Figure 54.

Infection from a *human bite* poses a somewhat different problem. The presence of anaerobes with the usual streptococci and staphylococci alters the pattern of treatment. The metacarpophalangeal joint and adjacent tissues and spaces are most commonly involved because the teeth of the opponent are struck with the knuckle of the clenched fist. When the hand is unclenched, the skin wound retracts proximally covering the deeper part of the wound within which the bacteria have been deposited. Obviously, this airless, traumatized area forms an ideal site in which anaerobic organisms can flourish.

Treatment calls for excising a few millimeters of devitalized skin and underlying traumatized tissue so as to lay the wound wide open for thorough surgical cleansing of the tissues with generous amounts of normal saline solution. Penicillin usually helps to subdue the streptococci and staphylococci but exerts no effect upon the anaerobes. Based on the theory that nascent oxygen helps overcome the anaerobes, Meleny has suggested the use of moistened zinc peroxide powder. The other principles of treatment are the same as outlined for tendon sheath and fascial space infections, *i.e.,* adequate heat, elevation, and rest with the hand splinted in the position of function, Figure 39.

If a tendon has been severed, no attempt should be made to repair it at the time of the cleansing procedure. It is best to wait until several weeks after the wound has completely healed.

If a bone has been involved, no attempt should be made to curette the infected part. It is better to let the sequestrum separate spontaneously, thereby minimizing the chances of spreading the infection.

TREATMENT OF HAND INJURIES

It goes without saying that the detailed treatment of the various types of injuries which beset the hand cannot be included in this article; but, as in the paragraphs dealing with the treatment of hand infections, the general principles involved will be briefly described.

The **ideal time** to clean any recently sustained wound is the **first time.** Therefore, the immediate emergency treatment should consist of no more than the application of a sterile dressing (with pressure if there is bleeding) and immobilization with a splint. The patient should be taken at once to a well-equipped dressing room or operating room, where gloved, gowned, and masked, the surgeon can do a thorough job of cleansing so as to permit primary closure, if conditions warrant it.

Before the advent of antibiotics, the duration of the so-called "Golden Period" for treatment of an average lacerated or incised, contaminated wound was six to eight hours after the injury. During this period, a wound with no devitalized tissue or gross foreign bodies (or a wound in which the devitalized tissue and foreign bodies can be removed with certainty) should be given a thorough surgical cleansing with generous amounts of normal saline solution sloshed gently in the wound with a piece of gauze (not a brush or anything hard). If there are no contraindications, a *primary closure* can then be made. While antibiotics have permitted extension of the "Golden Period" by several hours, the general principle of removal of devitalized tissue and foreign bodies, followed by thorough, gentle surgical cleansing of the wound still applies.

Within the "Golden Period," severed tendons or nerves can usually be sutured if the wound has been satisfactorily cleansed. Because of loss of tissue, the tendon or nerve ends sometimes cannot be approximated with the hand in the position of function. The hand or fingers may then have to be flexed or extended, as the case may be, in order to approximate the ends of these structures without tension.

The sutures approximating the skin edges should not be under tension. It is safer to apply a split graft over the raw surface than to have tension on the suture line.

The so-called *secondary closure* can be used if the wound is seen *just after* the "Golden Period" has elapsed. If seen at this time, the wound is gently and thoroughly cleansed with generous amounts of normal saline solution (soap and water if there is grease in the wound) and then a gauze pack moistened in normal saline is placed in the wound. After 24 to 48 hours, the pack is removed and the wound inspected. If the tissues look clean and viable, closure is then made with fine silk sutures.

Following either primary or secondary closure, the hand is adequately dressed and put in the position of function in a comfortably applied splint. The treatment of extensive injuries with much loss of skin or segments of tendons, nerves, or muscles is much more complicated. Hence, the reader is referred to articles and books by the authors mentioned in the conclusion below.

CONCLUSION

Regardless of the pathologic change that one encounters in the hand, it is quite obvious that intelligent treatment demands, first of all, a sound knowledge of structure. Therefore, this article has been designed simply as a review of the surgical anatomy. The author has mentioned only enough of the pathology and surgery to assist in visualizing the pertinent anatomy.

The reader who expects to be charged with responsibility for surgical procedures involving the hand is referred to the works of Kanavel, Auchinchloss, Koch, Mason, Bunnell, Littler, and others who have outlined in far greater detail the management of infections and the various complicated procedures that are necessary for the rehabilitation of hands that have been badly damaged.

Brief as this article has been, the author hopes that it will help the reader to visualize, and to remember, the rather intricate details of the surgical anatomy of the hand.

SECTION B

C I B A

PULMONARY EMPHYSEMA
Seymour M. Farber, M.D.
Roger H. L. Wilson, M.D.

PULMONARY EMPHYSEMA

SEYMOUR M. FARBER, M.D.
In Charge of University of California Tuberculosis and Chest Service, San Francisco Hospital
Head of Continuing Education in Medicine and the Health Sciences,
University of California Medical Center

ROGER H. L. WILSON, M.D.
Assistant Clinical Professor of Medicine
University of California Medical Center

The importance of early diagnosis is less stressed and adequate treatment is more rarely prescribed than is the case with practically any other disabling condition coming to the physician's attention.

Emphysema is by far the most common chronic disease of the lungs. More frequent than tuberculosis, more frequent than lung cancer, it is the major single cause of disability having a pulmonary origin. Certainly more than a million people in our country are living restricted lives because of this condition.

To those who may consider this estimate an overstatement, we should like to point out that emphysema is the basic therapeutic problem in most patients with asthma and in most patients with chronic bronchitis past the age of 40. Then we have a group of patients whose shortness of breath has been attributed to cardiac trouble, when in fact their difficulty is really bronchial in origin. When we put all these groups together, we can safely estimate a total number in excess of the arthritic population of the country!

Emphysema has other unfortunate distinctions. Pulmonary physiology has received far less attention than has cardiovascular physiology, for example. Thus, the importance of early diagnosis is less stressed, and adequate treatment is more rarely prescribed than is the case with practically any other disabling condition coming to the physician's attention.

The onset of emphysema is insidious. The course is deceptively yet relentlessly progressive, particularly in the absence of adequate therapy. These patients do not die quickly. Rather they live for years, a trial and a tribulation to themselves, their families, and also their physicians, with whom they come to share a feeling of frustrated hopelessness. Unlike the patient with a broken arm who can assume a position of comparative comfort, the patient with emphysema must breathe 20,000 times each day, and he suffers with each and every breath.

The respiratory difficulty of the emphysematous patient can often be visualized by the way in which he seats himself in the physician's office (Plate I). Since he must utilize every inch of thoracic space and most of the accessory muscles of respiration, he will never slump in a chair or even sit comfortably. Instead, he will lean forward, placing his elbows on the arms of the chair or even on the desk, thus assuming the most favorable position in which to carry on his respiratory efforts.

If we are to provide a longer and more productive life for patients with emphysema, it is necessary to gain an understanding of the basic pathology that is involved, to employ the most practical diagnostic methods that have been developed, and then to plan a therapeutic campaign that utilizes all of the presently known methods of improving pulmonary function. We shall attempt to present this total approach on the pages that follow.

DEFINITION

Emphysema may be defined as enlargement of the whole or a part of the lung due to loss of inherent elasticity. The alveoli themselves have very little elastic tissue. The main elastic system of the lungs is therefore contained in the bronchi, bronchioles, alveolar ducts, and blood vessels. Thus the problem of emphysema is primarily a pre-alveolar problem. The alveolar stretching and rupture are secondary developments, contributing further to the disability.

Localized Emphysema

Only an isolated area of a lung may be involved. This may follow infection, a developmental defect, or a localized bronchial obstruction from a tumor or foreign body. Under any of these conditions, the bronchus may be so occluded that air passes only at the peak of inspiration. As soon as the peak of negative pressure is passed, when expiration begins, the bronchus closes completely, thus acting like the check valve in an automobile tire. The air can pass in one direction only — into the alveoli but not out. This produces single or multiple *bullae*, or rounded tension cysts. Alveolar rupture into the subpleural space may produce a *bleb*. Recognition of the presence of a bleb is important because it presents the threat of spontaneous pneumothorax. These localized conditions do not commonly cause confusion in diagnosis, and therapy consists of surgical intervention when necessary.

A simple atrophic condition, *senile emphysema*, causes chronic shortness of breath. On the other hand, shortness of breath may be found in *compensatory emphysema*, where a portion of the lung expands to make up the thoracic volume after a pneumonectomy or a lobectomy, or in pulmonary atelectasis or fibrosis. Senile emphysema and compensatory emphysema are not in themselves seriously disabling diseases, except where the obstructive element develops due to loss of elasticity. Therefore, we shall confine our discussion to chronic generalized obstructive emphysema.

CHRONIC GENERALIZED OBSTRUCTIVE EMPHYSEMA

This is a condition in which expiration is chronically embarrassed. Chronic bronchial allergy and/or chronic infection is commonly present. Here, recoil of alveoli is impeded and elasticity destroyed with consequent enlargement, coalescence, and loss of alveolar function. The picture is that of chronic wheezing dyspnea, variable it is true, but remorselessly progressive over the years, leading to respiratory failure with embarrassment or failure of the right side of the heart.

The normal lung has an immense amount of functional reserve. Not until about one-half of functional reserve is lost does the patient complain of any breathlessness. Indeed, many patients do not seek medical advice until their breathing reserves are reduced to one-third of normal or less.

ETIOLOGY

The two most frequent precursors of emphysema are *allergic asthma* and *chronic infectious bronchitis*. If persistent,

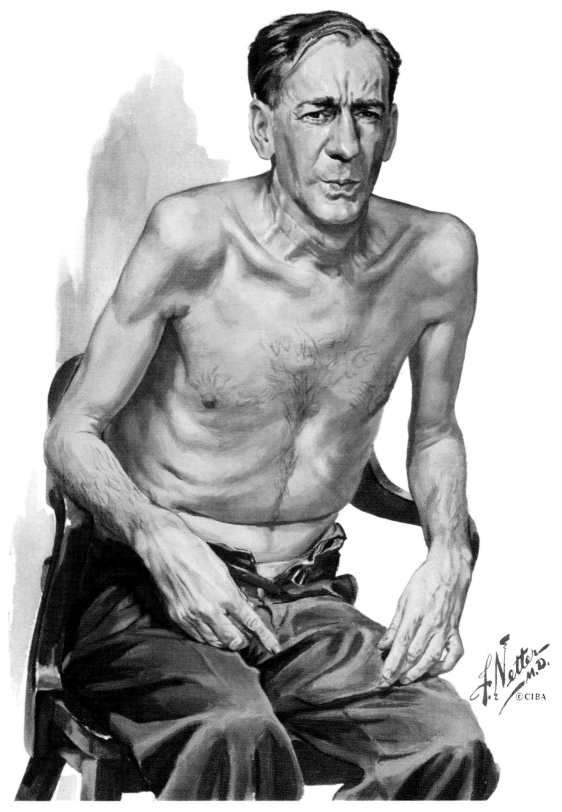

PLATE I   POSITION OFTEN ASSUMED BY PATIENT IN THE OFFICE

both of these conditions will inevitably lead to varying degrees of emphysema.

Once emphysema has been produced, a recurrent vicious circle results. As will be explained in more detail later, the bronchi and bronchioles in the emphysematous area tend to trap and retain allergens and/or bacteria. Retained mucus is an excellent culture medium. Therefore, the mere presence of emphysema tends to encourage exacerbations. These lead to further tissue destruction and degeneration. Around and around the spiral goes on a progressively downward course!

While *smoking* has been implicated in the production of emphysema, our own experience leads us to doubt that this is ever the sole factor, or even a major factor, in the loss of lung elasticity. However, in certain patients it may produce chronic irritation.

In some cases *intrinsic tissue weakness* may be involved. We believe that even without pathologic insult certain people will tend to develop degenerative changes in small bronchi before others. We accept individual differences of tissue susceptibility to degeneration in the heart and great vessels, or in the skin where some people develop earlier wrinkling, and in other tissues. Thus it seems only reasonable to believe that the same sort of individual difference in susceptibility to degeneration may exist in the bronchi. Although we are unable to present definite evidence that this is true, the fact that such a concept is not well defined should not blind us to the possibility of its importance.

The association of emphysema with old tuberculous or histoplasmous lymphadenopathy is under investigation. These diseases, as well as recurrent pneumonitis, may play a part etiologically.

A specific disease leading to emphysema is *mucoviscidosis*, sometimes called cystic fibrosis of the pancreas. Ordinarily, patients with this condition do not reach adult life. However, we have now discovered that this disease exists in mild form in adults, who can in turn transmit it to their children. These people have very viscid secretions, which are difficult to bring up. Therefore, they develop three things: (1) chronic bronchitis, (2) small areas of bronchiectasis, and (3) generalized obstructive emphysema. Often these patients are called asthmatics because of their tendency to wheeze. The same thing happens in *other pulmonary fibroses*, where inadequacy of cough and drying of secretions by mouth breathing convert an original compensatory emphysema into an obstructive one.

So long as the emphysema is simply compensatory, the patient gets along fairly well, but when the obstructive factor is added, the result may be true respiratory failure with cor pulmonale.

Vascular disease in the pulmonary and bronchial arteries may be involved in certain cases. Some authors have described localized endarteritis in these vessels which is not present elsewhere. Whether this is a primary condition caused by the localized effect of an allergen on the vascular shock organ or whether it is due to infection, we do not know. However, this condition does exist, and we should be aware of the possibility that it may be an important primary cause.

Essential pulmonary hypertension, either on arteriosclerotic, thromboangiitic, or multiple embolic grounds, is a separate problem. Although cardiorespiratory failure is the sequel, obstructive emphysema is not the main pattern.

CLINICAL COURSE

One of the earliest symptoms of emphysema is wheezing on effort. This is sometimes interpreted as being a symptom of asthma and the patient treated with antihistaminics, usually without success. The shortness of breath may be thought to be an indication of heart trouble and the patient treated with rest, digitalis, and diuretics — again unsuccessfully.

Of course, one must keep the possibility of spasmodic asthma or cardiac dyspnea in mind and take appropriate measures to rule them out. In the case of asthma, failure to respond adequately to bronchodilators and sympathomimetics should raise very serious doubt that spasm has a major rôle in causing the wheezing. Even in known asthmatics, medications directed solely at the spasmodic or allergic element will rarely prove effective, as will be pointed out later under "Treatment." Where a cardiac cause is suspected, one must find other evidence of heart trouble before one is justified in attributing wheezy dyspnea on exertion to "cardiac failure." It must be remembered that peripheral edema and some orthopnea may be seen in severe pulmonary emphysema, in which involvement of the right heart has become an important part of the pattern. Moreover, the coexistence of cardiac failure with pulmonary disease may produce a mixed syndrome, in which the treatment of only one of the factors will prove inadequate.

It is important to understand the meaning of a wheeze. This may be demonstrated by blowing through a reed. No sound is produced until the sides of the reed are compressed. So it is in the bronchi. When the lumen is narrowed either by spasm or loss of elasticity, a wheeze is produced. Therefore, one must remember that "All that wheezes is *not* asthma." What is even more important, considering the laws of probability, "When one hears a wheeze, the *first* diagnosis to consider is emphysema."

As the disease progresses and more lung tissue becomes involved, the symptoms become more severe and are brought on by less and less exertion. As we have said previously, the disease is insidiously progressive. In addition, it is subject to exacerbations whenever the patient gets a respiratory infection. For this reason, as will be pointed out under "Treatment," it is essential to protect the patient by all possible means against such infections.

The final stage is the development of cor pulmonale with pulmonary artery hypertension and right heart failure and of respiratory acidosis. Death of most of these patients is due to respiratory acidosis in the presence of heart failure.

PATHOGENESIS

Although the nature and rôle of many of the etiologic factors remain obscure at the present time, the sequence of events leading to the full-blown pathologic picture of obstructive emphysema is relatively clear. A series of mechanisms causing bronchial narrowing can be defined.

Bronchial narrowing is *not* synonymous with *bronchospasm*. Often this latter word is used with unfortunate looseness to describe all forms of wheezing. However, spasm can refer only to the bronchial musculature. This is smooth muscle, having a slow, rhythmic peristalsis and a natural tonus. Chronic increase of tonus due to chronic allergies or infectious processes will narrow the bronchial lumen and at the same time give rise to hypertrophy of the muscle layer. It is common to see hypertrophy of the bronchial musculature at autopsy in emphysema, but this is much less marked in the middle aged and elderly emphysematous patient than in the younger individual with spasmodic asthma. Also, in emphysema misleading appearances of hypertrophy may be found on gross inspection, which histologic examination will prove to be due to a closer approximation of individual muscle fibers (because of loss of elasticity) rather than actual hypertrophy. Thus the histologic picture is much different in obstructive emphysema than it is in spasmodic asthma. However, it is only fair to say that any allergic or infectious process in a

AT END OF INSPIRATION AT END OF EXPIRATION

NORMAL

EMPHYSEMA

PLATE II

GROSS PATHOLOGIC CHANGES IN EMPHYSEMA

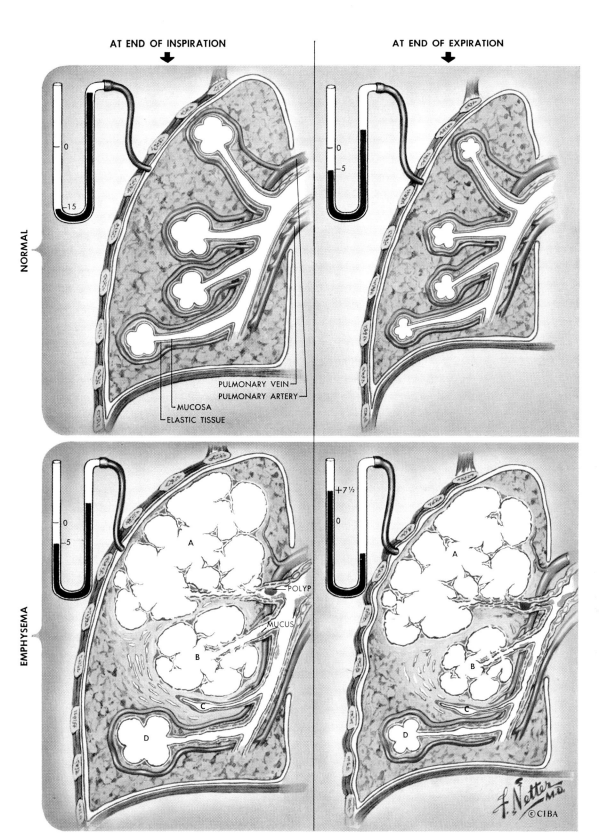

NORMAL

PULMONARY VEIN
PULMONARY ARTERY
MUCOSA
ELASTIC TISSUE

EMPHYSEMA

POLYP

MUCUS

F. Netter, M.D.
©CIBA

bronchus will produce reflex vagal activity that can only increase tonus and narrow the bronchial lumen.

Far more important than the bronchial musculature are the changes that take place in the *mucosa* and within the *bronchial lumen*. These are illustrated in Plates II and IV.

Allergy or infection produces edema and cellular infiltration of the mucosa as well as an increase in secretion of mucus. With the narrowing produced by changes in the mucosa and submucosa, cough becomes less efficient. This leads to retention of excessive mucus, which is thickened by desquamation of the endothelium. When dyspnea develops, mouth breathing further thickens and inspissates the mucus. This makes it still more difficult to dislodge and additionally compromises the area of the bronchial lumen. As in any inflammatory process, papillary outgrowth of a polypoid nature frequently develops.

The importance of the lining of the bronchus in the production of dyspnea is emphasized by the effect of air pollution on patients with chronic generalized obstructive emphysema. We have been able to show in our laboratories that an increase in the level of irritants in the atmosphere is associated with an easily demonstrated worsening of the patient's ability to breathe air out of the lungs.

The retention of mucus, which is a good culture medium, encourages the continued growth of bacteria. Leukocyte migration into the inspissated mucus is minimal. Thus, although the mucus may contain a considerable number of organisms (for example, Neisseria catarrhalis and Streptococcus viridans), the leukocyte migration necessary to deal with these organisms does not occur. This suggests the possibility that autogenous bacterial allergy may be an important factor in the maintenance of the bronchial inflammatory state.

In the presence of inflammatory disease of the bronchi, disturbances of blood supply to the bronchial wall may occur. As a result, bronchial fragmentation may take place with rupture of a small bronchus into adjacent alveoli. Finally, bronchial sequestration may occur, the fragmentated bronchus losing all continuity with the bronchial tree. This is accompanied by local coalescence of alveoli and cyst formation.

With increasing difficulty in expiration a more and more inflated position of the lung is adopted. The lung slowly becomes larger, until finally it is impossible to enlarge the thoracic cage without considerable structural alteration. Thus the patient develops the kyphotic increase of the anteroposterior chest diameter with flattened depressed diaphragms, and still the lung continues to enlarge.

As the lung becomes larger, it is less efficient from a functional point of view. Also, the pulmonary blood supply may be compromised. Cough becomes markedly less efficient, and dyspnea increases, further tending to increase the disability. Again we can describe the situation as a vicious spiral, in which various factors influence each other in a continual worsening of the patient's condition.

PATHOLOGY

The loss of elasticity of the lungs in generalized emphysema is far from uniform. The various changes in gross appearance are illustrated in Plate II. The changes in intrathoracic pressure on inspiration and expiration, both in the normal and in the emphysematous patient, are shown in the manometers (see also "Pneumodynamics," Plate IV).

It will be seen that in the emphysematous patient the chest cage is enlarged both on expiration and inspiration. The diaphragm is flattened and does not rise as high on expiration.

In the normal, the alveolar pattern is

rather uniformly sponge-like. However, in the emphysematous lung many different changes are apparent. Even when emphysema is generalized, some alveoli or even some lobules may be entirely normal. Others may have partially lost their elasticity. Still others will be found completely and irrevocably destroyed from a functional standpoint.

In Plate II a large cyst is shown in the upper lobe, which changes in size very little between inspiration and expiration. The elasticity having been almost completely lost and a papillary outgrowth in the bronchus acting like a check-valve, this area is functionless, and by occupying space in the chest cavity it actually impairs the function of more normal areas.

Below this will be seen a cyst that retains some elasticity, being somewhat reduced in size on expiration. This cyst retains some ventilating function, but its capacity for gaseous exchange is greatly decreased because of impairment of its blood supply and the breakdown of alveolar walls.

Around this cyst is an area of atelectasis. This latter region is white because the lymphatics have washed all the carbon away — evidence that the contained alveoli have been functionless for a very long time. This atelectatic area probably contains the very best alveoli in the lungs, having excellent elastic tissue. However, other areas of the lung, with little or no elasticity, have prevented the development of a sufficient amount of negative pressure to expand any normally elastic alveoli. Thus, in spite of the fact that this area would be capable of good function in a normal lung, placed as it is in an emphysematous lung, the relatively normal alveoli are completely functionless.

Below, and medial to this region, the lung is fairly normal. However, even here some areas are semi-atelectatic.

The non-ventilating, functionless cyst at the apex is served by a large bronchus, which has become fragmented, rupturing into an alveolus. This alveolus in turn has ruptured into other alveoli so that the entire cyst is composed of broken alveoli. In the bronchus subserving the large cyst A, the muscle and mucosal layers are somewhat hypertrophied. The lumen contains a papillary outgrowth which may have caused obstruction. The submucosa is thickened by edema and infiltration. There is also a plug of mucus containing some incompletely detached desquamated cells in alveolus A, which must act as a block even to inspiration.

Cyst B has some elasticity and a fairly large bronchial opening. Therefore it ventilates. However, it is relatively useless from a functional point of view.

Pulmonary Blood Vessels (Plate III)

A functionless area of the lung will lose its blood supply because a minimum oxygen tension in the capillary blood is necessary if perfusion by way of the pulmonary arteriole is to continue.

Thus the large non-ventilating cyst (A) previously shown in Plate II has almost completely lost its blood supply. In the partially functioning cyst (B), only a small blood supply remains. This cyst also is practically useless from the standpoint of gaseous exchange.

Below this the alveolus C in the atelectatic area has also lost its blood supply. Although this is one of the least affected alveoli in the lung, it has become functionless. The lung having become voluminous, the normal elasticity of this alveolus has caused it to contract so that it no longer is being used for ventilation. Deprived of oxygen, vessels have constricted and finally disappeared, and circulation of blood has ceased.

Alveolus D represents a damaged broncho-alveolar unit that is the main functional unit remaining. Having impaired elasticity, it has enlarged. Definite bronchial changes are present. However, a sufficient degree of elasticity remains for it

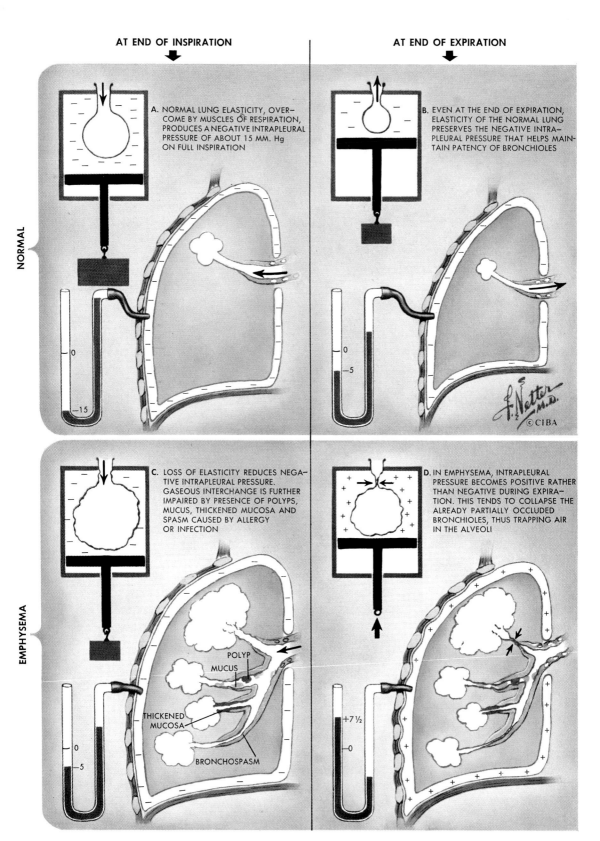

AT END OF INSPIRATION

AT END OF EXPIRATION

NORMAL

A. NORMAL LUNG ELASTICITY, OVER-COME BY MUSCLES OF RESPIRATION, PRODUCES A NEGATIVE INTRAPLEURAL PRESSURE OF ABOUT 15 MM. Hg ON FULL INSPIRATION

B. EVEN AT THE END OF EXPIRATION, ELASTICITY OF THE NORMAL LUNG PRESERVES THE NEGATIVE INTRA-PLEURAL PRESSURE THAT HELPS MAIN-TAIN PATENCY OF BRONCHIOLES

EMPHYSEMA

C. LOSS OF ELASTICITY REDUCES NEGA-TIVE INTRAPLEURAL PRESSURE. GASEOUS INTERCHANGE IS FURTHER IMPAIRED BY PRESENCE OF POLYPS, MUCUS, THICKENED MUCOSA AND SPASM CAUSED BY ALLERGY OR INFECTION

D. IN EMPHYSEMA, INTRAPLEURAL PRESSURE BECOMES POSITIVE RATHER THAN NEGATIVE DURING EXPIRA-TION. THIS TENDS TO COLLAPSE THE ALREADY PARTIALLY OCCLUDED BRONCHIOLES, THUS TRAPPING AIR IN THE ALVEOLI

POLYP

MUCUS

THICKENED MUCOSA

BRONCHOSPASM

PLATE IV

PNEUMODYNAMICS OF EMPHYSEMA

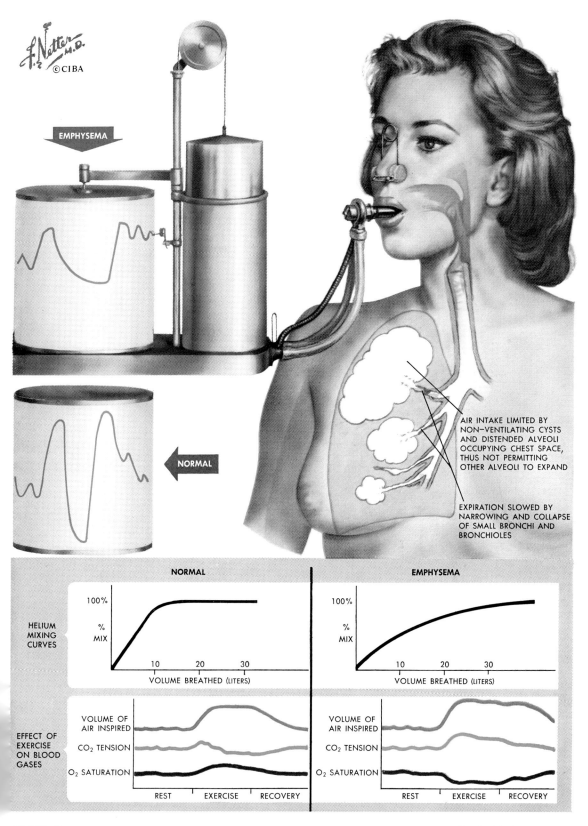

EMPHYSEMA

NORMAL

AIR INTAKE LIMITED BY
NON-VENTILATING CYSTS
AND DISTENDED ALVEOLI
OCCUPYING CHEST SPACE,
THUS NOT PERMITTING
OTHER ALVEOLI TO EXPAND

EXPIRATION SLOWED BY
NARROWING AND COLLAPSE
OF SMALL BRONCHI AND
BRONCHIOLES

NORMAL	EMPHYSEMA

HELIUM
MIXING
CURVES

100%

%
MIX

10   20   30

VOLUME BREATHED (LITERS)

100%

%
MIX

10   20   30

VOLUME BREATHED (LITERS)

EFFECT OF
EXERCISE
ON BLOOD
GASES

VOLUME OF
AIR INSPIRED

CO₂ TENSION

O₂ SATURATION

REST   EXERCISE   RECOVERY

VOLUME OF
AIR INSPIRED

CO₂ TENSION

O₂ SATURATION

REST   EXERCISE   RECOVERY

PLATE V   PHYSIOLOGIC TESTING

to function in ventilation, and therefore its blood supply is rather well preserved.

PNEUMODYNAMICS
(PLATE IV)

In the illustrations on page 180, the suspended balloons represent the lungs; the weighted plungers represent the muscles of respiration, and the cylinder represents the thoracic cage. In the normal, the elasticity of the balloon opposed by muscle contraction and muscle tone combines to maintain a negative pressure during expiration as well as during inspiration.

In contrast, the balloon in emphysema has lost its elasticity. It is, therefore, larger both on inspiration and expiration as is the total content of the cylinder. Also, due to loss of elasticity the excursion of the cylinder is much reduced in emphysema. In addition, during expiration pressure must be exerted upward in the piston to force air from the flaccid balloon.

This pressure may constrict or even completely obstruct the neck of the balloon so that it is difficult or impossible to expel air from the balloon, regardless of the degree of pressure exerted.

The lung diagrams in Plate IV schematically depict the bronchial changes that contribute to loss of elasticity in impairing ventilation. These factors include thickening of the mucosa and submucosa by edema and cellular infiltration, collection of mucus which tends to become dessicated, development of polypoid growths, and bronchospasm.

The manometers indicate the intrapleural pressure on inspiration and expiration in both normal and emphysematous subjects. In the normal there is a negative intrapleural pressure even on expiration, due to the elasticity of the lung. On inspiration this negative pressure is increased to about 15 mm. of mercury.

In the emphysematous chest, where elasticity is greatly reduced, there is very little negative pressure even on inspiration. On expiration the pressure may become positive, reaching 7.5 mm. of mercury or more above atmospheric pressure. In other words, whereas in the normal person expiration is a passive act, the air leaving the lungs because of elastic recoil as it would from a tire after the valve stem has been removed, in emphysema the patient must literally squeeze the air from his chest, producing a positive intrapleural pressure.

To maintain an adequate bronchial lumen, air pressure on the inside must be greater than on the outside of the bronchial wall. This is especially true in the finest radicals. The bronchi in the normal lung remain patent even in forced expiration, because the intrathoracic pressure on the outer walls of the bronchi is less than the atmospheric pressure within the lumen.

In the emphysematous lung, on the other hand, the lungs have lost much of this negative pressure along with their elasticity, and bronchi tend to collapse. During inspiration in emphysema the bronchioles contain air at atmospheric pressure (760 mm. Hg). On the outside of the bronchi there is a negative pressure (perhaps 755 mm. Hg). This pressure difference of 5 mm. Hg is sufficient to keep the bronchioles expanded.

However, on expiration this differential is reversed, the intrathoracic pressure going from negative to positive. This causes the relatively flaccid bronchioles partially to collapse.

When dyspnea is present, this bronchiolar collapse is intensified. The patient who is literally fighting for breath, trying his best to force air through flattened bronchioles, merely succeeds in flattening them further as he increases the positive pressure in his chest by muscular effort. Indeed, with enough effort he can even succeed in squeezing some of the bronchioles completely flat.

The Spirograph

The recording spirometer is a simple apparatus that will record the volume of air and the time used to complete both inspiration and expiration. Plate V compares the typical recording of the normal individual with that of the patient with emphysema.

In the normal individual, the line goes up more or less steeply as the patient inspires. As the breath is let out completely, the line falls away sharply, about 95 per cent of the air being expelled in the first three seconds. Then comes a very short period of rest before a second inspiration.

In the emphysematous patient, the air is inspired almost as quickly but fails to attain nearly the height reached in the normal. The major difference in emphysema is the prolongation of expiration caused by collapse of the bronchi that we have described earlier. In this case, eight to twelve seconds or more are required for total expiration. This leaves the patient breathless so that without any waiting period he hastens to inhale the succeeding breath.

The period of quiet breathing that follows is closer to the level of full inspiration than before the test. The fastest component of expiration is near the point of fullest inflation, since the bronchi are kept open most widely when the lungs are fully inflated, and the negative pressure in the pleura is greatest. A patient with emphysema can only breathe rapidly in the position of full inflation.

This test takes less than five minutes. It provides immediate information as to the patient's respiratory status, practically making the diagnosis. *If the patient has the type of expiration shown in the upper tracing on Plate V, and it fails to improve with bronchodilators, that patient has em-*

physema and must be treated accordingly.

Also on Plate V are shown the changes in the mixing of gases that occur in the lungs of patients with emphysema. To determine the rate of mixing, a closed-circuit spirometer containing helium is used. As the patient breathes into this spirometer, the content of helium can be determined continuously. From this can be found the rate at which helium mixes with the air in the lungs.

In the patient with normally functioning alveoli, the helium will mix rather rapidly with the air already present in the lung. Within two minutes of quiet breathing the normal lung may be within 20 per cent of complete equilibration. On the other hand, as will be seen in the curve on the right, mixing takes place much more slowly in the patient with emphysema. This is due to the many poorly ventilating areas in the emphysematous lung. Indeed, where a large non-ventilating cyst is present, complete mixing may take as long as an hour. While this test need not be used routinely, it does indicate quite graphically what an inefficient mechanism for gaseous exchange is the emphysematous lung.

Another method of determining the rate of mixing is to have the patient take a full inspiration of pure oxygen and measure the nitrogen concentration of the expired air. This test is not quantitative, but it is a rapid means of determining the presence of mixing difficulty.

The curves at the bottom of Plate V show the effect of exercise on blood gases in emphysema. In the normal individual the volume of air inspired increases on exercise but falls toward normal fairly rapidly during the recovery phase. On the other hand, due to the poor facility for gaseous exchange in the emphysematous lung, the patient with this condition increases his volume of inspired air more sharply; it reaches a higher level and returns to normal far more slowly.

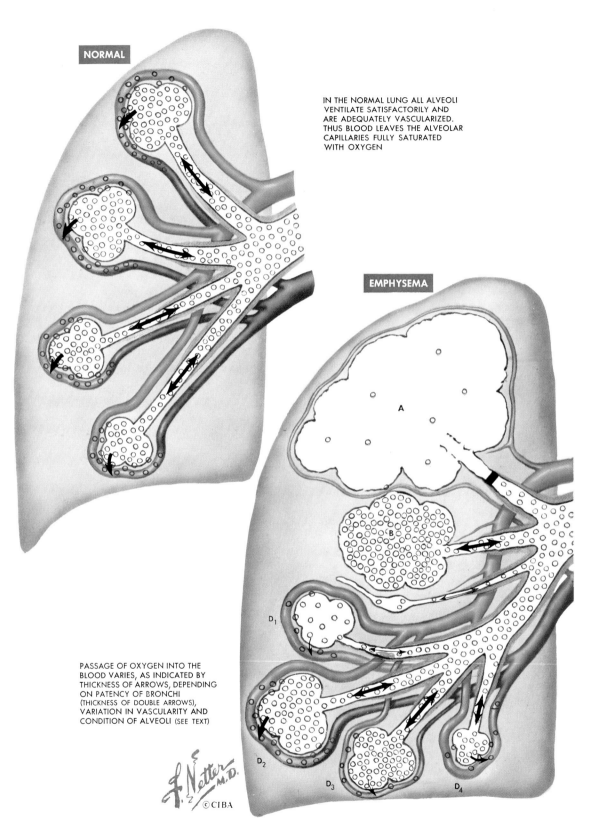

NORMAL

IN THE NORMAL LUNG ALL ALVEOLI
VENTILATE SATISFACTORILY AND
ARE ADEQUATELY VASCULARIZED.
THUS BLOOD LEAVES THE ALVEOLAR
CAPILLARIES FULLY SATURATED
WITH OXYGEN

EMPHYSEMA

A

B

D$_1$

D$_2$

D$_3$

D$_4$

PASSAGE OF OXYGEN INTO THE
BLOOD VARIES, AS INDICATED BY
THICKNESS OF ARROWS, DEPENDING
ON PATENCY OF BRONCHI
(THICKNESS OF DOUBLE ARROWS),
VARIATION IN VASCULARITY AND
CONDITION OF ALVEOLI (SEE TEXT)

F. Netter M.D.
©CIBA

PLATE VI   OXYGEN EXCHANGE IN NORMAL AND EMPHYSEMATOUS LUNGS

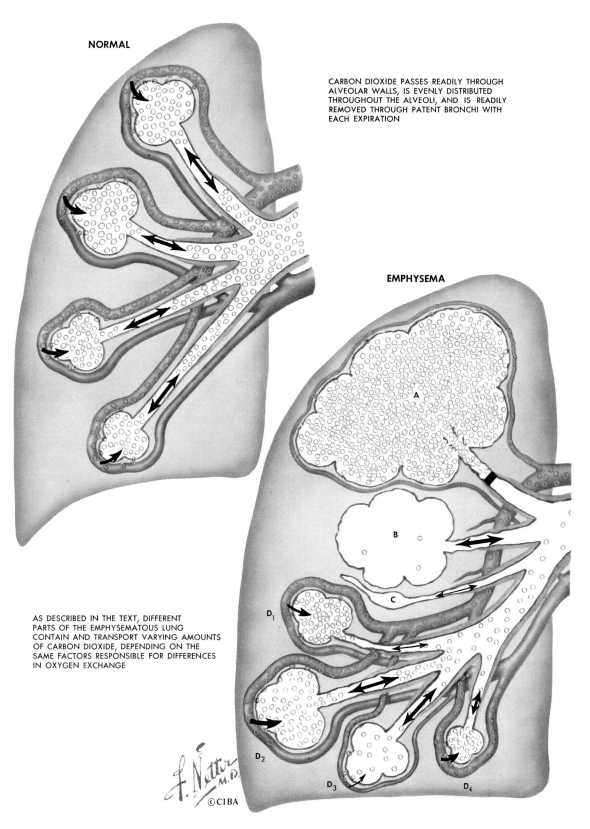

NORMAL

CARBON DIOXIDE PASSES READILY THROUGH
ALVEOLAR WALLS, IS EVENLY DISTRIBUTED
THROUGHOUT THE ALVEOLI, AND IS READILY
REMOVED THROUGH PATENT BRONCHI WITH
EACH EXPIRATION

EMPHYSEMA

AS DESCRIBED IN THE TEXT, DIFFERENT
PARTS OF THE EMPHYSEMATOUS LUNG
CONTAIN AND TRANSPORT VARYING AMOUNTS
OF CARBON DIOXIDE, DEPENDING ON THE
SAME FACTORS RESPONSIBLE FOR DIFFERENCES
IN OXYGEN EXCHANGE

PLATE VII   CARBON DIOXIDE EXCHANGE IN NORMAL AND EMPHYSEMATOUS LUNGS

At the same time, in the normal with plenty of respiratory reserve, the CO_2 level goes up only slightly and very transiently on exercise. The oxygen saturation is actually increased. In emphysema, on the other hand, despite the increased ventilation the CO_2 tension in the blood increases and the oxygen saturation falls, both returning slowly to normal on rest.

It must be remembered that there is a limit to the increase in ventilation that is possible to the emphysematous patient. Also, the range of respiratory movements is in a more inflated position, thus making the dilution of the air in the lungs less adequate with each breath. In addition, the increased ventilation requires a considerable increase of effort by the patient. This effort increases the production of CO_2, as well as requirement of oxygen, so the net gain from each breath is further reduced. Lastly, there may be ventilating areas in the lung which have lost their blood supply and which take up part of the breath for no useful purpose. All of these factors contribute to the oxygen desaturation and the increased accumulation of CO_2, despite the increased ventilatory rate that occurs on effort.

OXYGEN AND CARBON DIOXIDE EXCHANGE

Referring to Plates VI and VII the interrelationships of oxygen and carbon dioxide exchange in different areas of the emphysematous lung can be visualized. Looking at the oxygen and CO_2 situations of normal lung, one sees that all alveoli ventilate easily and are of such a size that at the end of expiration the blood flowing in the pulmonary capillaries is almost fully saturated, and CO_2 is still passing into the alveoli. However, in emphysema great disorders exist.

Alveolus A in the case of emphysema has a very low oxygen content and a high CO_2 content. It fails to ventilate and, therefore, makes no contribution to gaseous exchange in either direction. Alveolus B ventilates well. However, it has no blood supply. Therefore, it contains a normal inspired level of oxygen but practically no CO_2. This alveolus also contributes to the respiratory dead space. Alveolus C in the atelectatic area does not ventilate, nor does it have a blood supply. Therefore, it makes very little, if any, contribution to gas exchange. In the series of alveoli D_1, D_2, D_3, and D_4, one sees the following changes:

Alveolus D_1 does not ventilate well but has a normal blood supply. Therefore, it is low in oxygen and high in CO_2. Blood from this alveolus will thus tend to decrease the oxygen saturation and increase the CO_2 tension of the pulmonary return to the heart.

Alveolus D_2 is a fairly normal alveolus, except that it is rather large. It is ventilating adequately and is well perfused. Thus this alveolus returns blood to the heart that is fully saturated and contains little CO_2.

Alveolus D_3 is a normally ventilating alveolus but has a small blood supply. Therefore, it will be high in oxygen concentration since oxygen is not removed as completely as in D_2, and it will be low in CO_2 content because the possible CO_2 take-up is limited by the decreased blood flow. Although the blood coming from this alveolus will be fully saturated and will have less CO_2 than normal, it will not contribute as much as it should to the total flow of blood from the lung.

Alveolus D_4 is a small one. At the end of expiration the oxygen is almost completely used up. It is well ventilated. Through a whole respiratory cycle, such an alveolus will give rise to some incompletely saturated blood, although by and large most of the CO_2, but perhaps not enough, will have been taken off.

These are some of the permutations and combinations of ventilation and blood perfusion that give rise to the abnormalities of gaseous exchange in pulmonary emphysema.

RADIOGRAPHY

Radiography is of tremendous help in the study of the emphysematous. However, used alone it cannot be depended upon for diagnosis in more than 50 per cent of cases.

We routinely obtain x-rays both on inspiration and expiration in the postero-anterior position as well as for a lateral view. By actual measurement of the movement of the lung between inspiration and expiration, or by simply placing one film on top of the other, one gets a reasonably clear idea of the degrees of expansion and contraction of the different areas of the lung that occur during inspiration. The volume of the lung at the end of deep expiration can also be estimated from a view taken on full forced expiration.

This radiologic method of determining the amount of residual air in the lungs, while not quantitative, is nevertheless quite informative. A rough working classification of this radiologic residual air volume can be classified as: (1) normal, (2) slightly increased, (3) markedly increased, and (4) very grossly increased.

An adjunct of radiography, the fluoroscope, can make a great contribution to the study of these patients. Under the fluoroscope the movement of the diaphragm can be readily observed. In early cases one may notice that the diaphragm rises more slowly at the end of expiration. When an emphysematous patient is asked to breathe rapidly, the diaphragm will become almost immobile. When asked to breathe out forcibly, a lag in diaphragmatic movement will be noticed, or it may jump back and then go on up. This latter movement is diagnostic of air trapping in the bronchi, which is the characteristic difficulty of emphysema.

In the determination of whether or not a sufficient degree of localized disease exists to alter the therapeutic approach, such aids as bronchography, tomography, and pulmonary angiography may be required. Where there are large cystic areas shown by any of these techniques, surgical intervention may be considered.

RESPIRATORY ACIDOSIS AND CARBON DIOXIDE NARCOSIS

Chemical control of respiration in mammals is governed by the levels of carbon dioxide in the blood, an excess of oxygen always being available. Normally, when the carbon dioxide level rises, breathing becomes deeper and more rapid, and the excess CO_2 is "washed away." However, with the development of respiratory insufficiency in emphysema, the patient is unable to keep the carbon dioxide level within normal limits, despite all his efforts.

The effect of an excess of almost any stimulant is depression. So it is with the respiratory stimulant, carbon dioxide. When the medulla becomes overloaded with CO_2 (almost twice normal concentration), the respiratory center becomes depressed, and breathing becomes more shallow rather than deeper. (In this connection it is interesting to recall that carbon dioxide was used as an anesthetic agent at the end of the last century.)

When the respiratory center becomes depressed or anesthetized by the overload of carbon dioxide, the secondary mechanism, fall of arterial blood oxygen tension, takes over. This is probably a relic of those amphibia in which respiratory regulation depends primarily on the oxygen tension of the blood. It is relatively much less efficient, capable of only barely meeting the needs of the patient.

As the respiratory center and other parts of the brain become more and more depressed or anesthetized by the overabundance of carbon dioxide, the phy-

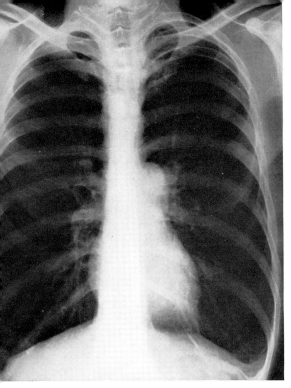
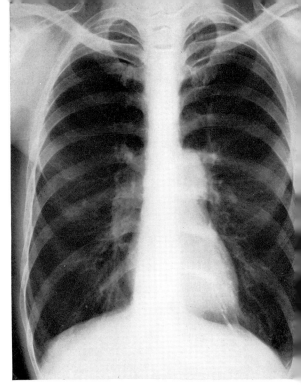

Inspiration and expiration P. A. films of patient with emphysema. The process is radiologically diffuse, with fixed chest cage and diaphragm and hyperaeration. However, this represents pathologically the same process, ranging from air cysts to normal tissue, that is shown in the type case discussed in this monograph.

X-rays showing emphysema of the type discussed and illustrated. Right lung contains a non-ventilating cyst in upper lobe, a ventilating cyst in right midzone, and increased density at right pericardiophrenic angle.

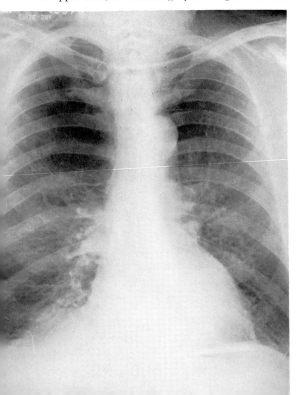
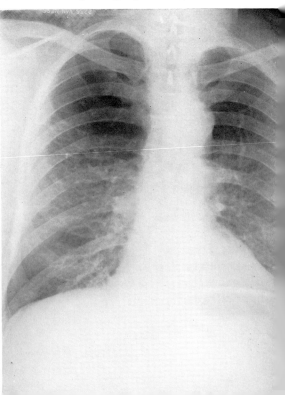

sician must be more careful in the administration of oxygen since this may remove the only stimulus to breathing which is left.

Since carbon dioxide retention or respiratory acidosis is always serious and is a common cause of death in these patients, it must be detected early, adequately treated, and prevented if possible.

Diagnosis

The earliest thing one notices is a *slight cyanosis with hyperventilation at rest.* Then as the respiratory insufficiency progresses over a period of days, weeks, months or years, the next thing observed is *a little mental vagueness.* With further progress there comes one of the most important signs, *twitching of the fingers.* This occurs only at rest. It disappears on movement. One notices a definite sleepiness with some apparent drunkenness. Next the patient becomes more and more sleepy and more and more deeply cyanosed, but respiration is not accelerated.

At this point, on clinical grounds alone, one is justified in making a diagnosis of carbon dioxide narcosis. The proof lies in determination of the carbon dioxide content of the blood. Also, one should determine the pH of the arterial blood. The determination of the pH of arterial blood is a simple procedure. The technique of arterial puncture is illustrated in Plate VIII. Unless promptly and heroically treated, this respiratory acidosis and the associated carbon dioxide narcosis will rapidly lead to a fatal termination.

If elevation of CO_2 content is gradual, chloride is excreted by the kidney. This conserves base, allowing most of the retained carbon dioxide to be converted to bicarbonate so that the blood pH is not altered. However, if the increase in CO_2 is rapid, there is no time to develop a so-called "compensated respiratory acidosis." In this situation the CO_2 acts in solution as a dissociated acid, and the acidity of the blood increases. The pH of the blood, which is normally about 7.40, will fall, and the excretion of acid from the cells of the body will be materially disturbed.

COR PULMONALE (PLATE IX)

The pulmonary vascular bed is normally a lower pressure circuit than the systemic circulation. The right ventricle is a thinner-walled organ than the left ventricle and the pulmonary artery thinner walled than the aorta. Loss of alveoli by rupture, stretching, or failure to take part in ventilation reduces the pulmonary vascular bed. Since the same volume of blood (about 5 liters per minute) must pass through a smaller vascular bed, the pressure must be increased to accelerate blood flow. Thus when the pulmonary vascular bed is reduced to less than half of that normally present, the pressure in the pulmonary artery has to rise considerably to maintain circulation. In early stages the rise of pressure is more marked on effort and later is considerably elevated even at rest. This causes hypertrophy of the right ventricle. With hypoxia there will be a rise in the hematocrit.

The electrocardiogram will first show changes in cardiac position because the heart becomes more vertical than normal. Later, delayed transmission across the chest leads is seen, and finally the picture of right ventricular strain and right bundle-branch block develops. In these later stages, filling of the right ventricle requires more pressure, and changes in the P waves are seen, connotating a right auricular hypertrophy.

In the final stages there is considerable cardiac dilatation, and a tricuspid insufficiency develops. Throughout the whole of these late phases, there may be evidence of increased venous pressure as seen by enlargement of the liver and peripheral edema. The electrocardiogram and the hematocrit are exceedingly useful signs of the existence of marked increase of pulmonary artery pressure and cor pulmonale. The exaggeration of the pulmonary conus in the x-ray further assists one in making the diagnosis.

The septum in cor pulmonale is illustrated as invaginated into the left ventricle. This is a possibility, although its existence is not yet proven. However, it would seem that there may be some interference with left ventricular filling due to alteration of the septum, the reverse Ebstein phenomenon.

TREATMENT

Instructions to the Patient

The first thing that must be done about the patient with emphysema is to explain carefully to him the nature of his illness. The changes in his lungs are irreparable. They will tend to get worse. Thus the more he learns about his disability and the measures that must be used for his relief, the more cooperative he will be in carrying out prolonged therapy.

Our patients receive written instructions. The introduction reads as follows:

"Normally the lungs are like very elastic balloons within the chest. The individual inhales simply by expanding the chest. The lungs expand to fill up the extra space and thereby draw in the air. Breathing out is accomplished by relaxing the muscles of the chest. The air is forced out of the lungs, not by the pressure of the chest wall but by the elastic quality of the lungs themselves. You possibly are having difficulty in breathing because your lungs have lost some of this elastic quality. You are still able to inhale normally, although it may seem difficult. However, when you exhale, the air is not forced out as completely as it should be due to the loss of stretch. Therefore, you have to push it out by compressing the chest cage and forcing the lungs to contract. This is inefficient, as you can demonstrate for yourself by trying to squeeze the air out of a plastic bag with a small opening.

"We cannot put the stretch back into your lungs. However, we can do a great deal to keep this lack of stretch from unduly interfering with your usual activities. For one thing, we can help you meet the abnormal demand made upon your breathing apparatus. This is done by special exercises designed to strengthen the muscles chiefly affected. In the second place, we shall be concerned to keep the many openings within the lungs through which the air must be forced as large as possible. There has already been some reduction in the diameter of at least some of these passages. This can be corrected by the use of special dilator drugs.

"In the next place, there must be a special effort made to keep these passages free of sputum. Such sputum narrows lung passages. Lastly, great care must be taken to keep you free from even minor lung infections since these often produce large quantities of sputum, and in any case they cause swelling of the passage walls.

"Therefore, this is a program of maintenance and will obviously require your cooperation. The instructions which follow are not as complicated as they might seem at first glance. If you follow them faithfully, they will very soon become a part of a normal routine and will hardly be noticed except insofar as you may find it easier to breathe."

From this we go on to a section on breathing exercises which we divide into those for the diaphragm and the chest muscles, and then a section on special devices and medication, and finally general instructions. The patients take this home and read it over and over, and their families read it over and over. It is one of the most useful things we can give them.

With this approach the patient quickly gets the idea that the therapeutic attack is not merely a matter of taking pills; rather it has many facets, each of which must have careful attention.

Breathing Exercises

As we have pointed out earlier, the lungs are not involved uniformly. Some portions ventilate far better than others. The purpose of our breathing exercises, therefore, are threefold:

(1) They help the patient to get maximum ventilation from all parts of his lungs and therefore to breathe more efficiently.

(2) They strengthen the muscles of respiration.

(3) They reinforce the patient's realization of his disability and his determination to prevent progression.

These exercises are illustrated in Plate X. The first exercise assists the patient to elevate his diaphragm. Sitting erect on the side of the bed, the patient inhales deeply while holding a small pillow or book against his abdomen. He then exhales slowly, at the same time bending over and pressing the pillow as firmly as possible against the abdomen.

This maneuver is repeated ten times each morning and evening after first clearing the lungs as completely as possible of sputum. By thus forcing the diaphragm upward by pressure from below, it encourages aeration of the lower parts of the lung and may dislodge sputum that the patient cannot raise by any other means.

The second exercise strengthens the abdominal muscles. Each leg is raised alternately, bringing it as near the vertical as possible. This is done slowly, the patient exhaling as the leg is lifted. This should be repeated ten times for each leg. However, the debilitated patient may have to modify the exercise both in the extent the legs are raised and the number of times the exercise is repeated. As strength improves, the legs will be raised more easily. Then after a few minutes rest, the patient raises his head and shoulders from the bed, at the same time exhaling. He inhales again as his head is dropped back on the bed. This is repeated five times in a leisurely fashion.

While the patient lies upon the bed, a fourth exercise is carried out. This exercises both the abdominal muscles and the diaphragm. A small book is placed upon the abdomen. First the patient breathes in, puffing out the abdomen, so as to raise the book as far as possible. He then exhales slowly, emptying the lungs as much as possible, at the same time pulling in the abdomen so that the book is brought as close to his vertebral column as pos-

sible. This is repeated ten times. Like the first exercise, this one increases aeration of the lower portions of the lung and helps to dislodge mucus. Synchronization of abdominal and diaphragmatic muscles with respiration is also improved.

Several other exercises which we have found helpful have not been illustrated. These help in the expansion and contraction of the chest. Therefore, they improve aeration and help to dislodge sputum.

In the first of these, the hands are placed lightly on the lower ribs, the fingers well around in front. The patient inspires as deeply as possible. Then with slow expiration the hands are pressed firmly together compressing the lower ribs. This is repeated ten times.

After a few minutes rest, the same exercise is carried out ten times with pressure this time on the upper ribs, the pressure being exerted and relaxed by lowering and raising the elbows.

Pursed-Lip Breathing (Plate XI)

As explained earlier, the chief difficulty in emphysema is the tendency of the bronchi to collapse during expiration due to (1) their loss of elasticity, and (2) the positive intrathoracic pressure that is necessary to force air from inelastic lungs.

If the lips are pursed during expiration, the pressure within the bronchi is increased because the air must be forced through the narrow opening between the lips. This encourages the bronchi to remain open during expiration, thus improving this most difficult phase of respiration for the emphysematous patient.

As indicated in Plate XI, the spirometer tracing is quite different when the emphysematous patient breathes through pursed lips. The period of expiration is shorter, and the line does not level out because of progressive collapse of bronchi during the expiratory phase. In addition, the line of expiration falls further, indicating that a greater volume of air has been expelled

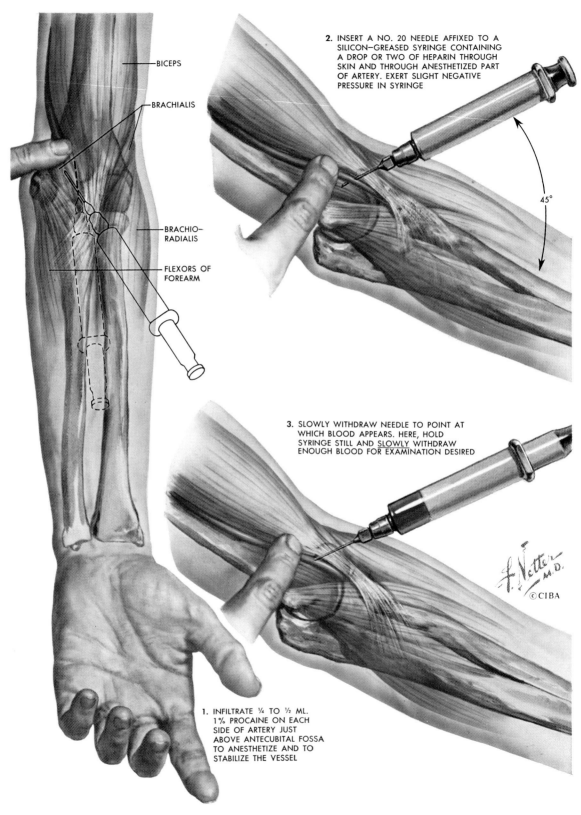

BICEPS

BRACHIALIS

BRACHIO–
RADIALIS

FLEXORS OF
FOREARM

2. INSERT A NO. 20 NEEDLE AFFIXED TO A
SILICON–GREASED SYRINGE CONTAINING
A DROP OR TWO OF HEPARIN THROUGH
SKIN AND THROUGH ANESTHETIZED PART
OF ARTERY. EXERT SLIGHT NEGATIVE
PRESSURE IN SYRINGE

45°

3. SLOWLY WITHDRAW NEEDLE TO POINT AT
WHICH BLOOD APPEARS. HERE, HOLD
SYRINGE STILL AND SLOWLY WITHDRAW
ENOUGH BLOOD FOR EXAMINATION DESIRED

1. INFILTRATE ¼ TO ½ ML.
1% PROCAINE ON EACH
SIDE OF ARTERY JUST
ABOVE ANTECUBITAL FOSSA
TO ANESTHETIZE AND TO
STABILIZE THE VESSEL

F. Netter M.D.
©CIBA

PLATE VIII

TECHNIQUE OF ARTERIAL PUNCTURE

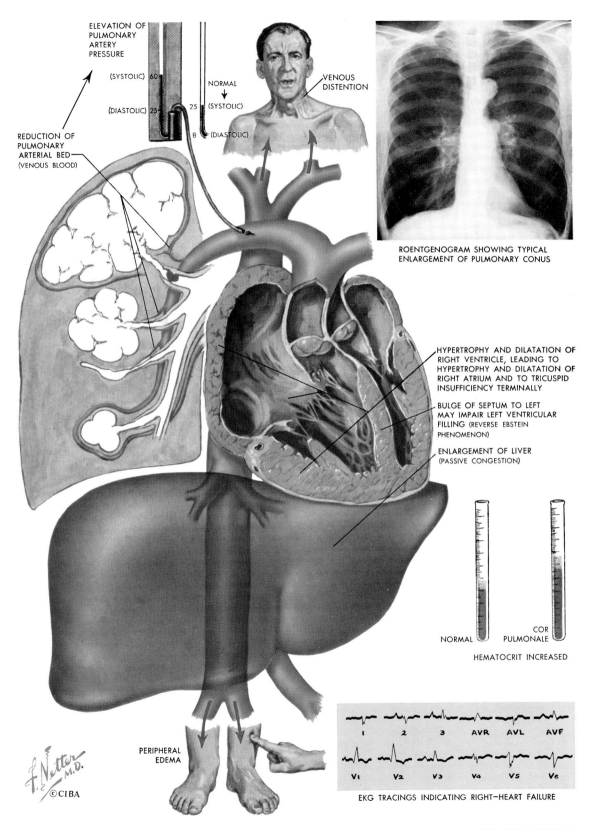

ELEVATION OF PULMONARY ARTERY PRESSURE

(SYSTOLIC) 60
(DIASTOLIC) 25
NORMAL
25 (SYSTOLIC)
8 (DIASTOLIC)

VENOUS DISTENTION

REDUCTION OF PULMONARY ARTERIAL BED (VENOUS BLOOD)

ROENTGENOGRAM SHOWING TYPICAL ENLARGEMENT OF PULMONARY CONUS

HYPERTROPHY AND DILATATION OF RIGHT VENTRICLE, LEADING TO HYPERTROPHY AND DILATATION OF RIGHT ATRIUM AND TO TRICUSPID INSUFFICIENCY TERMINALLY

BULGE OF SEPTUM TO LEFT MAY IMPAIR LEFT VENTRICULAR FILLING (REVERSE EBSTEIN PHENOMENON)

ENLARGEMENT OF LIVER (PASSIVE CONGESTION)

NORMAL

COR PULMONALE

HEMATOCRIT INCREASED

PERIPHERAL EDEMA

1   2   3   AVR   AVL   AVF
V1   V2   V3   V4   V5   V6

EKG TRACINGS INDICATING RIGHT-HEART FAILURE

F. Netter M.D.
©CIBA

PLATE IX

COR PULMONALE

from the lungs. This is also indicated by the schematic drawing of the piston and balloon.

Bronchodilators

Since one of the main defects in emphysema is the bronchial narrowing, particularly during expiration, therapy aimed directly at increasing the bronchial caliber must have highest priority.

Bronchodilators fall into two groups, the direct bronchodilators and the indirect bronchodilators. The indirect bronchodilators we shall deal with later.

Direct bronchodilators, acting chiefly upon the smooth muscle of the bronchi, have limited action in emphysema, even though in asthma their effect may be quite profound. Such substances as ephedrine, propylamine, and epinephrine derivatives, orally or parenterally, will produce some relaxation in emphysema, not necessarily of spasm but perhaps of the tone of the smooth muscle of the bronchial tree, and thus permit some degree of dilation. The same may be said of intravenous or rectal aminophylline. However, the oral preparations of aminophylline have been disappointing. The parasympatheticolytic agents, such as belladonna and its derivatives, are also of limited action in emphysema, although they have some usefulness.

The reason for these parenteral or oral preparations being disappointing lies in the fact that their generalized systemic effect may be disadvantageous to the patient, thus limiting the benefit they may produce. These substances (with the exception of aminophylline) have antisecretory and vasoconstricting actions on the mucosa. Also, one cannot get the full effect without other systemic symptoms ranging from tachycardia for the sympatheticomimetics to dryness of the mouth in the case of the parasympatheticolytics. Therefore, these compounds are more useful as basal medications, given in small quantity to produce relaxation of bronchial muscle tonus, than they are when used in full dosage as the main bronchodilator effort. Aminophylline as a suppository is useful, but its routine use tends to cause a granular proctitis to develop. Thus, this method of administration should be reserved for exacerbations.

Nebulized Vasodilators: One of the most effective ways to utilize the dilating effect of epinephrine-like drugs is direct application to the bronchi by use of a hand nebulizer as shown in Plate XII.

To be effective it is essential that the kind of nebulizer used should produce droplets of a very small size, preferably averaging three microns or below. Otherwise the spray will not pass much beyond the larynx, trachea, and very large bronchi which are not particularly involved. Even in the presence of systemic hypertension, epinephrine-like drugs are safe to use frequently and in large doses by the nebulized route since systemic absorption is limited. Some useful preparations for this method are: Racemic epinephrine (Vaponefrin), isopropyl norepinephrine (Isuprel), N-substituted arterenol derivative (Caytine), and isoproterenol with Phenyl-ephrine (Nebu-Prel).

It is important that the patient be carefully instructed on the proper use of his nebulizer. Our own instructions are as follows:

"Your hand nebulizer is to become your most constant companion. It should be by your bed when you go to sleep at night and on your person whenever you leave the house. By now you probably know very well when an attack of difficult breathing is about to begin. For most patients a feeling of tightness in the chest is the first sign of trouble. This tightness represents a reduction in the diameter of your air passages. The fluid in your nebulizer is a dilator: it enlarges these passages. Therefore, if you will use it at the first feeling of tightness, you will generally be able to avoid altogether attacks of difficult breathing. In any case such attacks will be less severe. You should also get into the habit of foreseeing the kind of activity which may bring on an attack of difficult breathing.

"You should use your nebulizer before you undertake such activities since it is much easier to prevent trouble than to stop it after it is under way. However, do not use the nebulizer more often than you have been told since, if it is used too often, it may gradually lose its effect. In any case do not use it carelessly.

"Open your mouth widely and put the nozzle of the nebulizer well into the back of the mouth. Then pump the hand bulb vigorously while you breathe in through the mouth six times. Give a cough and raise any sputum that has accumulated; then repeat the treatment. Remember, take your time and give yourself a full treatment every time you use the nebulizer; do not get into the habit of 'taking a whiff or so now and then.' "

After a time it is often found advisable to switch to another nebulizing agent and then back to the original one. It must be remembered that the effects of the bronchodilator are not so much to reduce bronchial muscle spasm as to act as a vasoconstricting agent, reducing edema, widening the air passages, and permitting the expectoration of mucous plugs.

One of the most important times to use the hand nebulizer is on arising in the morning since during the night mucus accumulates due to the shallower breathing and diminished cough reflex.

Intermittent Positive Pressure Breathing (IPPB)

The intermittent positive pressure valve is one of the most significant advances in recent years in the treatment of chronic bronchitis. Designed to supply a controlled pressure during inspiration, to cycle at the patient's will, and to apply aerosolized medication, it is a major triumph of medical engineering (Plate XIII). As soon as the patient starts to breathe in, a counterpoised valve opens and provides air or oxygen at a constant flow that has been determined as being optimum for the individual patient. When inspiration stops the pressure goes on being applied until it reaches a pre-set point at which the valve turns off and an exhaust opens. Thus at the end of the

patient's breath, additional air is forced in, and the patient breathes much more deeply than he would or could otherwise.

The effects are obvious: Flaccid bronchi are directly dilated, ventilation is increased, cough is promoted, and with an attached nebulizer the bronchial mucous membranes are medicated more completely than is possible with any other technique. By means of such equipment, patients who have been severe respiratory cripples have become moderately active.

Intermittent positive pressure equipment is also invaluable in dealing with or warding off complications. Not the least of its services is the aid it gives to the cough reflex, since the difficulty that patients with chronic bronchitis ordinarily have in coughing up sputum makes even a common cold a potential threat to life. Also it can be used at regular intervals throughout the day to forestall the development of carbon dioxide retention, and in acute exacerbations it may be the only means of saving the patient's life.

A number of valves are on the market which have a sufficient background of trial for the mechanism to have been perfected. In choosing between them, one of the most important factors to consider is the availability of local service facilities. Actually, very little service is necessary. The valves are metal and usually operate satisfactorily with no more attention than a simple washing about once a year. However, as with any mechanical device, occasional servicing may be required and with equipment as important as IPPB, it is essential that it be available without undue delay.

Whatever model is preferred, intermittent positive pressure therapy is an important tool in the management of chronic bronchitis and emphysema. It is an indispensable item in hospitals, and its simplicity and relative inexpensiveness make it feasible for use in the home of the patient as well as in a physician's office.

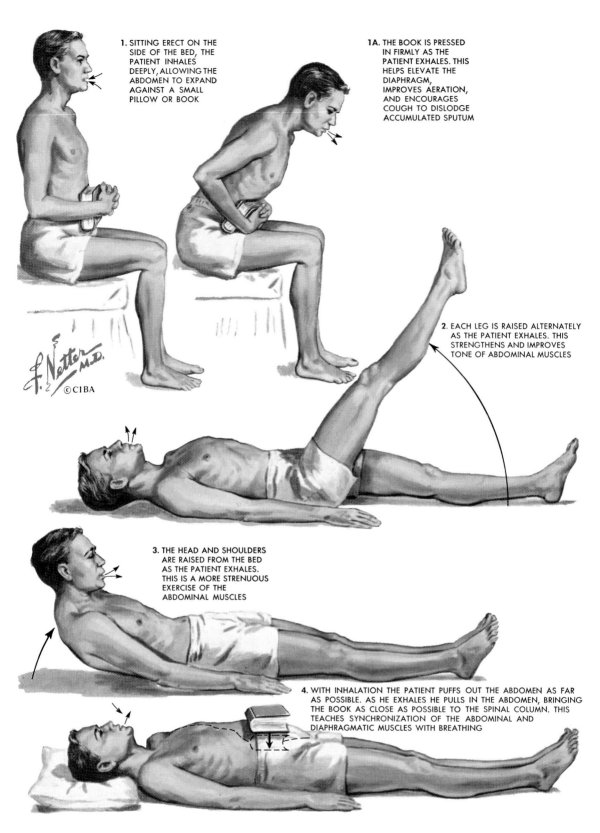

1. SITTING ERECT ON THE SIDE OF THE BED, THE PATIENT INHALES DEEPLY, ALLOWING THE ABDOMEN TO EXPAND AGAINST A SMALL PILLOW OR BOOK

1A. THE BOOK IS PRESSED IN FIRMLY AS THE PATIENT EXHALES. THIS HELPS ELEVATE THE DIAPHRAGM, IMPROVES AERATION, AND ENCOURAGES COUGH TO DISLODGE ACCUMULATED SPUTUM

2. EACH LEG IS RAISED ALTERNATELY AS THE PATIENT EXHALES. THIS STRENGTHENS AND IMPROVES TONE OF ABDOMINAL MUSCLES

3. THE HEAD AND SHOULDERS ARE RAISED FROM THE BED AS THE PATIENT EXHALES. THIS IS A MORE STRENUOUS EXERCISE OF THE ABDOMINAL MUSCLES

4. WITH INHALATION THE PATIENT PUFFS OUT THE ABDOMEN AS FAR AS POSSIBLE. AS HE EXHALES HE PULLS IN THE ABDOMEN, BRINGING THE BOOK AS CLOSE AS POSSIBLE TO THE SPINAL COLUMN. THIS TEACHES SYNCHRONIZATION OF THE ABDOMINAL AND DIAPHRAGMATIC MUSCLES WITH BREATHING

PLATE X   BREATHING EXERCISES

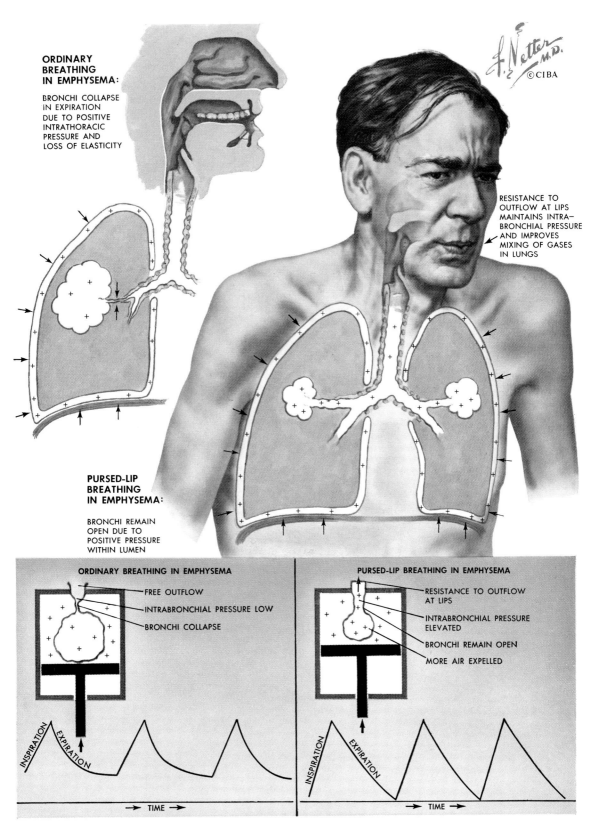

ORDINARY BREATHING IN EMPHYSEMA:

BRONCHI COLLAPSE IN EXPIRATION DUE TO POSITIVE INTRATHORACIC PRESSURE AND LOSS OF ELASTICITY

RESISTANCE TO OUTFLOW AT LIPS MAINTAINS INTRA– BRONCHIAL PRESSURE AND IMPROVES MIXING OF GASES IN LUNGS

PURSED-LIP BREATHING IN EMPHYSEMA:

BRONCHI REMAIN OPEN DUE TO POSITIVE PRESSURE WITHIN LUMEN

ORDINARY BREATHING IN EMPHYSEMA

FREE OUTFLOW
INTRABRONCHIAL PRESSURE LOW
BRONCHI COLLAPSE

INSPIRATION
EXPIRATION
TIME

PURSED-LIP BREATHING IN EMPHYSEMA

RESISTANCE TO OUTFLOW AT LIPS
INTRABRONCHIAL PRESSURE ELEVATED
BRONCHI REMAIN OPEN
MORE AIR EXPELLED

INSPIRATION
EXPIRATION
TIME

PLATE XI

PURSED-LIP BREATHING

For IPPB to be effective, the patient must permit his lungs to expand fully. The design of the equipment is such that when pressure becomes equalized the valve will turn off, but many patients tend to blow, which cuts off inspiration at or before the peak of vital capacity. If the patient will cooperate, larger volumes can be inspired. A value of as much as 675 ml. above the inspiratory reserve was recorded in one of our patients. This appears to result from depressing the diaphragm farther than normal and also from preventing whatever paradoxical elevation occurs in some patients at full inspiration.

If used properly, patients will cough up mucus with this therapy; otherwise, an important advantage of the hyperventilation produced by this technique will be missed.

With regard to the use of bronchodilator drugs with IPPB, it is our experience that a much smaller dose of nebulized bronchodilator appears to be necessary when IPPB is administered simultaneously. For this purpose a small aerosol gun containing the bronchodilator is inserted in the IPPB circuit. This may deliver the bronchodilator continuously or only during inspiration, depending on the type of equipment.

If viscid sputum is a factor, intermittent positive pressure appears to afford more relief than a bronchodilator drug alone. In patients with inefficient cough and uneven ventilation, there is considerable benefit in the long-term application of intermittent positive pressure breathing as a mechanism for clearing away secretions. Many patients find IPPB of the greatest use in the morning on arising, to aid in expectoration of mucus. The relief they obtain from this therapy is commonly greater than they had obtained from any bronchodilator drug used alone.

Use of IPPB should be regulated according to the amount of improvement shown and the severity of the disease. In early cases it is sufficient to apply it at the office or clinic only when the patient has a cold. In more advanced cases a patient may wish to have an apparatus in his home and to use it particularly on arising in the morning and at night before retiring. In some cases active work can only be carried on by having such an apparatus mobile and freely available at his work, in the car, and at home.

We prefer patients to use 40 per cent oxygen, but IPPB may be run on either 100 per cent oxygen or on compressed air. Our reasons for preferring the 40 per cent oxygen are: This concentration represents a reasonable economy in oxygen with the advantages of adequately oxygenating the patient from time to time during the day, while avoiding any possible cardiovascular complications from increasing the amounts of bronchodilator drugs.

Where patients have developed respiratory acidosis, it becomes very much more important that they should use IPPB in full treatments several times during the day to blow off accumulating carbon dioxide. It is also important that when patients are prescribed such apparatus, they should realize that benefit is obtained by the combined therapy of oxygen, careful hyperventilation, and medication of the bronchi. In carbon dioxide narcosis the apparatus may have to be fitted to the opening of a tracheotomy tube which has to be inserted to control bronchial secretion and improve ventilation.

Selection of Patients for IPPB: It is important to establish whether or not intermittent positive pressure breathing should or should not be used in any particular patient. This is best done by obtaining a spirogram, treating the patient for 10 to 15 minutes with IPPB, and immediately repeating the spirogram. A few patients with check valve cystic disease as a major component will respond unfavorably to this form of treatment. Some patients show little obvious improvement.

However, the majority of patients after such treatment for 10 to 20 minutes will show a marked improvement of their timed expiratory capacity and a marked improvement of their exercise tolerance which may last some hours. If any improvement is shown, then it is obvious that this is a beneficial form of therapy. If no improvement is shown, it must be kept in mind that at a subsequent time, when perhaps a respiratory infection is present, it may do a great deal of good. It should be retried when such a situation exists.

The Indirect Bronchodilators

Antibacterial Agents: Since mucus is an excellent culture medium, and since recurring bouts of infection represent one of the greatest hazards to these patients, prompt adequate therapy with antibiotics from time to time is essential. Whether one's choice should be a low-level constant medication with such a substance as tetracycline or a sulfonamide, or whether large doses should be given intermittently to combat exacerbations, is a moot point.

On the whole we prefer to use large doses of antibiotics intermittently, switching from one to another according to changes in the flora of the sputum.

Nebulized antibiotics, particularly penicillin and streptomycin, are used by many physicians. However, there is some tendency to develop hypersensitivity with this use as well as for overgrowth of monilia in the mouth and lower respiratory tract. For these reasons we feel that the oral or parenteral route is preferable to the nebulized route. It should be remembered that the very viscid secretions may contain quite a large bacterial flora without becoming obviously purulent. This is because the fibrous structure of drying mucus prevents leukocyte migration into it. For this reason a Gram's stain and culture of sputum are more useful than symptoms in determining the presence of infection.

Sputum Liquefying Agents

Oral sputum liquefacients, such as the iodides, are somewhat disappointing in chronic obstructive emphysema. Again the problem arises that a very large dose is necessary for any considerable bronchorrhea to be produced. Thus, with the iodides, effective dosage for a normal adult is between one and one and one-half grams of calcium iodide per day, which may be sufficient to produce mild soreness of the throat and loss of taste and smell. Occasionally such dosage also may produce a cutaneous acneform eruption.

By far the most useful liquefying agent is water, both by mouth and by inhalation, the latter in the form of hot steam or cold nebulized water. However, to be satisfactory the output of a water nebulizer must be more than 20 ml. of water per hour. To the water may be added wetting agents, of which there are several on the market, and exosmotics-cum-wetting agents, such as glycerol or propylene glycol. It is our impression that it is the water itself that is the most useful part of this therapy, although much research remains to be done in this area.

The routine use of enzymes, such as trypsin or desoxyribonuclease, in these patients appears to have some risk. We have frequently observed hypersensitivity to these enzymes. In the case of trypsin there is a definite change produced on the bronchial mucosa, which is thought to be undesirable. We reserve these agents for emergency use in exacerbations. One must remember that bronchial mucosa, when it is at its healthiest, is a very delicate mucous membrane; when it is suffering the assaults of a disease process, great care must be taken not to insult it any further.

The Treatment of Cough

One of the most distressing symptoms of these patients is cough. Since cough is inadequate and excess mucus is present,

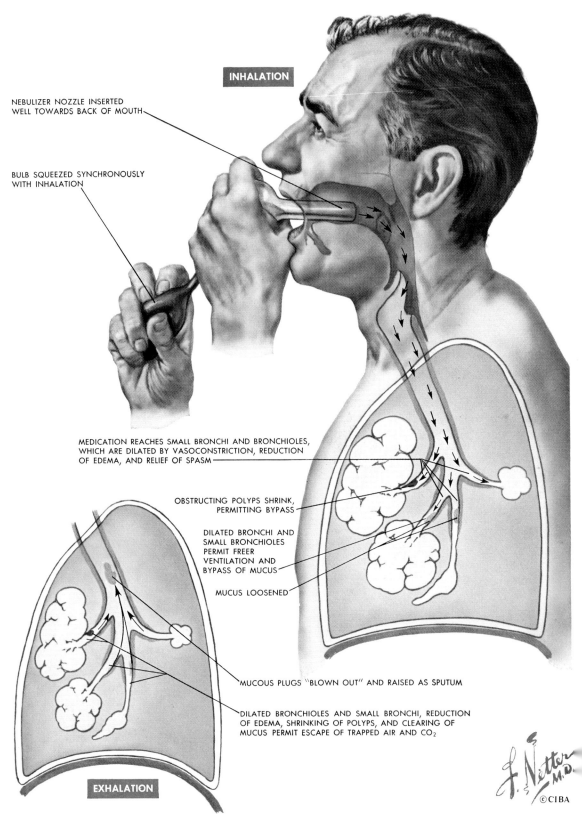

INHALATION

NEBULIZER NOZZLE INSERTED
WELL TOWARDS BACK OF MOUTH

BULB SQUEEZED SYNCHRONOUSLY
WITH INHALATION

MEDICATION REACHES SMALL BRONCHI AND BRONCHIOLES,
WHICH ARE DILATED BY VASOCONSTRICTION, REDUCTION
OF EDEMA, AND RELIEF OF SPASM

OBSTRUCTING POLYPS SHRINK,
PERMITTING BYPASS

DILATED BRONCHI AND
SMALL BRONCHIOLES
PERMIT FREER
VENTILATION AND
BYPASS OF MUCUS

MUCUS LOOSENED

MUCOUS PLUGS "BLOWN OUT" AND RAISED AS SPUTUM

DILATED BRONCHIOLES AND SMALL BRONCHI, REDUCTION
OF EDEMA, SHRINKING OF POLYPS, AND CLEARING OF
MUCUS PERMIT ESCAPE OF TRAPPED AIR AND CO_2

EXHALATION

PLATE XII

USE OF THE HAND NEBULIZER

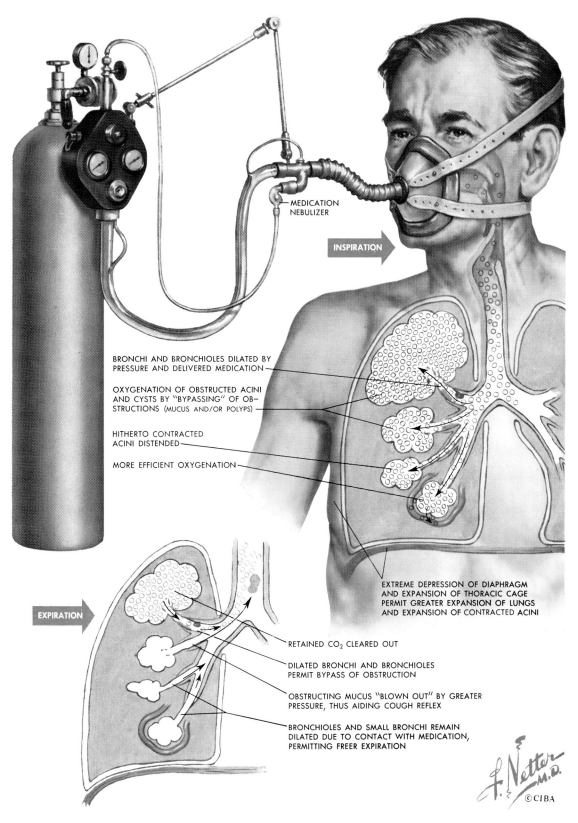

MEDICATION
NEBULIZER

INSPIRATION

BRONCHI AND BRONCHIOLES DILATED BY
PRESSURE AND DELIVERED MEDICATION

OXYGENATION OF OBSTRUCTED ACINI
AND CYSTS BY "BYPASSING" OF OB-
STRUCTIONS (MUCUS AND/OR POLYPS)

HITHERTO CONTRACTED
ACINI DISTENDED

MORE EFFICIENT OXYGENATION

EXTREME DEPRESSION OF DIAPHRAGM
AND EXPANSION OF THORACIC CAGE
PERMIT GREATER EXPANSION OF LUNGS
AND EXPANSION OF CONTRACTED ACINI

EXPIRATION

RETAINED CO_2 CLEARED OUT

DILATED BRONCHI AND BRONCHIOLES
PERMIT BYPASS OF OBSTRUCTION

OBSTRUCTING MUCUS "BLOWN OUT" BY GREATER
PRESSURE, THUS AIDING COUGH REFLEX

BRONCHIOLES AND SMALL BRONCHI REMAIN
DILATED DUE TO CONTACT WITH MEDICATION,
PERMITTING FREER EXPIRATION

F. Netter
M.D.

©CIBA

PLATE XIII

INTERMITTENT POSITIVE PRESSURE BREATHING

direct suppression by codeine and its analogues is not desirable, particularly considering the effect of such drugs on the respiratory center. On the other hand, excessive coughing is harmful to the bronchi by the mechanical squeezing, and to weak alveolar structures by stretching on sudden inspiration. Thus cough itself may worsen the emphysema and perpetuate the bronchitis.

A considerably useful preparation in safely controlling cough in these patients is Tessalon, acting chiefly on the afferent arm and central mechanism of the Hering-Breuer and associated reflexes. The oral dosage necessary is from 300 to 600 mg. daily in divided doses, or 5 mg. intramuscularly up to every four hours. This preparation appears to have an advantageous effect directly upon the breathing of many of these patients.

Antihistaminics

Although not comparable to the corticoids in their effects upon the bronchial mucosa, these preparations, such as Pyribenzamine, may markedly assist in reducing the frequently associated rhinitis and postnasal drip which exacerbate both cough and bronchitis. In more severe cases the use of nasal sprays containing corticoids and vasoconstrictors may further assist in controlling the nasal aspect.

Corticosteroid Therapy

In the presence of bronchial inflammation, any anti-inflammatory substance acts as an indirect bronchodilator. Thus there is a real usefulness in many of these cases for corticosteroid therapy which, of course, must be covered from time to time with antibiotics. Fortunately, the dosage required to produce improvement in these patients is little more than their normal output from the adrenals. As a rule, after an initial loading dose, some 10 to 15 mg. of prednisone in the morning will reduce the sputum very considerably and increase the expiratory vital capacity. On the whole it appears that there is no advantage in using ACTH gel in place of the oral corticoid. As with all cases where prolonged corticoid therapy is envisaged, one should be careful to control negative nitrogen balance by using androgens as required. Also one should watch for decalcification. Sodium restriction on this dosage is not usually necessary unless it is thought desirable from the point of view of cor pulmonale.

Although corticoid therapy should not be embarked on lightly, it is of considerable use intermittently to control exacerbations. In the more severe cases continuous therapy may be necessary to maintain well-being. We have studied the effects of nebulized soluble hydrocortisone but have been rather disappointed in the results obtained. Although some initial benefit appears to occur, it is often followed by some degree of bronchorrhea. Thus the benefit ceases to exist.

Cor Pulmonale with Emphysema

Cor pulmonale represents an additional need for those therapeutic measures already in operation. If ventilation can be improved, perfusion of blood through the lungs will also improve as a general rule. Thus pressure will be lowered in the pulmonary artery, and strain taken off the right ventricle. Therefore, such findings as a rising hematocrit or a change in the electrocardiogram should be regarded first of all as an indication to increase the efficiency of respiration by the various means already described.

In addition, specific therapy for cor pulmonale will commonly be necessary. The earlier controversies having been resolved, it appears now that digitalis is a very useful drug. This is particularly true in those patients with a low cardiac output, which is relatively easily detected by the presence of cold cyanosed extremities. If the extremities are warm and the pulse is a bounding one, the use of digitalis is more controversial; however, it should be tried. We prefer slow digitalization with a preparation that is excreted rather rapidly. Chiefly this is because of the greater ease of controlling the digitalization. Although the effects of digitalis are not dramatic, there does appear to be evidence that it will improve a falling cardiac output and thus benefit the patient.

In the presence of an increased hematocrit, *phlebotomy* is of considerable importance. When the hematocrit rises above 55 per cent there is a definite increase in the viscosity of blood, which means an increase in cardiac work required to circulate the same blood volume. With this will appear problems of the sludging of red cells in the pulmonary capillaries, which will further reduce effective circulation through the lung.

Except in emergency, phlebotomy should not exceed 250 ml. per day. The hematocrit should be controlled at approximately 50 per cent. By removing 250 ml. per day, the hematocrit should be reduced to this level in four or five days. Withdrawing more than this at one time may invite the possibility of shock, particularly if dehydration is contributing to the elevated hematocrit.

Salt restriction is of considerable importance, either used alone or with diuretics, to reduce the total blood volume, thus reducing the work of the right heart. As a diuretic agent acetazolamide (Diamox) is perhaps the drug of choice, since this compound acts as a carbonic anhydrase inhibitor and will increase the excretion of bicarbonate and thus help prevent respiratory acidosis. Where the patient is already in acidosis, it should be used with care (see "Treatment of Carbon Dioxide Narcosis"). Also one must keep in mind that Diamox may superimpose a metabolic acidosis by increasing potassium and sodium excretion, and this may be sufficient to cause a transient CO_2 narcosis.

The desirable dose of this agent varies from 375 to 625 mg. per day, best used for a period of three days a week. In the presence of a low plasma chloride associated with a compensated respiratory acidosis, it is undesirable to use agents, such as the mercurials, which will cause chloride excretion.

Treatment of the Acute Episode of Carbon Dioxide Narcosis

In the presence of suspected carbon dioxide narcosis, it is necessary to be most energetic in one's therapy. Any delay may give rise to deepening of the narcosis with the increased risk of a fatal outcome.

The most important thing for the patient is the elimination of CO_2 by improving ventilation. To accomplish this it may be necessary to do a tracheotomy and to institute intermittent positive pressure breathing around the clock. Coughing will not only be inadequate but may be absent. Therefore, to assist in the evacuation of secretions, mechanical aids, such as suction and a cough machine (OEM Coflator), will be required from time to time.

Energetic antibiotic therapy, as well as therapy for cor pulmonale (which is almost certain to be present at some time), must be instituted. Adequate hydration is all-important.

The use of oxygen in emphysema has been a matter for much discussion in recent years. Provided that ventilation and thus CO_2 excretion is maintained, there is little doubt that improving the patient's oxygenation is of real value. Moreover, shortage of oxygen in the medulla increases the narcotic effect of CO_2 in excessive amounts. Therefore, the use of oxygen at a flow sufficient to give a concentration between 30 and 40 per cent is often beneficial. It must be carefully supervised and adequately humidified.

In the presence of CO_2 narcosis, particular care in the use of oxygen is needed because this may remove the only remaining stimulus to respiration. However, it may be possible to supply a very slow flow with careful watch of the patient by the physician. The main drive must be to the establishment of as much alveolar hyperventilation as is possible and as complete and careful bronchial toilet as can be maintained. Those agents which will help both as direct and indirect bronchodilators should be used freely. Corticoids are almost always indicated. When no improvement is noted, it may be desirable to use a respirator to assist the patient's breathing. We have had the best success using the chest cuirass type rather than the "iron lung."

To evaluate the patient's condition and the effect of therapy, one must determine at intervals the blood pH as well as the total CO_2 content. When these two factors are known, the CO_2 tension of the arterial plasma can be determined from a chart available in Peters and Van Slyke's textbook, *Quantitative Clinical Chemistry*, or by the formula:

$$P_{CO_2} = \frac{\text{Total } CO_2 \text{ content (mM/1)}}{0.0301 \ (1 + 10 \ \text{pH} - 6.1)}.$$ This

formula is easily worked out with a circular slide rule. The normal values are: arterial pH — 7.41; total CO_2 content in plasma — 56 to 60 volumes per cent; CO_2 tension — 40 mm. of mercury.

In respiratory acidosis the CO_2 may be built up quite rapidly. Under such circumstances it may be impossible for available base to unite with a sufficient amount of carbon dioxide to keep the pH within normal limits. The ratio $B.HCO_3/H.HCO_3$ is 20/1 at pH 7.4. As the numerator in this ratio falls, the pH is reduced and the blood becomes more acid. Although the CO_2 content has only risen by a very small amount, within laboratory error in some cases, the CO_2 tension has risen a great deal. This causes a serious retention of CO_2 in body cells. Therefore, to know the CO_2 content of blood is not sufficient; only by knowing the exchange limits between cells and blood (the CO_2 tension) can one evaluate the severity of acidosis and the effects of therapy. For example, the patient may come in with a CO_2 content elevated to about 85 volumes per cent, his pH reduced to 7.3, and CO_2 tension raised to nearly 100 mm. Hg.

After hyperventilation with IPPB for four or five hours, possibly assisted by a respirator, a repetition of these tests may show the CO_2 content to be relatively unchanged. However, if the pH has risen, indicating that the CO_2 in solution has been blown off and thus the carbonic acid in blood reduced, one knows that progress is being made. Thus the importance of determining pH *as well as* CO_2 content!

In the event that efforts to improve ventilation are unsuccessful in eliminating the excess CO_2, the kidney can be called into play. One of the chief actions of the carbonic anhydrase inhibitor, Diamox, is that it increases excretion of bicarbonates in the urine. By this action it reduces the plasma bicarbonates and, therefore, the CO_2 content of the blood. In doing this it creates a metabolic (hyperchloremic) acidosis. However, the main problem is the CO_2 content rather than the blood pH. Therefore, even in the presence of the metabolic acidosis, the patient will be improved, once his respiratory center has been rendered more sensitive by elimination of excessive CO_2.

It must be emphasized that one cannot depend on the presence or absence of cyanosis, either for diagnosis of carbon dioxide narcosis or as a guide to therapy. Even when alveolar CO_2 is doubled and the patient is in severe acidosis, the blood may be fairly well saturated with oxygen. So great is the margin of safety where oxygen is concerned, that the blood will be fully saturated when alveolar oxygen tension is reduced to two-thirds of normal.

One last factor that should be mentioned at this point is the effect of increased CO_2 tension on cerebral vessels and the secretion of spinal fluid. The rise of arterial CO_2 tension causes cerebral vasodilatation. This increases production of cerebrospinal fluid. Since the reabsorbing surface of the subarachnoid villi is limited, there will be a rise of cerebrospinal fluid pressure and often a complaint of headache. This is a very useful guide to the patient who is passing fairly rapidly into acidosis and may be confirmed by examination of the fundus oculi. The vasoconstrictive effect of excess oxygen is much less powerful. Thus, if the patient becomes pink on oxygen therapy but has headaches or visual trouble, the oxygen should be discontinued. In older patients with cerebral arteriosclerosis, vasodilatation is limited. Not only is this useful guide to therapy lost, but because of slow blood flow through the medulla it may be necessary for the arterial blood to be more alkaline (lower CO_2 tension) than normal to remove the amount of CO_2 necessary to maintain the normal pH of the cells in the respiratory center.

The use of intravenous sodium lactate or carbonate, providing no cor pulmonale is present, has a temporary usefulness in acute acidosis, but sodium excess must be avoided. Where all other measures fail, it may be necessary to resort to the surgical approach previously discussed.

SURGERY IN EMPHYSEMA

This is a new and rapidly expanding field of endeavor. Although considerable interest has been shown in operations on the sympathetic and parasympathetic nervous supply of the lungs, we personally have been little impressed by this approach. In our own research on this subject we have been more interested in the problem of removing space-occupying lesions or ventilating devascularized cysts.

As we have pointed out previously, the better the alveolus from the point of view of its elastic structure and its bronchial integrity, the more likely it is to be completely collapsed; the worse the alveolus from these points of view, the more space it will occupy in the already enlarged thorax. Thus, as the disease progresses, the less useful parts of the lung expand in volume; the potentially more useful ones contract. Moreover, as an alveolus ceases to ventilate, it cuts off its own blood supply by a chemical reflex dependent upon the alveolar oxygen tension. This will cause marked reduction of the pulmonary vascular bed and increase the strain upon the right ventricle, thus increasing pulmonary hypertension.

Our concepts of the aims of surgery in this disease are to plicate and resect space-occupying lesions and to remove ventilating cysts, thus permitting the less damaged parts of the lung to re-expand and re-establish ventilation and perfusion with blood. The effects of such surgery are to increase the total volume of ventilation, ventilation at the alveolar level and the vascular bed of the lung, with a resulting fall in pulmonary artery pressure.

It is still early to assess such results adequately, but it is sufficient to say that there have been some striking improvements in patients in whom these procedures have been done, both from the ventilation and from the cardiac standpoints.

The operation is hazardous. It requires scrupulous technical supervision and a very careful preoperative work-up to make certain of the indications for surgery. However, operative intervention holds considerable promise as a palliative procedure. Theoretically, although other cystic areas will enlarge with time, the need of a second operation has not yet come up in our cases. The preoperative evaluation of the patient includes a complete pulmonary physiologic study both of ventilation and perfusion, as well as localizing radiologic studies, to determine the areas to be obliterated.

SECTION C

C I B A

DEVELOPMENT OF GASTROINTESTINAL TRACT

EDMUND S. CRELIN, Ph.D.

Associate Professor of Anatomy
Yale University School of Medicine
New Haven, Connecticut

As illustrated in Plate I, the flat entodermal roof of the yolk sac, which underlies the embryonic disk, becomes incorporated within the human embryo in the form of a tube, the primitive gut, as the embryonic disk folds into a cylindrical embryonic body. The cranial end of the yolk sac roof invaginates into the developing embryonic head fold to become the foregut. Then the caudal end of the yolk sac roof invaginates into the developing tail fold to become the hindgut.

Before the hindgut develops, a tubular diverticulum of the caudal end of the yolk sac roof (the allantois) invaginates into the body stalk. It is drawn into the tail fold along with the hindgut to become a hindgut diverticulum.

Within the body of the embryo, the roof of the yolk sac, intervening between the fore- and hindguts (the midgut), originally has a wide communication with the extra-embryonic portion of the yolk sac. Along the periphery of this midgut-yolk sac communication, the body of the embryo becomes bounded by definite folds, which increase in depth and undercut the embryo to decrease gradually the size of the midgut-yolk sac communication, as shown in Plate II. Before the communication is ultimately lost, it is reduced to a long slender tube, the yolk stalk, passing from the tubular midgut into the umbilical cord, as indicated in Figures 11 to 13, Plate III. The approximation of the body folds forms the ventral body wall and is associated with the formation of the umbilical cord.

The blind cranial end of the foregut forms the inner entodermal layer of the buccopharyngeal membrane, the outer layer of which is the ectodermal floor of a surface depression in the oral region, the stomodeum (Figure 5, Plate II). Disintegration of this membrane establishes the cranial gut opening (Figure 8, Plate II). The blind caudal end of the hindgut forms the inner entodermal layer of the cloacal membrane, the outer layer of which is the ectodermal floor of a surface depression in

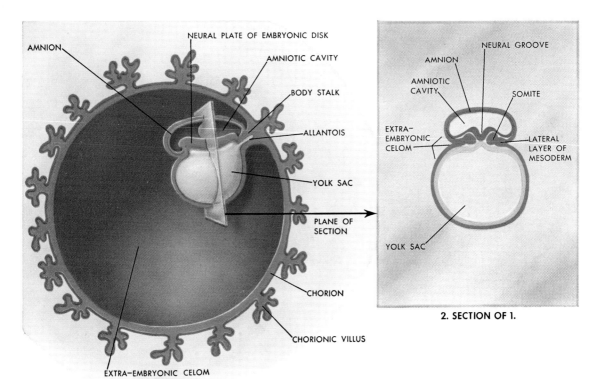

1. FOURTEEN DAYS

2. SECTION OF 1.

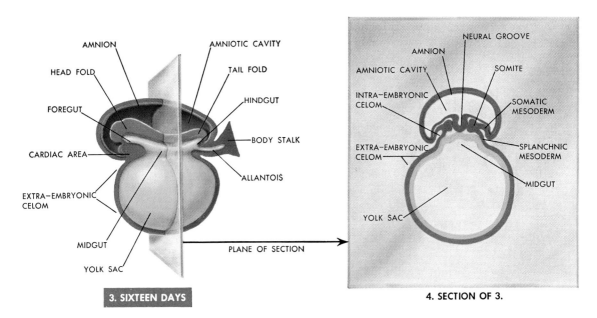

3. SIXTEEN DAYS

4. SECTION OF 3.

KEY

ENTODERM

MESODERM

ECTODERM

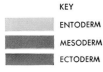

PLATE I

DEVELOPMENT OF GASTROINTESTINAL TRACT AT 14 AND 16 DAYS

the anal region, the proctodeum (Figures 5, 8, and 11). Disintegration of the cloacal membrane establishes the caudal gut opening (Figure 13, Plate III).

The gut entoderm gives rise to the mucosal lining as well as the secretory cells of the glands of the following organs: From the foregut are derived the pharynx, respiratory tract, esophagus, stomach, first part and upper half of the second part of the duodenum. From the midgut comes the lower half of the second part and the third and fourth parts of the duodenum, the jejunum, ileum, cecum, appendix, ascending colon, and right and middle thirds of the transverse colon. The hindgut gives rise to the left third of the transverse colon as well as the descending and sigmoid colon, the rectum, upper part of the anal canal, and a greater part of the urogenital system from its allantoic diverticulum.

Before the primitive gut develops into a tube, a flat layer of mesoderm, continuous with the somites located on each side of the midsagittal plane of the embryonic disk, intervenes between the disk ectoderm and the entodermal yolk sac roof (Figure 2, Plate I). A split occurs in each of these lateral mesodermal layers throughout their length, within the boundaries of the embryonic disk, to produce a slitlike cavity, the intra-embryonic celom (Figure 4, Plate I). It communicates with the relatively large chorionic cavity, the extra-embryonic celom, beyond the boundaries of the embryonic disk. The intra-embryonic celom becomes the pericardial, pleural, and peritoneal cavities. The dorsal sheets of intra-embryonic mesoderm, the somatic (parietal) mesoderm, resulting from the split in the lateral mesodermal layers to form the intra-embryonic celom, become closely associated with the disk ectoderm, and ultimately give rise to the parietal peritoneum of the abdominal cavity (Figures 6, 7, 9, and 10, Plate II). The ventral sheets of the

intra-embryonic mesoderm, the splanchnic mesoderm, resulting from the split in the lateral mesodermal layers, become closely associated with the primitive gut. They give rise to the musculature of the gut, its serosal covering (visceral peritoneum), and its primary ventral and dorsal mesenteries.

When the body folds at the periphery of the midgut-yolk sac communication have completely undercut the embryo to form the ventral abdominal wall and umbilical ring, the communication between the intra- and extra-embryonic celoms is greatly reduced in size as the extra-embryonic celom becomes a tubular cavity within the umbilical cord (Figure 12, Plate III).

Faulty closure of the body folds to form the umbilical ring can result in most of the abdominal viscera developing outside of the body cavity in a transparent sac of amnion. The sac is directly attached to the placenta, with only a portion or no true ventral abdominal wall present. This is one type of omphalocele, also known as eventration of the abdominal viscera or abdominal hernia.

During the closure of the body folds, the two layers of splanchnic mesoderm approach each other and come into direct contact at the midline of the embryonic body. In so doing, they enclose the now tubular gut and form the dorsal and ventral divisions of the primary mesentery, which suspends the gut from the dorsal and ventral body walls (Figures 4, 6, 7, 9, and 10). This mesentery completely separates the celomic cavity into right and left divisions in the abdominal area. However, the two abdominal divisions of the cavity at this developmental stage each extend cephalad as pleural canals, one on each side of the esophagus dorsal to the transverse septum, to become continuous with the single pericardial celom surrounding the developing heart (Figure 11, Plate III). The pericardial celom is later subdivided into the pleural and pericardial cavities as the lungs develop.

The transverse septum is a shelf of somatic mesoderm extending from the ventral body wall, which partitions off the pericardial region from the abdominal region (Figure 11, Plate III). It becomes the ventral part of the diaphragm as shown in Figure 16, Plate IV. The pleural canals become closed by folds of somatic mesoderm, the pleuroperitoneal membranes, arising from the posterolateral body wall on each side. They extend toward the midline of the body, being continuous with the dorsal border of the transverse septum, to meet and fuse with the midline visceral mesoderm, in which the esophagus is embedded, to complete the formation of the diaphragm. Later, the musculature of the diaphragm develops as a secondary ingrowth from the body wall.

The phrenic innervation from the cervical spinal cord to the diaphragm originates when the transverse septum first develops at the cervical level of the embryo. As the septum shifts to a low thoracic level, the phrenic nerves keep pace with the change in position by elongating.

The commonest developmental abnormality of the diaphragm is a faulty development of the left pleuroperitoneal membrane, leaving an opening through which abdominal viscera tend to herniate into the left pleural cavity.

As indicated in Figure 8, Plate II, the portion of the foregut caudal to the origin of the tracheal outgrowth (lung bud) becomes narrowed to form the esophagus. The primary dorsal mesentery, suspending the esophagus to the dorsal body wall, never develops to the extent it does along the gut caudal to the esophagus. Therefore, the mesoderm of the esophageal portion of the dorsal mesentery remains relatively thick and contributes to the formation of the mediastinum (Figure 16, Plate IV).

The esophagus is at first a short tube, immediately caudal to which the gut undergoes a dilatation, the stomach. Originally, the stomach is situated cranial to the transverse septum. As it passes to the abdominal position caudal to the septum, the esophagus elongates. During this elongation, the lumen of the esophagus becomes occluded by extensive growth of its epithelium. This is followed by later recanalization.

Failure of proper recanalization of the lumen results in congenital atresia of the esophagus. Also, faulty development of the tracheal outgrowth results in the commonest anomaly of the trachea, in which an abnormal opening between the trachea and esophagus occurs below the level of the larynx, known as a tracheo-esophageal fistula. Atresia of the esophagus ranks second to imperforate anus as a cause of obstruction of the alimentary canal in newborn infants, and is usually accompanied by a tracheo-esophageal fistula.

In the abdominal area the gastrointestinal tract is at first suspended between the ventral and dorsal body walls by the primary ventral and dorsal mesenteries, as shown in Figures 7 and 9, Plate II. The more caudal part of the ventral mesentery disintegrates very early after its formation, bringing the right and left divisions of the abdominal celom into confluence to establish the unpaired condition of the peritoneal cavity (Figures 8 and 10, Plate II).

As shown in Plates II and III, the liver develops within the persisting cranial portion of the ventral mesentery. The portion of the ventral mesentery between the developing liver and the ventral body wall becomes the falciform ligament. When the single umbilical vein is formed, it passes within the caudal free edge of the falciform ligament (Plates V and VI). After birth the vein becomes a fibrous cord, the ligamentum teres (Figure 20).

The portion of the persisting ventral mesentery between the liver, the developing stomach, and the upper first part of the duodenum becomes the lesser omentum, the development of which is shown in Figures 9, 11, 12, and 17. In contrast, almost the entire primary dorsal mesentery persists. It not only supports the gut in the abdominal cavity but serves as a pathway through which vessels and nerves pass to reach the gut from their main trunks along the dorsal body wall.

When the subdivisions of the gastrointestinal tract are first established, the different portions of the continuous dorsal mesentery receive distinct names. Thus, that part of the dorsal mesentery attaching to the stomach is known as the dorsal mesogastrium. The part attaching to the duodenum is called the mesoduodenum. The mesocolon attaches to the colon, while only that portion attaching to the jejunum and ileum retains the name, dorsal mesentery (Figure 11, Plate III).

During the early stages of the formation of the duodenum, a small hepatic diverticulum arises from a thickened ventral area of duodenal entoderm. This is destined to form the parenchyma of the liver, the liver tubules, their duct system, and the gallbladder. The young hepatic tubules grow out from the diverticulum, extending between the two layers of the ventral mesentery toward the transverse septum (Figures 8 and 9). As the liver grows, the surrounding layers of the ventral mesentery become its serosal covering, with which it is incompletely encapsulated. The reflections of the serosal covering from the liver onto the transverse septum constitute the coronary ligament. The area between these reflections, where the liver is in direct contact with the transverse septum without an intervening serous layer, constitutes the bare area of the liver, as shown in Figures 18 to 20, Plates V and VI. The term, coronary ligament, is quite appropriate

early in the development when the bare area is the shape of a crown. However, its shape later becomes more crescentic. The lateral extensions of the anterior and posterior layers of the coronary ligament constitute the right and left triangular ligaments. The anterior layer is continuous with the falciform ligament.

The caudal portion of the original hepatic diverticulum becomes demarcated early from the main hepatic mass and gives rise to the gallbladder and cystic duct. The single hollow stalk of attachment to the duodenum of the developing hepatic ducts and cystic duct elongates to form the common bile duct, which lies in the free caudal edge of the persisting portion of the ventral mesentery (lesser omentum), Figures 11, 12, and 17.

When the caudal portion of the ventral mesentery disintegrates, the future intestines are represented by the part of the primitive gut tube extending from the stomach to the proctodeum. It lies in the midsagittal body plane parallel to the dorsal body wall, to which it is suspended by the dorsal mesentery.

The first departure from this condition is a rapid elongation of the gut. This results in the formation of a horizontal U-shaped or hairpin-shaped loop that extends into the proximal portion of the umbilical cord (Figure 12, Plate III). The connection of the yolk stalk with the gut lies at the bend of this primary loop. The part of the gut between the stomach and the yolk stalk is the cranial limb of the loop. The part between the yolk stalk and future anus is the caudal limb.

The yolk stalk connection is just proximal to the point of transition between the small and large intestines. Therefore, the cranial limb of the loop forms the 18 to 20 feet of small intestine comprised of the duodenum, jejunum, and upper part of the ileum. The caudal limb forms the terminal 2 to 3 feet of the ileum and all of the large intestine. When the primary gut

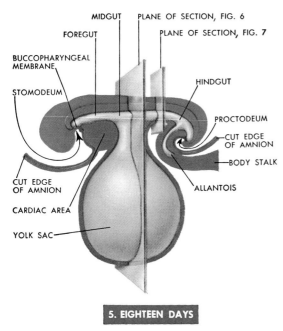

5. EIGHTEEN DAYS

MIDGUT
FOREGUT
PLANE OF SECTION, FIG. 6
PLANE OF SECTION, FIG. 7
BUCCOPHARYNGEAL MEMBRANE
STOMODEUM
HINDGUT
PROCTODEUM
CUT EDGE OF AMNION
BODY STALK
CUT EDGE OF AMNION
CARDIAC AREA
ALLANTOIS
YOLK SAC

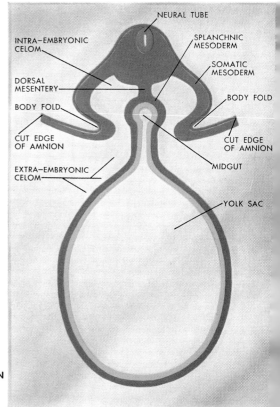

6. SECTION OF 5.

NEURAL TUBE
INTRA—EMBRYONIC CELOM
SPLANCHNIC MESODERM
SOMATIC MESODERM
DORSAL MESENTERY
BODY FOLD
BODY FOLD
CUT EDGE OF AMNION
CUT EDGE OF AMNION
EXTRA—EMBRYONIC CELOM
MIDGUT
YOLK SAC

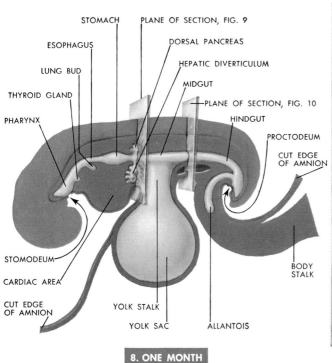

8. ONE MONTH

STOMACH
PLANE OF SECTION, FIG. 9
ESOPHAGUS
DORSAL PANCREAS
LUNG BUD
HEPATIC DIVERTICULUM
THYROID GLAND
MIDGUT
PLANE OF SECTION, FIG. 10
PHARYNX
HINDGUT
PROCTODEUM
CUT EDGE OF AMNION
STOMODEUM
CARDIAC AREA
CUT EDGE OF AMNION
YOLK STALK
YOLK SAC
ALLANTOIS
BODY STALK

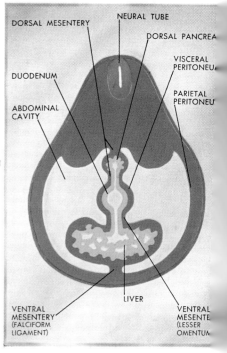

9. SECTION OF 8. (ANTERIOR)

DORSAL MESENTERY
NEURAL TUBE
DORSAL PANCREAS
VISCERAL PERITONEUM
DUODENUM
PARIETAL PERITONEUM
ABDOMINAL CAVITY
VENTRAL MESENTERY (FALCIFORM LIGAMENT)
LIVER
VENTRAL MESENTERY (LESSER OMENTUM)

PLATE **II**   DEVELOPMENT OF GASTROINTESTINAL TRACT AT 18 DAYS AND 1 MONTH

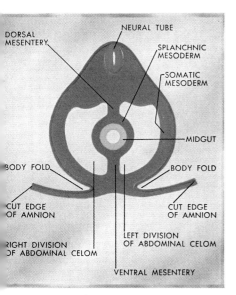

DORSAL MESENTERY

NEURAL TUBE

SPLANCHNIC MESODERM

SOMATIC MESODERM

BODY FOLD

MIDGUT

BODY FOLD

CUT EDGE OF AMNION

CUT EDGE OF AMNION

LEFT DIVISION OF ABDOMINAL CELOM

RIGHT DIVISION OF ABDOMINAL CELOM

VENTRAL MESENTERY

7. SECTION OF 5.

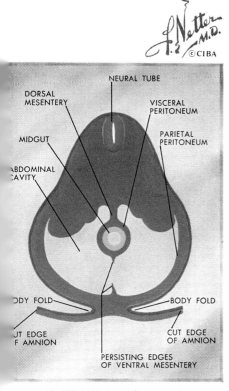

DORSAL MESENTERY

NEURAL TUBE

VISCERAL PERITONEUM

MIDGUT

PARIETAL PERITONEUM

ABDOMINAL CAVITY

BODY FOLD

BODY FOLD

CUT EDGE OF AMNION

CUT EDGE OF AMNION

PERSISTING EDGES OF VENTRAL MESENTERY

10. SECTION OF 8. (POSTERIOR)

loop develops, a small local dilatation in its caudal limb appears, which becomes the cecum (Figure 12). The cecal dilatation enlarges as a whole, but in time its distal end develops less rapidly, so that an extension of smaller diameter is formed. This slender extremity becomes the vermiform appendix (Figures 13 to 15).

The part of the gut which is to become the large intestine is at first of a smaller diameter than the part which becomes the small intestine. Later in development the large intestine acquires a greater diameter.

The changes in position which bring about the adult relationships of the intestines are initiated by a twist or rotation in the horizontal primary gut loop situated in the umbilical cord. The rotation is in a counterclockwise direction when one views the ventral aspect of the embryo (Figure 13). The central axis of the twist is the superior mesenteric artery passing through the dorsal mesentery directly from the dorsal body wall to the yolk stalk (Plate III).

As the cecal dilatation begins to rotate in a counterclockwise direction, it passes above the original cranial limb or right half of the horizontal primary loop. Meanwhile, the original cranial limb of the loop rapidly increases in length and undergoes coiling. Since this coiling of the small intestine begins while the partially rotated loop of gut is still in the umbilical cord, it produces the normal umbilical hernia of development. However, when the abdomen has enlarged sufficiently to accommodate the entire intestinal tract, the protruding part of the tract passes back through the umbilical ring into the abdominal cavity, and the yolk stalk begins to disappear (Figure 14, Plate IV). During this retraction, the coils of small intestine tend to slip into the abdominal cavity ahead of the protruding part of the colon. In so doing, they crowd the lower part of the colon, which had always remained

73

within the abdominal cavity, to the left. This establishes the descending colon in its adult position close against the left side of the dorsal body wall. When the upper part of the colon, which had protruded into the umbilical cord, is drawn at last into the abdominal cavity, its cecal end continues its rotation in a counterclockwise direction toward the right side of the abdominal cavity and then downward to the lower right quadrant of the abdomen (Figure 15). This establishes the transverse colon in a position above the jejunum and ileum and the ascending colon close against the right side of the dorsal body wall.

As the ascending colon approximates the dorsal body wall, the original left side of its mesocolon fuses with the parietal peritoneum dorsal to it in a triangular fashion (Figure 15). The base of this triangle is the ascending colon from the ileocecal junction to the right colic flexure. The apex is at the duodenojejunal flexure. The upper border of the triangle runs from the right colic flexure to the apex, thus forming the right half of attachment between the transverse mesocolon and the dorsal body wall.

The lower border of the triangle passes from its apex to the ileocecal junction to form the attachment (root) of the mesentery of the small intestine to the dorsal body wall.

In the adult, the attachment or root of the mesentery of the small intestine, which is 6 or 7 inches long, runs on an angle from the level of the left side of the second lumbar vertebra to the right iliac fossa anterior to the right sacro-iliac joint.

When the original left side of the serous covering of the ascending mesocolon meets with the parietal peritoneum, the approximated serous surfaces are lost to form a fusion fascia, which is a double plane of connective tissue. Likewise, a plane of fusion fascia develops behind the surface of the ascending colon, which

had fused with the peritoneum of the body wall (the bare area of the ascending colon).

Since the vessels and nerves supplying the ascending colon were originally within its mesocolon, they pass to its left surface after fusion of its mesocolon to the body wall. Therefore, the ascending colon in the adult can be freed from its attachment to the body wall, by first incising its visceral peritoneum as it is reflected off its lateral surface to become the parietal peritoneum all along its right border. Following the incision, blunt dissection along the plane of fusion fascia toward the midline of the body allows extensive elevation of the ascending colon and its nerve and blood supply away from the dorsal body wall.

When the descending colon closely approximated the dorsal body wall on the left side, as the intestines returned to the abdominal cavity from the umbilical cord, the original left side of its mesocolon fused with the parietal peritoneum of the dorsal body wall in a quadrangular fashion (Figure 15, Plate IV). The right border of this fusion quadrangle is the original attachment of the descending mesocolon along the midsagittal plane of the dorsal body wall from the level of the duodenojejunal flexure down to the rectum. The upper border of the quadrangle passes from the duodenojejunal flexure to the left colic flexure, to form the attachment of the left half of the transverse mesocolon to the dorsal body wall. The left border of the quadrangle is the descending colon from its left colic flexure down to its junction with the sigmoid colon. The lower border of the quadrangle passes from the junction of the descending and sigmoid colon to the rectum, to form the attachment of the sigmoid mesocolon to the dorsal body wall.

This quadrangular fusion of the original left side of the descending mesocolon to parietal peritoneum of the dorsal wall forms a fusion fascia, in the same manner previously described for the ascending mesocolon. Also, a plane of fusion fascia develops between the surface of the descending colon and the body-wall peritoneum (the bare area of the descending colon). Since the vessels and nerves supplying the descending colon were originally within its mesocolon, they pass to its right surface, following fusion of its mesocolon to the body wall.

Therefore, the descending colon can be freed from its attachment to the body wall by first incising its visceral peritoneum, as it is reflected off its lateral surface to become the parietal peritoneum all along its left border. Following the incision, blunt dissection along the plane of fusion fascia toward the midplane of the body allows extensive elevation of the descending colon and its nerve and blood supply away from the dorsal body wall.

Concomitant with the formation of the triangular and quadrangular fusion fascias, certain constant, and a number of inconstant, folds of peritoneum develop. Some of the folds conduct blood vessels, whereas others do not. Since a cul-de-sac type of fossa occurs under each fold, it is possible for a loop of intestine to burrow into and enlarge a fossa to form an intraperitoneal hernia. Such fossae occur chiefly at the duodenojejunal flexure (superior, inferior, retro- and paraduodenal); ileocecal junction (superior and inferior ileocecal); dorsal to the cecum (retrocecal); between the dorsal surface of the sigmoid mesocolon and the body-wall peritoneum (intersigmoid).

The portions of the gut which protrude into the umbilical cord during development may not return to the abdominal cavity, as they normally do. This results in a type of umbilical hernia (omphalocele) in which the proximal portion of the umbilical cord at birth is actually a sac of amnion containing nearly all or part of the small intestine and the proximal portions of the large intestine. A similar type of umbilical hernia can be the result if the intestines return normally to the abdominal cavity, only to herniate secondarily, either pre- or postnatally, through an inadequately closed umbilical ring.

The rotation of the intestine and its final positioning after it returns to the abdominal cavity from the umbilical cord may cease at any stage. If the intestines return to the abdomen as a single mass, no rotation occurs, and the jejunum and ileum lie on the right side of the peritoneal cavity and the large intestine on the left. More commonly, partial rotation (so-called malrotation) occurs. If so, the loops of the small intestine occupy the right side of the abdominal cavity and the large intestine the left side, with the cecum lying high in the abdomen near the midline. In this instance, the large intestine retains an extensive mesentery and is freely movable. Actually, the cecum may be located in any position between the middle portion of the upper abdomen and the lower right quadrant, depending on the degree of nonrotation.

A complication of malrotation of the gut, known as volvulus, is the result of having the cecal dilatation rotate clockwise instead of counterclockwise, and in so doing, loop one or more times around the superior mesenteric artery.

In this type of volvulus, the ascending colon is not fused to the body wall, and the transverse colon passes dorsal to the superior mesenteric artery, as it wraps around it to cause both intestinal obstruction and occlusion of the superior mesenteric artery.

One of the commonest anomalies of the intestines, known as Meckel's diverticulum, is due to the partial persistence of the yolk stalk. It is a sacculation of the ileum, occurring about 2 to 3 feet above the ileocecal junction in the adult. It may be a blind pouch or extend to the umbilicus, with or without a patent lumen.

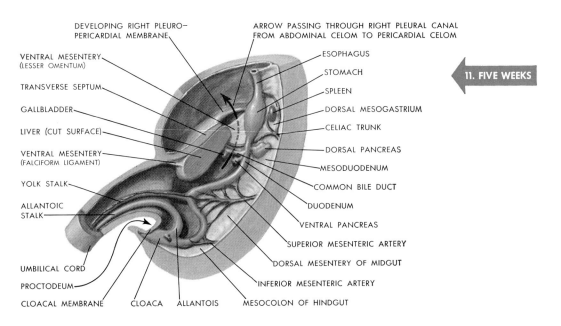

DEVELOPING RIGHT PLEURO-
PERICARDIAL MEMBRANE

ARROW PASSING THROUGH RIGHT PLEURAL CANAL
FROM ABDOMINAL CELOM TO PERICARDIAL CELOM

VENTRAL MESENTERY
(LESSER OMENTUM)

TRANSVERSE SEPTUM

GALLBLADDER

LIVER (CUT SURFACE)

VENTRAL MESENTERY
(FALCIFORM LIGAMENT)

YOLK STALK

ALLANTOIC
STALK

UMBILICAL CORD

PROCTODEUM

CLOACAL MEMBRANE   CLOACA   ALLANTOIS

ESOPHAGUS

STOMACH

SPLEEN

DORSAL MESOGASTRIUM

CELIAC TRUNK

DORSAL PANCREAS

MESODUODENUM

COMMON BILE DUCT

DUODENUM

VENTRAL PANCREAS

SUPERIOR MESENTERIC ARTERY

DORSAL MESENTERY OF MIDGUT

INFERIOR MESENTERIC ARTERY

MESOCOLON OF HINDGUT

11. FIVE WEEKS

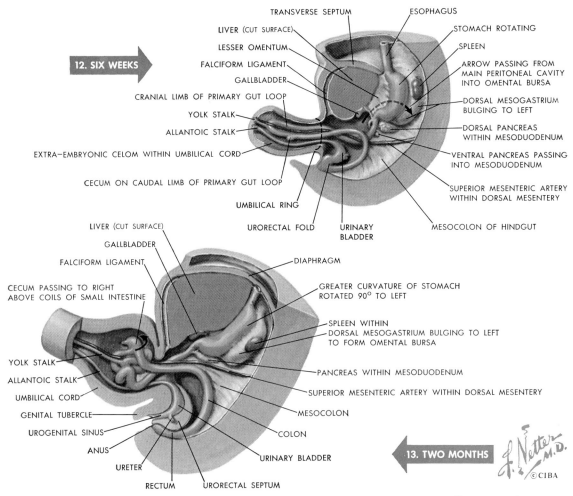

TRANSVERSE SEPTUM   ESOPHAGUS

LIVER (CUT SURFACE)

LESSER OMENTUM

FALCIFORM LIGAMENT

GALLBLADDER

CRANIAL LIMB OF PRIMARY GUT LOOP

YOLK STALK

ALLANTOIC STALK

EXTRA-EMBRYONIC CELOM WITHIN UMBILICAL CORD

CECUM ON CAUDAL LIMB OF PRIMARY GUT LOOP

UMBILICAL RING

URORECTAL FOLD   URINARY
BLADDER

STOMACH ROTATING

SPLEEN

ARROW PASSING FROM
MAIN PERITONEAL CAVITY
INTO OMENTAL BURSA

DORSAL MESOGASTRIUM
BULGING TO LEFT

DORSAL PANCREAS
WITHIN MESODUODENUM

VENTRAL PANCREAS PASSING
INTO MESODUODENUM

SUPERIOR MESENTERIC ARTERY
WITHIN DORSAL MESENTERY

MESOCOLON OF HINDGUT

12. SIX WEEKS

LIVER (CUT SURFACE)

GALLBLADDER

FALCIFORM LIGAMENT

CECUM PASSING TO RIGHT
ABOVE COILS OF SMALL INTESTINE

YOLK STALK

ALLANTOIC STALK

UMBILICAL CORD

GENITAL TUBERCLE

UROGENITAL SINUS

ANUS

URETER

RECTUM   URORECTAL SEPTUM

DIAPHRAGM

GREATER CURVATURE OF STOMACH
ROTATED 90° TO LEFT

SPLEEN WITHIN
DORSAL MESOGASTRIUM BULGING TO LEFT
TO FORM OMENTAL BURSA

PANCREAS WITHIN MESODUODENUM

SUPERIOR MESENTERIC ARTERY WITHIN DORSAL MESENTERY

MESOCOLON

COLON

URINARY BLADDER

13. TWO MONTHS

J. Netter M.D.
©CIBA

PLATE III   DEVELOPMENT OF GASTROINTESTINAL TRACT AT 5 WEEKS, 6 WEEKS,
AND 2 MONTHS

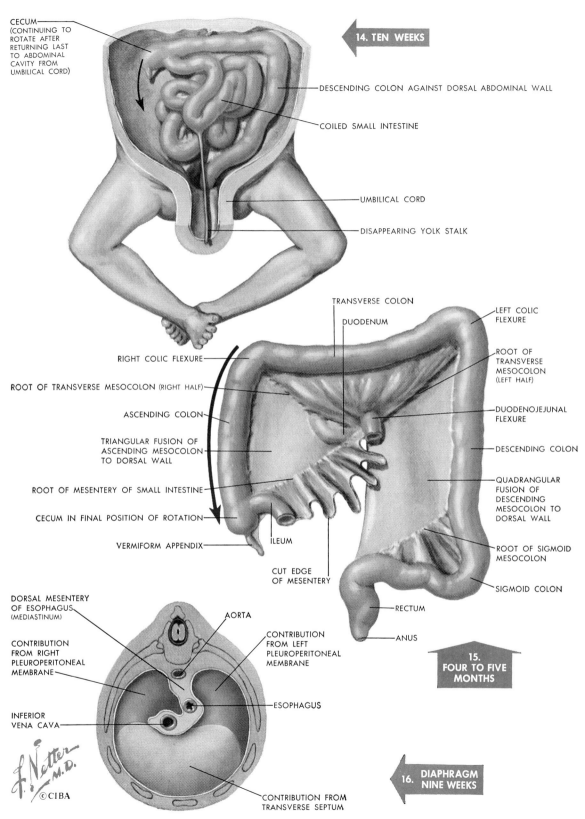

CECUM (CONTINUING TO ROTATE AFTER RETURNING LAST TO ABDOMINAL CAVITY FROM UMBILICAL CORD)

14. TEN WEEKS

DESCENDING COLON AGAINST DORSAL ABDOMINAL WALL

COILED SMALL INTESTINE

UMBILICAL CORD

DISAPPEARING YOLK STALK

TRANSVERSE COLON

DUODENUM

LEFT COLIC FLEXURE

ROOT OF TRANSVERSE MESOCOLON (LEFT HALF)

RIGHT COLIC FLEXURE

ROOT OF TRANSVERSE MESOCOLON (RIGHT HALF)

ASCENDING COLON

DUODENOJEJUNAL FLEXURE

TRIANGULAR FUSION OF ASCENDING MESOCOLON TO DORSAL WALL

DESCENDING COLON

ROOT OF MESENTERY OF SMALL INTESTINE

QUADRANGULAR FUSION OF DESCENDING MESOCOLON TO DORSAL WALL

CECUM IN FINAL POSITION OF ROTATION

VERMIFORM APPENDIX

ILEUM

CUT EDGE OF MESENTERY

ROOT OF SIGMOID MESOCOLON

SIGMOID COLON

RECTUM

ANUS

15. FOUR TO FIVE MONTHS

DORSAL MESENTERY OF ESOPHAGUS (MEDIASTINUM)

AORTA

CONTRIBUTION FROM LEFT PLEUROPERITONEAL MEMBRANE

CONTRIBUTION FROM RIGHT PLEUROPERITONEAL MEMBRANE

ESOPHAGUS

INFERIOR VENA CAVA

16. DIAPHRAGM NINE WEEKS

CONTRIBUTION FROM TRANSVERSE SEPTUM

PLATE IV

DEVELOPMENT OF GASTROINTESTINAL TRACT AT 10 WEEKS AND 4 TO 5 MONTHS; DIAPHRAGM AT 9 WEEKS

While the intestines caudal to the duodenum were undergoing changes in shape and position, the stomach and duodenum were simultaneously undergoing changes. The dorsal border of the gut dilatation, which becomes the stomach, grows faster than its ventral border. This produces the convex greater curvature on the dorsal aspect of the stomach, in contrast to the slower-growing lesser curvature of the ventral aspect. The stomach fundus arises as a local bulge near its craniodorsal end (Figure 12). Once the greater and lesser curvatures become established, the stomach undergoes a 90° rotation about its longitudinal axis, which results in its lesser curvature facing to the right and its greater curvature to the left. The stomach rotation causes the lower end of the esophagus also to rotate. This shifts its closely associated right and left vagus nerves to dorsal and ventral positions as they pass toward the stomach. Assisting the stomach rotation is the rapid growth of the dorsal mesogastrium attaching the greater curvature to the dorsal body wall, and the relatively slower growth of the ventral mesentery (lesser omentum) attaching the lesser curvature to the liver (Figures 12 and 13). At the time of stomach rotation, the enlarging liver displaces the freely movable cranial end of the stomach to the left, whereas the caudal end is relatively anchored by the short ventral mesentery. As a result, the whole stomach extends obliquely across the abdomen from left to right.

While the stomach is assuming this position, the dorsal mesogastrium continues to expand to become the greater omentum by forming a large sac protruding to the left. The cavity developing within this increasingly voluminous greater omentum is the omental bursa. When the stomach has acquired its oblique position, the bursa continues to grow, but now in a caudal direction. In so doing it encounters the transverse mesocolon, which deflects it ventrally, so that it hangs over the transverse colon and covers the underlying coils of small intestine, like an apron (Plate VI).

While it is forming this apron, the original left side of the serous layer of the omentum dorsal to the stomach begins to fuse with the parietal peritoneum of the dorsal body wall. Also, once the apron is formed, the serous layer of the original left side of the omentum, which comes to lie against the transverse colon and its mesocolon, fuses with them. The two layers of the omentum beyond the transverse colon forming the apron then fuse with each other to obliterate the distal part of the bursal lumen (Figure 20).

Later, when fat begins to be laid down in the body, this omental apron becomes one of the important sites of fat storage, and also provides an insulating layer protecting the abdominal viscera.

During the early stages of formation of the duodenum, the pancreas develops from two separate primordia, which arise from the duodenal entoderm. The first primordium, the dorsal pancreas, appears on the dorsal duodenal wall opposite, but slightly cranial to, the hepatic diverticulum (Figures 8, 9, and 11). The other primordium, the ventral pancreas, arises immediately caudal to the hepatic diverticulum (Figure 11). Its cavity may communicate with that of the hepatic diverticulum, or may open separately into the duodenum. With the growth and elongation of the common bile duct, the ventral pancreas migrates around the right side of the duodenum by passing beneath its serosal covering to extend into the mesoduodenum (Figure 12). Simultaneously, the duodenum rotates about 90°, so that its original ventral surface is then directed to the right. These growth changes bring the ventral pancreas into contact with the dorsal pancreas within the mesoduodenum and the two merge (Figures 13 and 17).

The dorsal pancreas gives rise to all of the adult gland, except the caudal portion of the head and the uncinate process, which are derived from the ventral pancreas. In the coalescence of the primordial glandular tissue from the two independent sources, their duct systems fuse. The ventral duct, now communicating with the left side of the duodenum by way of the common bile duct, or in close relationship to it, persists, whereas the proximal portion of the dorsal duct usually atrophies. The distal part of the dorsal duct persists and drains the neck, body, and the tail of the pancreas by way of its anastomosis with the ventral duct (Figure 17).

Occasionally, however, the proximal portion of the dorsal duct persists as an accessory duct, opening separately into the duodenum cranial to the opening of the common bile duct.

As the pancreas grows within the mesoduodenum at the duodenal level, it extends cranially into the dorsal mesogastrium (greater omentum), which is continuous with the mesoduodenum, toward the spleen (Figure 18). The original left side of the part of the dorsal mesogastrium (greater omentum), now containing the neck, body, and tail of the pancreas, and the original right side of the mesoduodenum, containing the head of the pancreas, fuse with the parietal peritoneum of the dorsal body wall (Figures 18, 19, and 20). Thus, part of the head, the neck, body, and tail of the pancreas come to lie dorsal to the stomach beneath the serosal lining of the dorsal wall of the omental bursa.

While the stomach was in its early stages of rotation, the spleen began to form within the cranial part of the dorsal mesogastrium (greater omentum) (Figure 11). It grows rapidly and bulges out the left surface of the mesogastrium, forming the left lateral wall of the omental bursa (Figures 12, 13, and 17). The portion of the dorsal mesogastrium extending from the greater curvature of the stomach to the spleen becomes the gastrolienal ligament. The short portion of the dorsal mesogastrium, extending from the spleen to its point of fusion to the parietal peritoneum of the dorsal wall, becomes the lienophrenic ligament, where the point of fusion overlies the left dorsal aspect of the diaphragm, and the lienorenal ligament, where it overlies the left kidney.

As the ascending colon approximated the dorsal abdominal wall and its mesocolon fused with the parietal peritoneum, the upper part of its mesocolon came to overlie and fuse with the second and third parts of the duodenum, which had already fused with the original body wall peritoneum (Figure 15). Thus, the original peritoneal investment of the second and third parts of the duodenum is completely resorbed when it becomes covered by this secondary peritoneal covering of mesocolon. Also, the fusion of the ascending mesocolon results in the root of the transverse mesocolon crossing the head of the pancreas and the second part of the duodenum, and the root of the mesentery of the small intestine crossing the third part of the duodenum (Figure 15).

The entrance from the main peritoneal cavity into the omental bursa is at first a broad, slitlike opening in the midsagittal body plane facing to the left (Figures 12, 17, and 18). It later becomes reduced in size to become the epiploic foramen to the right of the midsagittal body plane. This occurs when the duodenum forms a U-shaped loop and swings to the right to fuse with the body wall, as the growth of the dorsal portion of the liver extends its inferior surface to a lower body level. Thus, the cranial boundary of the completed epiploic foramen is the caudate lobe of the liver (Figure 20). Its dorsal boundary is the dorsal body-wall peritoneum overlying the inferior vena cava. The caudal boundary is the point where the first part of the duodenum fused with

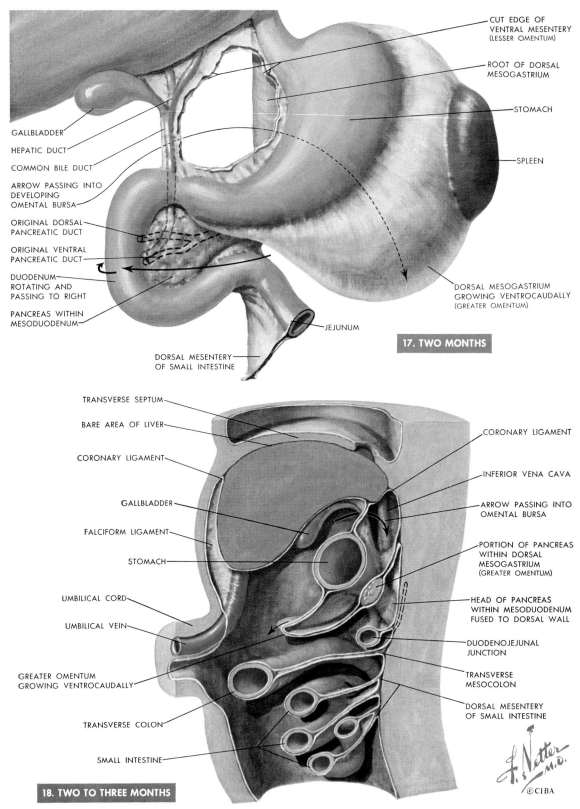

CUT EDGE OF VENTRAL MESENTERY (LESSER OMENTUM)

ROOT OF DORSAL MESOGASTRIUM

STOMACH

SPLEEN

DORSAL MESOGASTRIUM GROWING VENTROCAUDALLY (GREATER OMENTUM)

GALLBLADDER

HEPATIC DUCT

COMMON BILE DUCT

ARROW PASSING INTO DEVELOPING OMENTAL BURSA

ORIGINAL DORSAL PANCREATIC DUCT

ORIGINAL VENTRAL PANCREATIC DUCT

DUODENUM ROTATING AND PASSING TO RIGHT

PANCREAS WITHIN MESODUODENUM

JEJUNUM

DORSAL MESENTERY OF SMALL INTESTINE

17. TWO MONTHS

TRANSVERSE SEPTUM

BARE AREA OF LIVER

CORONARY LIGAMENT

GALLBLADDER

FALCIFORM LIGAMENT

STOMACH

UMBILICAL CORD

UMBILICAL VEIN

GREATER OMENTUM GROWING VENTROCAUDALLY

TRANSVERSE COLON

SMALL INTESTINE

18. TWO TO THREE MONTHS

CORONARY LIGAMENT

INFERIOR VENA CAVA

ARROW PASSING INTO OMENTAL BURSA

PORTION OF PANCREAS WITHIN DORSAL MESOGASTRIUM (GREATER OMENTUM)

HEAD OF PANCREAS WITHIN MESODUODENUM FUSED TO DORSAL WALL

DUODENOJEJUNAL JUNCTION

TRANSVERSE MESOCOLON

DORSAL MESENTERY OF SMALL INTESTINE

©CIBA

PLATE V

RELATIONSHIPS OF STOMACH AT 2 MONTHS; SAGITTAL SECTION AT 2 TO 3 MONTHS

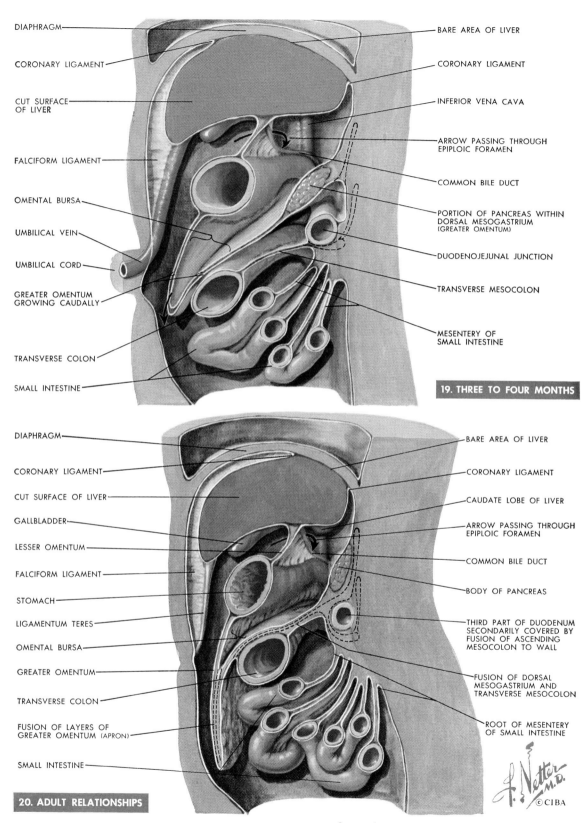

DIAPHRAGM

CORONARY LIGAMENT

CUT SURFACE
OF LIVER

FALCIFORM LIGAMENT

OMENTAL BURSA

UMBILICAL VEIN

UMBILICAL CORD

GREATER OMENTUM
GROWING CAUDALLY

TRANSVERSE COLON

SMALL INTESTINE

BARE AREA OF LIVER

CORONARY LIGAMENT

INFERIOR VENA CAVA

ARROW PASSING THROUGH
EPIPLOIC FORAMEN

COMMON BILE DUCT

PORTION OF PANCREAS WITHIN
DORSAL MESOGASTRIUM
(GREATER OMENTUM)

DUODENOJEJUNAL JUNCTION

TRANSVERSE MESOCOLON

MESENTERY OF
SMALL INTESTINE

19. THREE TO FOUR MONTHS

DIAPHRAGM

CORONARY LIGAMENT

CUT SURFACE OF LIVER

GALLBLADDER

LESSER OMENTUM

FALCIFORM LIGAMENT

STOMACH

LIGAMENTUM TERES

OMENTAL BURSA

GREATER OMENTUM

TRANSVERSE COLON

FUSION OF LAYERS OF
GREATER OMENTUM (APRON)

SMALL INTESTINE

BARE AREA OF LIVER

CORONARY LIGAMENT

CAUDATE LOBE OF LIVER

ARROW PASSING THROUGH
EPIPLOIC FORAMEN

COMMON BILE DUCT

BODY OF PANCREAS

THIRD PART OF DUODENUM
SECONDARILY COVERED BY
FUSION OF ASCENDING
MESOCOLON TO WALL

FUSION OF DORSAL
MESOGASTRIUM AND
TRANSVERSE MESOCOLON

ROOT OF MESENTERY
OF SMALL INTESTINE

20. ADULT RELATIONSHIPS

PLATE VI   SAGITTAL SECTIONS AT 3 OR 4 MONTHS COMPARED WITH ADULT

the body wall, and the ventral boundary is the free edge of the lesser omentum, enclosing the common bile duct, portal vein, and proper hepatic artery.

Since the fusion to the body wall of the rotated duodenum and its mesoduodenum occurs as it does, the common bile duct, pancreatic duct or ducts, and the nerve and blood supply of the second part of the duodenum all enter it on the left pancreatic surface. This allows the right side of the second part in the adult to be elevated from the dorsal body wall by blunt dissection, and reflected toward the midline of the body to expose the dorsal surface of the lower end of the common bile duct, which would otherwise be difficult to approach anteriorly because of the overlying head of the pancreas.

The lumen of the duodenum, jejunum, and ileum becomes occluded by masses of epithelial cells early in development with later recanalization.

Faulty recanalization of the lumen or its complete failure may result in localized or extensive areas of atresia.

When the midgut first began to form its primary loop and pass out into the umbilical cord, the caudal end of the hindgut began to undergo changes. The hindgut caudal to the point of origin of the allantois becomes enlarged to form the cloaca. An ectodermal depression, the proctodeum, extends toward the cloaca, being separated from it by the thin cloacal membrane (Figure 11).

A division of the cloaca into two parts is produced by the development of a crescentic fold of its entoderm (the urorectal fold), which cuts into the cranial part of the cloaca in the angle where the allantois and hindgut meet. It then extends caudally toward the cloacal membrane (Figures 11 and 12).

As the fold cuts deeper into the cloaca, a wedge-shaped mass of mesenchyme grows into the fold to produce the urorectal septum (Figure 13). The complete formation of the septum partitions the cloaca into a separate ventral division, the urogenital sinus, and a dorsal division, the rectum and upper part of the anal canal. Once the cloaca is completely divided, the cloacal membrane disintegrates to establish a separate opening into the urogenital sinus and a separate anal opening into the anorectal cloacal division.

The urogenital sinus and allantois give rise to the epithelium and secretory glandular cells of the greater part of the urogenital system. The portion of the proctodeal depression of ectoderm, in continuity with the anorectal division, gives rise to the lower part of the anal canal. The lumen of the rectum during its early stages of development is occluded by a proliferation of epithelial cells, and is later recanalized.

Partial or complete failure of the lumen to recanalize results in rectal stenosis or atresia. If the union fails to take place between the rectum and the proctodeal depression, an imperforate anus is the result. Abnormalities in the development of the urorectal septum, to divide the cloaca into two parts, are responsible for an anomalous communication between the rectum and the urinary bladder, the urethra, or the vagina. Many varieties are possible, but most common in males is a fistula between the rectum and urethra or between the rectum and the bladder. In females, fistulas are almost exclusively between the rectum and the vagina.

The basic formation and positioning of the various subdivisions of the gastrointestinal tract and their glandular derivatives are essentially completed by the end of the fifth month of intra-uterine development.

DISEASES OF THE LARGE INTESTINE

H. E. LOCKHART-MUMMERY, M.D., M.CHIR., F.R.C.S.

Surgeon, St. Thomas' Hospital, London,
and St. Mark's Hospital, London

DIVERTICULOSIS
(PLATE I)

Diverticulosis of the colon is an acquired condition which results from herniation of the mucosa through defects in the muscle coats. The defects are usually located where the blood vessels pierce the muscular wall. These vessels, the "long circular" arteries, always enter just on the mesenteric side of the two lateral taeniae coli. Therefore, diverticula commonly occur in two parallel rows along the bowel.

The appendices epiploicae are also situated in this same location. Thus, diverticula frequently enter the base of these structures.

The diverticula probably arise from pulsion as a result of increased intraluminal pressure from incoordinated peristalsis. However, the etiology is not exactly known. Obesity and constipation may be aggravating factors but are not primary causes.

Diverticula do not occur in the rectum, but they may be found throughout the entire length of the colon. They are much more common on the left side, and most frequently they affect the sigmoid colon.

Diverticulosis is rare under the age of 40. Its incidence increases with age, occurring in about 10 per cent of persons of middle age, more commonly in males.

Diverticula of the colon are flask-shaped, having a narrow neck through the muscle wall and a wider body. Because their walls have no muscular layer, fecal material that enters a diverticulum cannot be expelled and thus hardens into firm concretions.

If the mucosa of a diverticulum becomes ulcerated by the hard fecalith and then becomes infected, various forms of diverticulitis may be produced.

X-ray

The diagnosis of diverticulosis is made by radiologic examination after an opaque enema. The earliest radiographic change is a fine serration of the wall of the affected part of the colon, usually the sigmoid. This is called the "prediverticular state" and may be followed in time by the appearance of sacs and pouches aris-

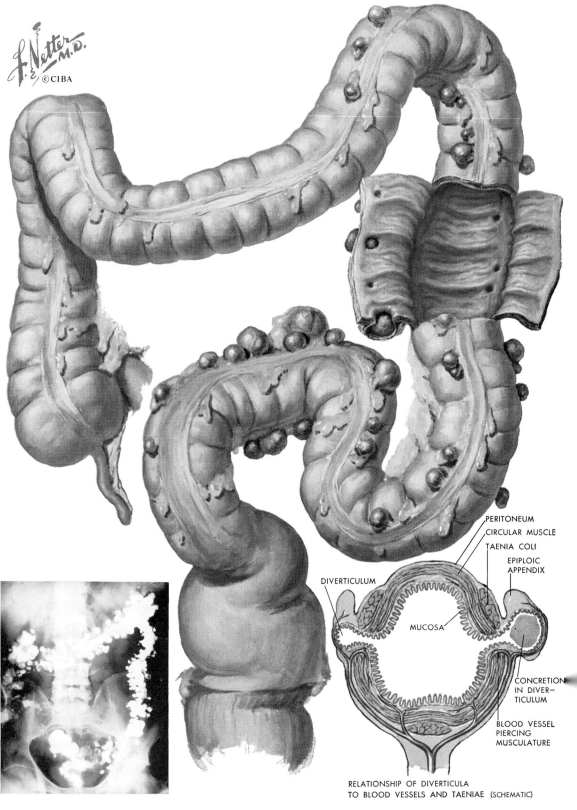

PERITONEUM

CIRCULAR MUSCLE

TAENIA COLI

EPIPLOIC APPENDIX

DIVERTICULUM

MUCOSA

CONCRETION IN DIVERTICULUM

BLOOD VESSEL PIERCING MUSCULATURE

RELATIONSHIP OF DIVERTICULA
TO BLOOD VESSELS AND TAENIAE (SCHEMATIC)

PLATE I

DIVERTICULOSIS

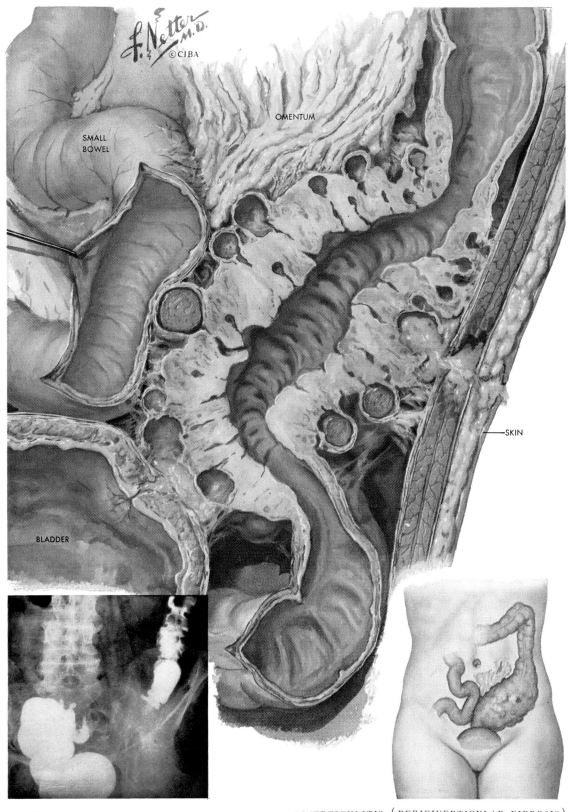

SMALL BOWEL

OMENTUM

SKIN

BLADDER

PLATE II

DIVERTICULITIS (PERIDIVERTICULAR FIBROSIS)

ing from the bowel, which are at first retractile. However, in fully developed diverticulosis they are permanently distended and extracolic.

Clinical Features

Clinically, diverticulosis is a symptomless condition, often detected incidental to the administration of an opaque enema given for investigation of symptoms arising from some other lesion. Usually, no active treatment is required, but the patient should be advised to take mineral oil regularly to ensure a soft stool, to avoid much roughage in the diet, and to avoid obesity.

Diverticulitis and its complications occur in only a small proportion of individuals with diverticulosis. Therefore, patients should not be alarmed unduly if diverticula are found on x-ray.

Sometimes a solitary diverticulum is found in the cecum or transverse colon, not associated with a generalized diverticulosis of the colon, and occurring in people of younger age. Should inflammation occur in such a solitary diverticulum, the patient may develop abdominal pain which mimics appendicitis.

The surgeon who operates usually finds a mass in the cecum, which is difficult to distinguish from carcinoma. However, if the correct diagnosis can be made at operation, excision of the diverticulum, with repair of the bowel wall, suffices for cure.

DIVERTICULITIS
(Peridiverticular Fibrosis)
(PLATE II)

As previously stated, ulceration with bacterial invasion leading to diverticulitis occurs in only a small percentage of patients with diverticulosis. Once infection develops around one or more diverticula, the subsequent course depends upon the virulence of the organism and the resistance of the patient. Occasionally, acute inflammation, in which all structures of the intestinal wall participate, may terminate in perforation, leading to general peritonitis. However, more commonly, an abscess will remain localized, walled off by other viscera, the omentum, and abdominal wall. A more usual course is that of a low-grade inflammatory process (peridiverticulitis), with formation of much fibrofatty tissue around the affected part of the bowel. This results in narrowing of the lumen, shortening of the loop, and adhesion to nearby structures. This thickening, which may extend over several inches of bowel, gives rise to a firm, tender mass along the line of the colon. Infection persists within this thickened tissue, and recurrent activity of the inflammation may lead to the further extension of small abscesses, which may open into the organs that wall off the infection. In this way fistulas may form, leading to the anterior abdominal wall, the bladder, small bowel, or female pelvic organs.

Complications

The complications that may follow diverticulitis are therefore: (1) obstruction of the colon, more often partial and chronic than complete; (2) free perforation with general peritonitis; (3) abscess formation; and (4) the development of internal or external fistulas. The most serious complication is the formation of a vesicocolic fistula, for this gives rise to persistent infection of the urinary tract. It occurs rarely in women, owing to the interposition of the uterus.

Clinically, acute diverticulitis causes pyrexia, with pain in the left lower quadrant of the abdomen. Examination will reveal a tender mass in that area, the lower edge of which may also be palpable by rectum.

Patients with chronic diverticulitis usually complain of dull or recurrent pain in this same region, often associated with some alteration of bowel habit, a sense of distention, and dyspepsia. Bleeding is unusual, but is said to occur in about 10 per cent of patients. Examination may reveal some tender enlargement of the sigmoid colon. Sigmoidoscopy may show rigidity and edema of the bowel above the rectosigmoid junction.

Should a vesicocolic fistula form, the classical symptom is pneumaturia, often associated with frequency and pain on micturition. An enterocolic fistula will give rise to severe diarrhea.

Radiologically, peridiverticulitis produces an irregular "filling defect." Diverticula can usually be seen in the colon near the defect. Diagnosis between such a defect and that caused by a carcinoma may be difficult, but in the latter the defect is usually shorter and has more abrupt margins.

Treatment

The milder forms of diverticulitis will respond to medical treatment, but surgery will be necessary if medical measures fail to control symptoms, if the disease progresses or recurs, or if complications arise.

If surgery should be needed, the aim should be resection of the diseased segment and anastomosis of normal colon to the rectum.

In patients having active inflammation, a staged operation with a preliminary transverse colostomy is usually wiser.

However, in the milder forms a one-stage operation can usually be done with safety. In a patient who is unfit for major surgery, a proximal defunctioning colostomy will usually allow the infection and symptoms to subside. It will probably have to be permanent.

VOLVULUS OF SIGMOID
(PLATE III)

Primary volvulus of the colon occurs only in the sigmoid colon and in the cecum. It is a comparatively rare form of intestinal obstruction in the Western world and usually occurs in middle-aged and elderly patients. However, it is more common in eastern Europe and Asia, probably because of different dietary habits. In less developed and poorer parts of the world, a bulky vegetable diet is more common; this results in a bigger fecal residue, which leads to a persistently loaded colon. In time, the loaded sigmoid colon may become chronically distended and elongated. As it elongates its two ends tend to approximate, producing a narrower mesenteric attachment. Some fibrosis often occurs in the base of the mesosigmoid, accentuating this narrow base. These are the essential predisposing features of a volvulus, and once they exist the actual precipitating cause is often trivial, such as straining or coughing.

In its early stages, a volvulus produces a "check-valve" effect, allowing flatus and some fluid feces to enter the loop, but preventing them from leaving. In this way, great and rapid distention is produced. If the twist becomes tighter, a complete "closed-loop" obstruction develops, and pressure on the vessels in the mesentery may lead to impairment of blood supply with gangrene of the bowel.

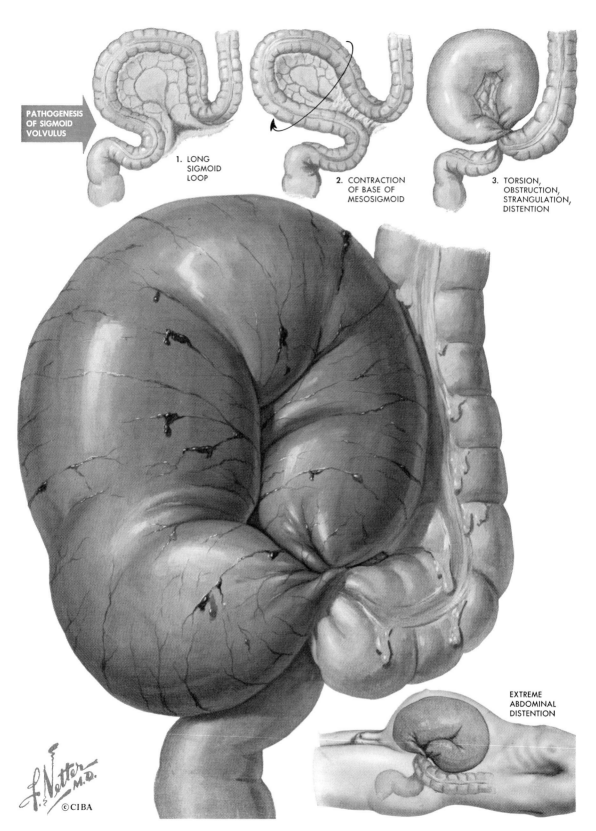

PATHOGENESIS OF SIGMOID VOLVULUS

1. LONG SIGMOID LOOP

2. CONTRACTION OF BASE OF MESOSIGMOID

3. TORSION, OBSTRUCTION, STRANGULATION, DISTENTION

EXTREME ABDOMINAL DISTENTION

PLATE III

VOLVULUS OF THE SIGMOID

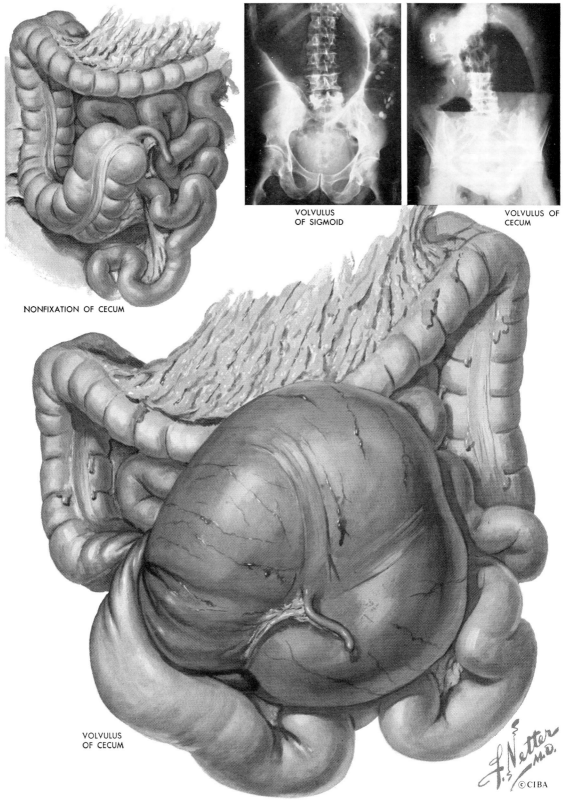

NONFIXATION OF CECUM

VOLVULUS
OF SIGMOID

VOLVULUS OF
CECUM

VOLVULUS
OF CECUM

PLATE IV

VOLVULUS OF THE CECUM

Clinically, the onset of the signs and symptoms of a sigmoid volvulus is usually sudden, with lower abdominal pain. Constipation is absolute, but sometimes tenesmus with passage of a little mucus may occur. Vomiting is unusual. The general condition is usually well-maintained unless gangrene of the loop has started, in which case loss of blood and fluid may soon lead to shock.

Distention occurs early and progresses rapidly, and is always a dominant part of the clinical picture. Within a few hours it may be so extreme that no other features are discernible on abdominal examination.

X-ray

The most valuable aid to diagnosis is a plain x-ray of the abdomen, both erect and supine. An enormous gas-filled loop containing a little fluid is usually revealed, giving a characteristic picture.

Treatment

In those patients who are not in shock, an attempt to pass a tube into the loop by the sigmoidoscope should first be tried. If intubation is successful, decompression usually leads to spontaneous reduction of the volvulus, and operation is avoided. If unsuccessful, an operation should be undertaken without delay.

In cases requiring surgery, a long left paramedian incision is made, and if the bowel is viable, it is then untwisted and fixed. If it is gangrenous, it will need to be resected. When this is required, immediate anastomosis is hazardous, and the operation may either be terminated as a double-barreled colostomy for later closure, or the distal end may be oversewed and the proximal end brought out as a colostomy.

Anastomosis can be undertaken later. Deflation of the loop by aspiration through a needle puncture or by a tube passed by rectum greatly facilitates the operation.

In cases of mild but recurrent volvulus, the patients complain of bouts of constipation, distention, and abdominal pain, which are relieved spontaneously after some hours with the passage of much flatus. In these cases, operation reveals a long sigmoid loop with a narrow base, as in the more severe forms of volvulus. The long loop should be resected, with immediate anastomosis to restore continuity.

VOLVULUS OF CECUM

(PLATE IV)

Volvulus of the cecum is an infrequent condition in the western part of the world and accounts for only about 1 per cent of the cases of intestinal obstruction. Like volvulus of the sigmoid colon, however, it appears to be more common in those parts of the world in which vegetables and roughage form a greater part of the diet, and it is thought that persistent loading of the bowel with a big fecal residue also may play a part in the etiology of this condition.

The predisposing factor is inadequate fixation of the cecum and ascending colon to the posterior abdominal wall. Normally, in the third stage of intestinal rotation during development, the cecum descends from the subhepatic region to lie in the right iliac fossa, and the ascending colon and most of the cecum become fixed to the posterior abdominal wall. If this last process is not fully completed, the cecum, a few inches of ascending colon, and a few inches of terminal ileum may be attached by a mesentery with a relatively short base and may then be free to rotate around this axis.

Should a twist occur, all these parts of the intestine are involved, and the condition should really be called "volvulus of the ileocecal segment."

As in volvulus of the sigmoid, the twist may not be tight at first and may untwist spontaneously. At this stage, the "check-valve" effect will tend to cause rapid distention of the cecum. If the twist becomes tighter, complete "closed-loop" obstruction is produced, and, finally, strangulation of the vessels will result in gangrene of the bowel, which is likely to occur more rapidly in this location than in volvulus of the sigmoid.

Volvulus of the cecum usually occurs at a younger age than does volvulus of the sigmoid colon, most patients being 20 to 40 years old.

The onset is sudden, with severe central abdominal pain. Vomiting soon follows. The pain is constant, but intermittent exacerbations due to spasm also occur.

Examination reveals some general abdominal distention caused by the low small intestinal obstruction. In most cases the distended cecum may be made out as a palpable tympanitic swelling in the central part of the abdomen. A feeling of emptiness in the right iliac fossa may be encountered.

X-ray

The most valuable aid to diagnosis is the plain x-ray, which will show the greatly distended central coil, with perhaps a fluid level within it if the x-ray study is made in an erect position.

Distention of the loops of ileum above the point of obstruction may also be recognizable.

Treatment

As soon as the diagnosis of cecal volvulus is made, a laparotomy is indicated, and the bowel should be untwisted if possible. Puncture and aspiration of the tensely distended cecum may be necessary before this can be attempted. If the bowel seems viable after untwisting and the patient's condition permits, it is advisable to try to fix the cecum in its correct position with a few carefully placed sutures. If the bowel is not viable or viability is doubtful, immediate resection and anastomosis is the wiser course.

Cases of partial volvulus with spontaneous untwisting also occur, giving rise to recurrent attacks of lower abdominal pain. In such cases, the diagnosis may be difficult, but the cause of the repeated attacks usually becomes apparent if laparotomy is undertaken. Fixation of the cecum will then prevent further attacks.

NONSPECIFIC ULCERATIVE COLITIS (PLATE V)

Pathology and Diagnosis

Ulcerative colitis is a disease of unknown etiology, characterized by diffuse inflammation of the large bowel. The disease is variable in its extent, its severity, and its clinical course, and our knowledge of many of its aspects is still incomplete.

In nearly all cases of ulcerative colitis, the rectum and rectosigmoid regions are involved. Indeed, in most cases the disease appears to start in this part of the bowel and to extend proximally. In the majority of severe cases, the entire colon is involved. However, sometimes only the descending and more distal colon takes part, the right colon remaining unaffected. In about 10 per cent of the cases, the disease not only involves the whole colon

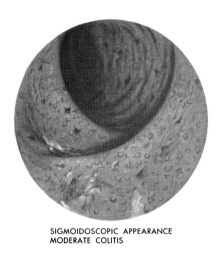

SIGMOIDOSCOPIC APPEARANCE
MODERATE COLITIS

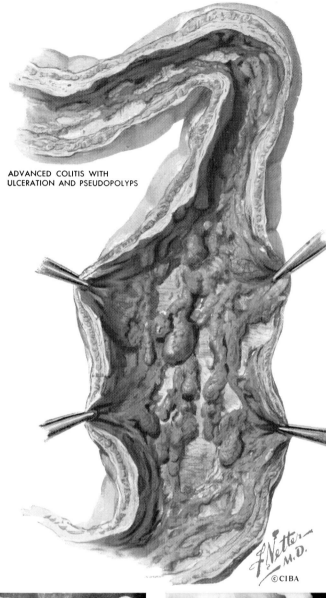

ADVANCED COLITIS WITH
ULCERATION AND PSEUDOPOLYPS

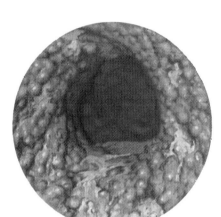

SIGMOIDOSCOPIC APPEARANCE
SEVERE COLITIS

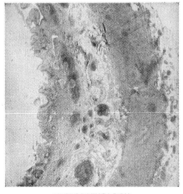

MICROPATHOLOGY

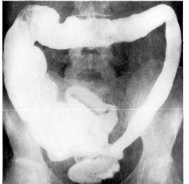

CONTRACTED BOWEL

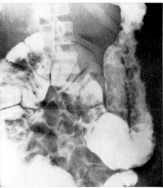

PSEUDOPOLYPOSIS

PLATE V   NONSPECIFIC ULCERATIVE COLITIS

but spreads in continuity to affect several inches of the terminal ileum. In such instances, the ileocecal valve always becomes dilated and incompetent.

The earliest microscopic changes in ulcerative colitis are confined to the mucosal layer, which becomes increasingly vascular and infiltrated with round cells. This leads to a rough and granular appearance of the mucosa, which bleeds easily on touch. This characteristic appearance of ulcerative colitis in its milder stages may be seen on sigmoidoscopic examination.

In more advanced cases, the round-cell infiltration extends, and abscesses form in dilated crypts, which discharge on the mucosal surface, with the formation of small ulcers. In this stage the changes in the bowel wall are still mainly superficial. However, all layers show an augmented blood supply and some round-cell infiltration, and the bowel is somewhat contracted.

In the most severe and active cases, abscesses burst through the walls of the crypts and spread in the submucosa. Areas of mucosa which are thus undermined and deprived of blood supply are shed. In this way extensive serpiginous ulcers are formed, which are often deep enough to expose the muscle coat. The remaining mucosa, being edematous and partly undermined, has a pseudopolypoid appearance.

In acute cases the bowel may be edematous and friable, and is sometimes dilated. In more chronic or recurring disease, the intestine tends to be both shortened in length and reduced in diameter. This is not the result of fibrosis but of hypertrophy and tonic contraction of the muscle coats.

The course of ulcerative colitis is commonly one of remissions and relapses. During remissions considerable repair and healing occur in the colon. The vascularity and edema subside, a thin epithelial covering grows over the granulation tissue of the denuded areas, and the rough and granular appearance of the mucosa may revert to normal. A contracted and shortened bowel may relax and haustrations reappear.

Sigmoidoscopy

The earliest sigmoidoscopic changes include loss of the normal vascular pattern, the mucosa being pink and finely granular. In more severe cases, the mucosa is a darker red, is more roughly granular, and bleeds easily. A variable amount of mucus, blood, and pus may be seen in the lumen of the bowel, which may be somewhat contracted. It is less common to see ulcers and pseudopolyps, but severe cases may show these changes even in the rectum.

X-ray

A barium enema will give information about the state of the colon above the reach of the sigmoidoscope. The changes to look for here are the loss of mucosal pattern, ulceration and pseudopolyps, loss of haustration, and contraction of the bowel.

The barium enema will help determine the severity and extent of the disease, guide the selection of therapy, and determine the prognosis.

SURGICAL MANAGEMENT OF NONSPECIFIC ULCERATIVE COLITIS

The treatment of nonspecific ulcerative colitis is primarily medical. However, surgical intervention may become necessary if the patient does not respond to medical management, or does so poorly as to be rendered a chronic invalid by the severity of the disease. A severe acute episode, which all efforts to treat medically have proved of no avail, may give the indication for an emergency operation to save the life of the patient.

The most frequent indications for operative treatment are intractable diarrhea, massive hemorrhage, chronic inanition, perforation of the distended colon, stricture or fistula formation, abscesses, increasing signs of pseudopolyposis or malignant changes (carcinoma), which may develop in long-standing cases, usually those of more than 10 years' duration. The chances of carcinoma developing increase with time, and are statistically more common in the younger patients in whom the disease started relatively early and who developed a marked pseudo-polypoidosis. Of the systemic complications in this disorder, a progressive or persistent arthritis may also be considered an indication for surgery.

Ileostomy and Subtotal Colectomy
(Plate VI)

Once the decision for surgery has been reached, it is usually advisable to remove the entire large bowel and to establish an ileostomy. In most cases it is desirable that this procedure be carried out in two stages; ileostomy and subtotal colectomy being done as a first stage, followed by excision of the remaining rectocolic segment a few months later. Total procto-colectomy can be done with safety in one stage in a very small number of patients, whose general condition is exceptionally good.

The operation of ileostomy and subtotal colectomy is best done through a long left paramedian incision. After explo-ration and assessment, the terminal ileum is mobilized and divided between clamps in healthy bowel as near to the cecum as possible, the blood supply to this future ileostomy being carefully preserved. The colon is then mobilized from its lateral attachments and from the stomach, by division between ligatures of the gastro-colic (greater) omentum. Mobilization of the splenic flexure may be difficult unless the entire colon has been much shortened by disease. Careful technique with good retraction and lighting are necessary if damage to the spleen is to be avoided.

Once mobilized, the colon may be removed, starting at the proximal end. By transilluminating the mesocolon with a strong light, the vessels are clearly seen and may be picked up easily with hemostats before division. The bowel is removed to the level of the lower sigmoid colon, preserving enough distally to allow the cut distal end to extend 2 inches above the surface of the abdominal wall without tension and with good blood supply. At this level it is again divided between clamps and the specimen removed.

The terminal ileum should be brought out as an ileostomy, through a separate "trephine" incision, in an area of smooth and healthy skin at least 2 inches away from the umbilicus or any bony prominence. As a belt will probably be worn to support an appliance, the ileostomy site should be on or only just below the belt line. At the point selected, a circle of skin three-quarters of an inch in diameter is removed, and the layers of the abdominal wall are then dissected and stretched, until a circular hole has been made through all layers. The terminal ileum is brought through this opening until about one and one-half inches protrude beyond the skin surface. The mesentery of the ileum should be sutured to the parietal peritoneum within the abdomen, and the space between the emerging ileostomy and the lateral abdominal wall should be closed by sutures if possible.

After closure of the abdomen and sealing of the main wound, the clamp on the ileostomy is removed, and the bowel is everted and sewed to the skin edges with interrupted catgut stitches, so that the final protrusion is only about three-quarters of an inch beyond the skin surface. The clamp on the distal colon is left in place for several days until sound fixation of the bowel to the abdominal wall has taken place.

Although patients usually improve rapidly in general health after subtotal colectomy and the establishment of an ileostomy, it is advisable to remove the remaining large bowel at a later date, because the persistence of the disease in the most distal part of the colon and rectum prevents a return to full health, and remains as a possible source of trouble and complication. It is usual to wait a few months before undertaking this second stage, allowing the patient to regain strength.

Removal of Sigmoid Colon and Rectum
(Plate VII)

Excision of the remaining sigmoid colon and rectum can be done most conveniently by the synchronous combined method of Lloyd-Davies (1939). With the patient in lithotomy-Trendelenburg position, using special supports to hold the legs in abduction with little flexion, an abdominal operator and a perineal operator work simultaneously, so that the operation can be completed quickly and with good control of bleeding.

The abdominal operator reopens the lower half of the previous left paramedian incision and extends it down to near the pubis. In doing this, the bowel is freed from the abdominal wall. A sterile swab is tied firmly over the upper end to prevent soiling. After gentle exploration and assessment, the small bowel is packed out of the pelvis, with the table tilted 10 to 15 degrees head-down. The peritoneum around the rectum is incised, and the superior hemorrhoidal vessels are defined, doubly ligated, and divided as they cross the pelvic brim.

Dissection then proceeds downward, first freeing the rectum posteriorly from the sacral curvature, then anteriorly from the cervix and vagina, or from the seminal vesicles and prostate. Lastly, the lateral attachments are divided. It is important, when excising the rectum for benign conditions, to keep the plane of dissection quite close to the bowel and to avoid taking too much perirectal tissue. In this way, damage to pelvic autonomic nerves can be avoided, and urinary and sexual functions left unaffected.

The perineal operator, having closed the anus with an encircling stitch, makes an oval incision around the anus, which is extended anteriorly and posteriorly an inch or so in the midline.

Dissection then proceeds through the fat of the ischiorectal fossa, the levator ani muscles are divided, and the fascia of Waldeyer posterior to the rectum is incised. A little further dissection posteriorly will lead to the same plane to which the abdominal operator has progressed. Similarly, dissection anteriorly, through the perineal body or recto-urethralis muscle, will lead to the plane between vagina and rectum or between prostate and rectum, and will also meet the field which the abdominal operator has dissected.

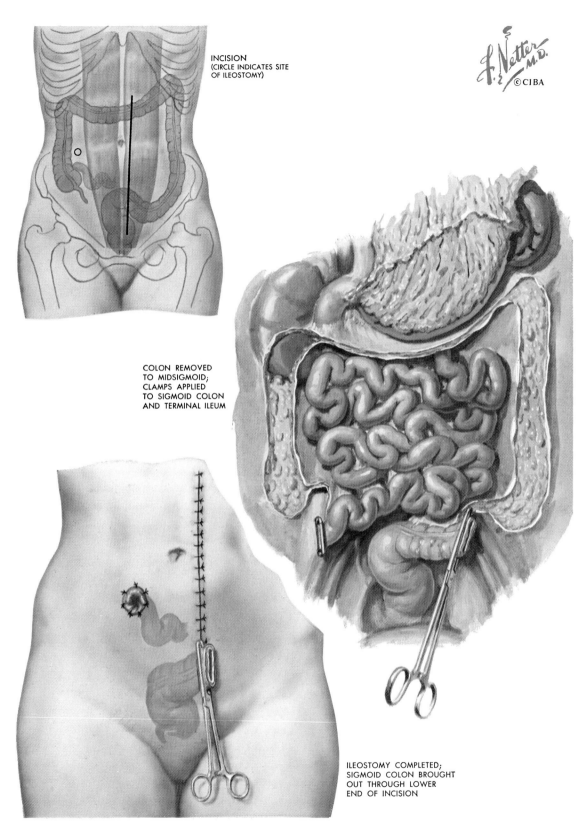

INCISION
(CIRCLE INDICATES SITE
OF ILEOSTOMY)

COLON REMOVED
TO MIDSIGMOID;
CLAMPS APPLIED
TO SIGMOID COLON
AND TERMINAL ILEUM

ILEOSTOMY COMPLETED;
SIGMOID COLON BROUGHT
OUT THROUGH LOWER
END OF INCISION

PLATE VI

ILEOSTOMY AND SUBTOTAL COLECTOMY

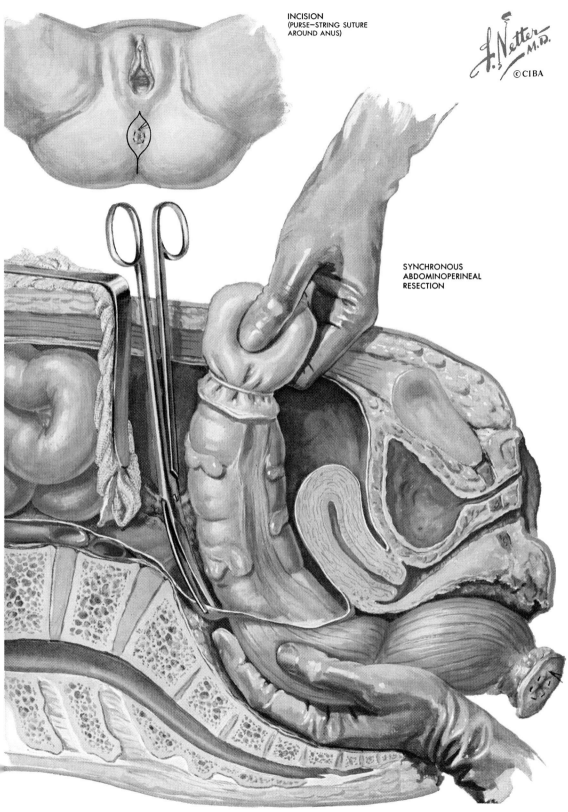

INCISION
(PURSE–STRING SUTURE
AROUND ANUS)

SYNCHRONOUS
ABDOMINOPERINEAL
RESECTION

PLATE VII

REMOVAL OF SIGMOID COLON AND RECTUM

The lower parts of the lateral attachments are then divided, again keeping close to the bowel, so that the entire specimen is completely free. Bleeding points are controlled easily by both surgeons working in cooperation.

The abdominal surgeon closes the pelvic peritoneal floor and then the abdominal wall.

The perineal surgeon closes the skin and subcutaneous tissues but leaves the central part of the wound open, with a large soft drain in the space anterior to the sacral curvature.

Ileostomy Alone

In certain toxic patients with severe, acute ulcerative colitis, considered too ill to withstand colectomy, ileostomy alone may be done as a first stage. A left paramedian incision is made, the terminal ileum is divided, and the distal end closed. The proximal end is brought out through a separate "trephine" incision and sewed to the skin, as already described. An ileostomy must always be most meticulously fashioned, otherwise complications are frequent, and in these sick patients any complication can be fatal.

Anastomosis of Ileum and Rectum

In a few patients the rectum may be preserved, and the ileum anastomosed to it after removal of the colon, the anastomosis being made about level with the sacral promontory. Selection of patients for this procedure is not easy, and the operation is sometimes unsuccessful, mostly because the retained rectum is involved in the pathologic process and absorption of toxic material continues. Such an ileosigmoid or ileorectal anastomosis may be attempted in young people and in those in whom the rectum has been proven to be not, or not badly, affected by the disease.

SECTION D

CIBA

SURVIVAL IN NUCLEAR WARFARE
Captain E. Richard King, MC, USN

SURVIVAL IN NUCLEAR WARFARE

CAPTAIN E. RICHARD KING, MC, USN[*]

The vast destructive power of a thermonuclear weapon has been widely publicized. Less well appreciated is the fact that tremendous as that released power may be, its capability for destruction by blast, heat, and direct radiation is definitely circumscribed. Except for burns of skin and eyes, even a 100 megaton detonation will produce severe damage over an area of less than 1,300 square miles, having a 20-mile radius.

Such an area, though large, is relatively insignificant compared with the 3,000,000 square miles of our total geographic area. Obviously, therefore, many such 100 megaton bombs would be required to paralyze our country *if* destruction were limited *only* to the direct effects of the explosion.

Of much greater importance, therefore, is the protection of our civil and military population in the thousands of square miles that will be subjected to lethal fallout, even from a single bomb of smaller size.

The purpose of this article is to provide our first line of civilian defense, the members of the medical profession, with data that will enable them to estimate the potential dangers at various distances from ground zero, so that they can make quick decisions as to the best means of insuring their own survival, and thus indirectly assuring the proper treatment and even survival of other members of their community.

VARIABLES

The effects of a thermonuclear weapon, both immediate and delayed, direct and indirect, will be subject to a number of variables that are impossible to assess in advance. Thus many of the rules of thumb that we shall provide can be considered as little more than rough approximations. These variables include:

The Power of the Bomb

Power is designated as an equivalent number of tons of TNT. Thus, the weapons used against Japan were called 10 and 20 kiloton (KT) bombs, equivalent to 10,000 to 20,000 tons of TNT. Available today are bombs of far greater power. Equivalent to millions of tons of TNT, they are rated in megatons (MT). The immediate effect of weapons of various KT and MT ratings are listed in Table I.

Site of Detonation

Exploded high above the ground, blast, heat, and immediate radiation will cover a wider area. If detonated on contact with the ground or under water, the total area

[*]Doctor King is currently Chairman, Division of Radiotherapy and Nuclear Medicine, Department of Radiation Therapy, Medical College of Virginia, Richmond 19, Virginia.

TABLE I

IMMEDIATE EFFECTS OF BOMBS OF VARIOUS POWER

POWER OF BOMB	RADIUS OF FIREBALL		BURNS OF SKIN (UNSHIELDED) MILES FROM GROUND ZERO			OVERPRESSURE POUNDS PER SQ. INCH (PSI) MILES FROM GROUND ZERO	
	Feet	Miles	First Degree	Second Degree	Third Degree	1.7 PSI	5.0 PSI
50 KT	900	0.16	3.5	2.6	2.1	2.5	1.4
100 KT	1,400	0.27	5.0	3.5	2.8	3.6	2.1
500 KT	2,200	0.41	10.0	7.0	6.0	5.6	3.6
1 MT	2,800	0.53	13.0	9.2	8.0	7.0	3.9
10 MT	7,000	1.33	34.0	23.0	21.0	15.4	8.6
20 MT	9,500	1.80	43.0	32.0	28.0	18.9	10.6
100 MT	20,000	3.79	90.0	60.0	54.0	32.2	18.0

EFFECTS OF OVERPRESSURE MENTIONED ABOVE ON BUILDINGS OF VARIOUS CONSTRUCTION

	TWO–STORY WOOD FRAME HOUSE	ONE–STORY WOOD FRAME RAMBLER	TWO-STORY BRICK HOUSE	REINFORCED ONE-STORY PRECAST CONCRETE HOUSE	REINFORCED ONE-STORY MASONRY BLOCK HOUSE
1.7 PSI	Badly damaged. Habitable if windows and doors covered and basement shored	Not too badly damaged except windows and doors	About same as frame house	Only minor damage except windows and doors	Minor damage except windows and doors
5.0 PSI	Totally destroyed	Damaged beyond repair. No damage to bathroom shelter	Damaged beyond repair. Basement partially filled with debris	Withstood shock well except for windows and doors. Habitable at small cost	Little damage except windows and doors

TABLE II

DAMAGE TO BUILDINGS SUFFERED AT VARIOUS DISTANCES IN MILES FROM GROUND ZERO

TOTAL DESTRUCTION

	Multistory Massive Wall Bearing Building		Multistory Reinforced Concrete, Small Window Area		Multistory Brick Apartment House Type		Wood Frame House		Light Corrugated Steel Arch 3' Earth Cover		Light Reinforced Concrete Shelter 3' Cover	
	Surface Blast	Air Blast	Surface Blast	Air Blast	Surface Blast	Air Blast	Surface Blast	Air Blast	Surface Blast	Air Blast	Surface Blast	Air Blast
50 KT	0.4	0.0	0.5	0.0	0.7	1.0	1.0	1.5	0.4	0.0	0.4	0.2
100 KT	0.5	0.0	0.7	0.0	0.9	1.3	1.3	2.0	0.5	0.0	0.6	0.3
500 KT	0.9	0.0	1.2	0.0	1.5	2.2	2.2	3.5	0.8	0.0	0.9	0.4
1 MT	1.2	0.0	1.5	0.0	2.0	2.7	2.7	4.5	1.1	0.0	1.1	0.6
10 MT	2.7	0.0	3.5	0.0	4.5	6.0	6.0	9.0	2.0	0.0	2.5	1.2
20 MT	3.2	0.0	4.3	0.0	5.5	8.0	8.0	12.0	2.7	0.0	3.1	1.5

DAMAGE NEEDING MAJOR REPAIRS

	Multistory Massive Wall Bearing Building		Multistory Reinforced Concrete, Small Window Area		Multistory Brick Apartment House Type		Wood Frame House		Light Corrugated Steel Arch 3' Earth Cover		Light Reinforced Concrete Shelter 3' Cover	
	Surface Blast	Air Blast	Surface Blast	Air Blast	Surface Blast	Air Blast	Surface Blast	Air Blast	Surface Blast	Air Blast	Surface Blast	Air Blast
50 KT	0.6 to 0.9	0.3 to 0.8	0.7 to 1.0	0.9 to 1.2	0.9 to 1.5	1.3 to 1.6	1.6 to 2.1	1.9 to 2.5	0.4 to 0.5	0.2 to 0.3	0.3 to 0.6	0.3 to 0.5
100 KT	0.7 to 1.2	0.4 to 1.0	0.9 to 1.4	1.1 to 1.7	1.2 to 1.9	1.7 to 2.0	1.9 to 2.8	2.2 to 3.2	0.5 to 0.6	0.3 to 0.4	0.5 to 0.7	0.3 to 0.7
500 KT	1.3 to 2.0	0.6 to 1.8	1.7 to 2.4	2.0 to 2.7	2.0 to 3.0	2.7 to 3.2	3.1 to 4.7	4.0 to 5.6	0.9 to 1.1	0.4 to 0.7	1.0 to 1.2	0.6 to 1.2
1 MT	1.6 to 2.5	0.8 to 2.2	2.2 to 3.0	2.5 to 3.4	2.6 to 4.0	3.5 to 4.2	4.0 to 6.0	5.0 to 7.0	1.2 to 1.4	0.6 to 0.9	1.3 to 1.6	0.7 to 1.5
10 MT	3.4 to 6.0	1.8 to 5.0	4.7 to 7.0	5.8 to 7.5	5.7 to 8.5	7.5 to 9.0	8.8 to 13.0	11.0 to 15.0	2.5 to 3.0	1.2 to 1.9	2.6 to 3.4	1.7 to 3.2
20 MT	4.5 to 7.0	2.2 to 6.0	6.0 to 8.5	7.0 to 9.5	7.0 to 11.0	9.5 to 12.0	12.0 to 14.0	13.5 to 19.5	3.2 to 3.7	1.7 to 2.5	3.6 to 4.4	2.1 to 4.1

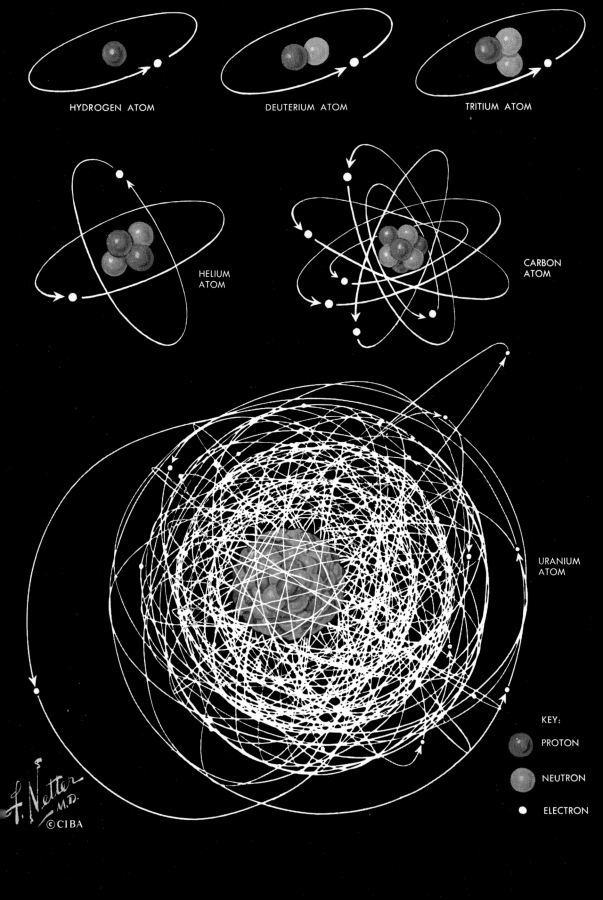

HYDROGEN ATOM

DEUTERIUM ATOM

TRITIUM ATOM

HELIUM ATOM

CARBON ATOM

URANIUM ATOM

KEY:

PROTON

NEUTRON

ELECTRON

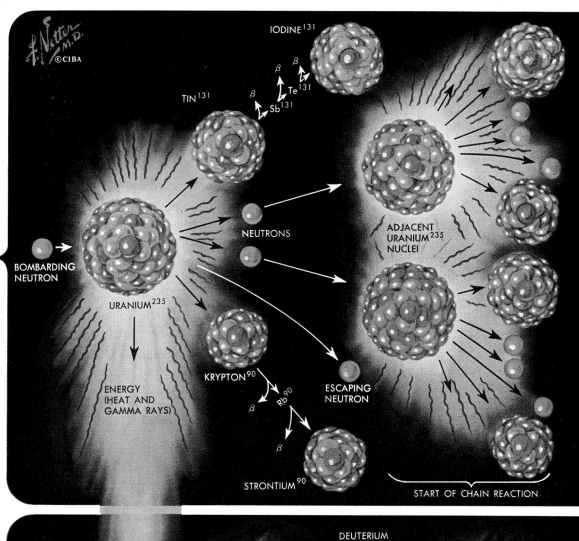

IODINE¹³¹

TIN¹³¹

Te¹³¹

Sb¹³¹

NEUTRONS

ADJACENT
URANIUM²³⁵
NUCLEI

BOMBARDING
NEUTRON

URANIUM²³⁵

ESCAPING
NEUTRON

KRYPTON⁹⁰

Rb⁹⁰

ENERGY
(HEAT AND
GAMMA RAYS)

STRONTIUM⁹⁰

START OF CHAIN REACTION

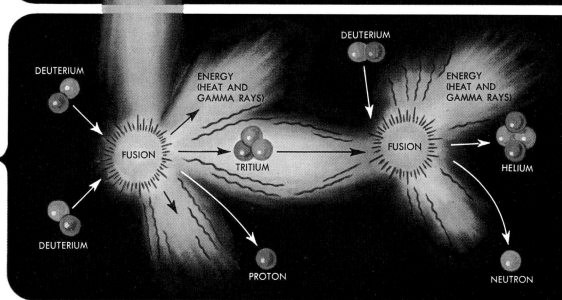

DEUTERIUM

DEUTERIUM

ENERGY
(HEAT AND
GAMMA RAYS)

ENERGY
(HEAT AND
GAMMA RAYS)

DEUTERIUM

FUSION

TRITIUM

FUSION

HELIUM

DEUTERIUM

PROTON

NEUTRON

immediately affected will be reduced. However, local induced radiation will be increased and fallout will be more intense, because radioactivated dust and debris from the ground will be borne upward in the cloud. In an underwater explosion, a dense mist of radioactive vapor will be spread about. Such an explosion, therefore, although causing less structural damage to buildings, may produce more lethal radioactivity, both immediate and delayed.

Atmospheric Conditions and Terrain

Thermal effects will be much reduced by haze, fog, or smoke in the air. All immediate effects will be reduced by intervening hills or mountains.

Direction and Velocity of Wind

If there is little or no wind, fallout will drop closer to the point of detonation, called ground zero. High winds will carry the fallout faster and farther. The more widespread the fallout, the less intense will be the effect on any one spot. Since the fallout pattern will be governed by both high and low altitude winds (the nuclear cloud may ascend as high as 20 to 25 miles), the direction and velocity of surface winds will not give a reliable indication of probable fallout pattern. Here, reliance must be placed upon information received after the explosion from Conelrad (radio 640 and 1240).

Shelter and Shielding

Thermal injury to the individual will be reduced by clothing, particularly if light in color and of several layers. Effects of direct radiation will be reduced by interposed buildings.

Building Construction

Damage by fire will depend upon the neighborhood. Slum areas with unpainted wooden buildings and combustible trash will be most affected. Industrial areas with fireproof, reinforced steel construction, and residential areas with widely separated houses, will suffer least. The effect of blast on buildings of various construction is shown in Tables I and II.

POWER OF THE BOMB
(Illustrated on pages 6 and 7)

The power of a thermonuclear weapon is due to the almost instantaneous transformation of atomic mass into energy. Utilizing Einstein's formula $E = mc^2$, or Energy equals mass times the square of the velocity of light, the fission of a single atom of uranium 235 will yield roughly 200 million electron volts (Mev). This permits the construction of a weapon having thousands of times the destructive force of TNT.

The terrific heat generated by such an explosion makes possible the fusion of isotopes of hydrogen (deuterium and tritium) with a yield of about 3.2 to 17.6 Mev per atomic fusion. Compared with uranium, hydrogen is extremely light so that on a weight for weight basis, the fusion of deuterium nuclei will produce nearly three times as much energy as the fission of uranium or plutonium. The coupling of fission and fusion in the same weapon will produce an explosion having far greater energy than either one alone.

In order to visualize the nuclear physics involved in fission and fusion, it must be recalled that each little atom is in fact a minuscule solar system, having a nucleus (like our sun) with electrons orbiting as do our planets. The nucleus is composed of protons and neutrons. The protons, each of which has one positive charge, are responsible for the "atomic number" of the element. The protons and neutrons together are responsible for almost the entire "atomic weight" or mass of the atom. Each of the orbiting electrons has a negative charge, balancing the positive charges of the protons.

8

The nucleus of the simplest element, hydrogen, contains no neutrons and only one positively charged proton (atomic weight and atomic number one), with one balancing negatively charged electron. The nucleus of helium contains two neutrons plus two protons^{++}, together giving an atomic weight of four, the two protons giving an atomic number of two. The nucleus of carbon contains six protons (atomic number six) plus six neutrons, giving an atomic weight of twelve.

The heavy nucleus of uranium is made up of 92 protons (the atomic number of the element) plus 146 neutrons, making an atomic weight of 238. Normally, the number of protons in the nucleus is more or less balanced by neutrons. However, where an imbalance exists, as it does in the uranium atom, the nucleus attempts to become more stable and in the process gives off energy in the form of alpha particles (identical with the helium nucleus), thus losing 4 units of atomic weight and 2 positive charges to become thorium 234, with release of beta particles (electrons), or gamma rays (similar to x-rays), or both.

The fission reaction responsible for the explosion and release of high amounts of energy is brought about by introducing an additional neutron into the already unstable nucleus of uranium 235. When this is accomplished, the nucleus splits into two unequal parts, and in the process two or three neutrons are thrown off (with two gamma rays) to bombard neighboring nuclei and set up a chain reaction, with the release of the tremendous amounts of energy referred to previously. For this chain reaction to be self-sustaining, certain technical steps must be taken to insure that neutrons are not lost by escape from the mass or captured by nonfissionable material faster than they are formed.

There are forty or more ways in which the atom of uranium may split, so that two hundred or more isotopes of thirty-five lighter elements are formed, each of which has an atomic weight close to 95 or close to 139. For example, uranium 235 may split into such isotopes as Sn (tin) 131 and Kr (krypton) 90, illustrated on page 7. Both of these isotopes rapidly decay with loss of beta particles to form isotopes of other elements having progressively longer half-lives. For example, Kr 90, with a half-life of 33 seconds, loses a beta particle to become rubidium 90, with a half-life of 2.7 minutes. This in turn loses a beta particle to become strontium 90, having a half-life of 28 years. Similarly, by successive loss of beta particles, tin 131 becomes antimony 131, tellurium 131, and then iodine 131.

The fusion reaction depends upon isotopes of hydrogen. As previously mentioned, the usual hydrogen nucleus contains only a single proton (H^1). However, an isotope may be formed which also contains a neutron (deuterium H^2 or D^2), as well as one containing two neutrons (tritium H^3 or T^3).

The following is an example of the reaction which may be brought about by fusing these isotopes: $H^2 + H^2 = H^3 + H^1 + 4$ Mev (million electron volts). The fusion of deuterium (H^2) with tritium (H^3) will yield 17 Mev.

The fission and fusion reactions complement each other. For fusion to take place, it is necessary to have an extremely high temperature that can only be attained by a fission explosion. Also, certain fusion reactions release neutrons, contributing to the fission of uranium or plutonium, thus adding to total energy release of the combined fission-fusion system present in a thermonuclear weapon.

IMMEDIATE EFFECTS

As stated previously, the power of a thermonuclear weapon is designated as an equivalent in tons of TNT. The energy

FIGURE 1

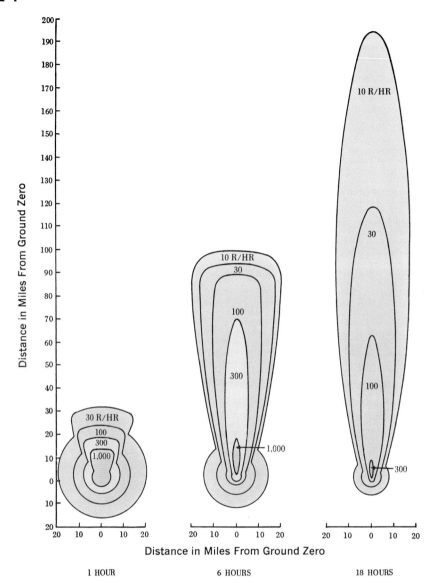

Distance in Miles From Ground Zero

1 HOUR   6 HOURS   18 HOURS

RATE PER HOUR AT 1, 6, AND 18 HOURS

	Cross and Upwind			Downwind		
Dose Rate	1000 r/hr.	300 r/hr.	100 r/hr.	1000 r/hr.	300 r/hr.	100 r/hr.
Effect in 1 hour	Lethal	Symptomatic Borderline	Asympto-matic	Lethal	Symptomatic Borderline	Asympto-matic
1 Hour	5 miles	8 miles	12 miles	15 miles	20 miles	25 miles
6 Hours	2 miles	2 miles	5 miles	20 miles	70 miles	90 miles
18 Hours	—	1 mile	2 miles	—	10 miles	60 miles

FIGURE 2

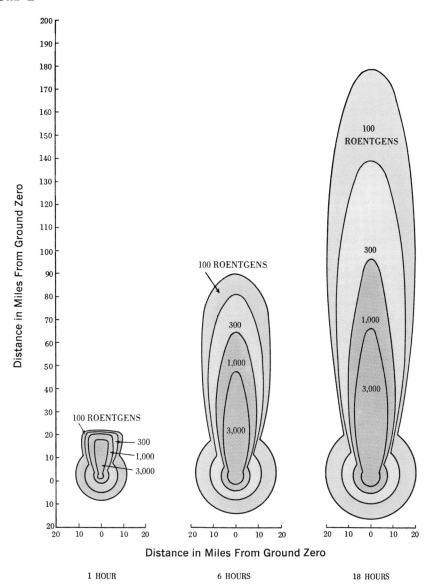

Distance in Miles From Ground Zero

1 HOUR   6 HOURS   18 HOURS

MEGATON RANGE
M.P.H.

ACCUMULATED DOSAGE WITHIN 18 HOURS

	Cross and Upwind			Downwind		
Dose	1000 r	300 r	100 r	1000 r	300 r	100 r
Cumulative Effect	Lethal	Symptomatic Borderline	Asymptomatic	Lethal	Symptomatic Borderline	Asymptomatic
1 Hour	2 miles	8 miles	12 miles	20 miles	22 miles	22 miles
6 Hours	8 miles	10 miles	18 miles	65 miles	80 miles	90 miles
18 Hours	8 miles	12 miles	20 miles	100 miles	140 miles	180 miles

of the explosion in a typical air burst will be distributed as follows: blast and shock 50 per cent; thermal radiation 35 per cent; initial nuclear radiation 5 per cent (residual nuclear radiation 10 per cent). The immediate effect of each of these, as it depends on the power of the bomb, is summarized in Table I.

Blast

From a typical air burst, three types of blast waves will converge upon surrounding structures. First is the direct or *incident wave*, which comes directly or diagonally downward from the fireball. This is closely followed by an upward *reflected wave* from the ground. Close-in buildings may be affected only by the incident wave. However, since the reflected wave travels through air that has been condensed by the incident wave, its rate of progression will be faster, so that farther away both waves may arrive together, producing a single horizontal "mach" reflection. Thus the upper part of a tall building at some distance from the blast may receive the downward incident wave, closely followed by the upward reflected wave, while the lower part may receive only a single horizontal "mach" reflection.

This positive overpressure will be closely followed by a negative (suction) phase. (Of course, a surface or underwater blast would produce only a single wave of horizontal pressure.)

In addition to the pressure waves just described, there will probably be a severe *ground shock*, similar to an earthquake, more severe in a surface blast. Immediately following will be an extremely high wind, known as a "drag," which will be of hurricane proportions.

The effect of all of these forces released by the blast will decrease rapidly with distance from ground zero.

In Table I will be found the distances from ground zero at which a pressure of 5 pounds per square inch (abbreviated p.s.i.) will be felt, as well as the distances receiving 1.7 pounds per square inch, each from bombs of various power. The structural damage (also tabulated) produced by both of these pressures has been determined by direct test in Nevada. The effect of blast on buildings of other construction is indicated in Table II.

As estimated from the effects on anthropometric dummies exposed to blast in Nevada, a man, if erect within the area having an overpressure of 5 p.s.i., may be hurled through the air for a distance of as much as 21 feet. If prone, he will not be displaced. Therefore, when the flash is seen, one should drop to the ground *immediately*. By so doing, it may be possible to avoid serious injury from flying objects, including oneself.

One of the greatest hazards in this day of picture windows is that of flying glass which, depending on the particle size and degree of overpressure, may attain a velocity enabling it to penetrate eyeball or peritoneal cavity.

Heat

Energy released in the form of heat would be equivalent to about 400,000 kilowatt hours per kiloton of the bomb. Temperature within the fireball of a 1 megaton weapon would range up to millions of degrees Fahrenheit, comparable with that in the center of the sun. Therefore, everything within the radius of the fireball (Table I) would be vaporized.

Again the effect of thermal radiation decreases with distance from ground zero. Table I outlines the degrees of burn of unshielded skin on a relatively clear day at various distances. These distances will be considerably decreased by haze, fog, or smoke in the air.

Depending upon the neighborhood and inflammability of structures, the area of thermal damage will probably far exceed that of blast destruction. The heat is received in a flash of very short duration.

12

Therefore, a painted frame structure may withstand temperatures of over 10 cal./sq. cm., sustaining nothing more than surface charring. On the other hand, inflammable material, such as curtains or trash, may be ignited by as little as 3 cal./sq. cm.

Once ignited, fires will be spread rapidly by the high winds. While the initial air blast or "drag" will spread fire outward from ground zero, the later and more persistent winds responsible for spread of fires will converge on the site of detonation because of the upward "draft" produced by ascent of the mushroom cloud.

Some idea of the velocity of winds to be expected from modern weapons can be gained from the fire storm produced by the relatively small bomb used at Hiroshima. There, about twenty minutes after detonation, wind commenced to blow toward the burning area, reaching a velocity of 30 to 40 m.p.h. about two or three hours after the explosion, decreasing to light and variable in about six hours. These winds could cause the spread of mass fires (fire storms) as far as 20 miles from the explosion of a 20 MT bomb.

During a fire storm, which may last for six hours, the street temperature may reach 1400° F., or almost three times the maximum heat in a kitchen oven. In addition, there will be an acute shortage of oxygen and a lethal concentration of carbon monoxide. Therefore, shelters in areas subject to fire storm, because of proximity to a likely target and the character of building construction, should contain a tank of oxygen if possible.

Nuclear Radiation

Received directly from the detonation, this will consist of a very intense, acute flash dose of gamma rays, all received within perhaps twenty seconds. In addition, these will be high energy gamma rays, requiring approximately double the shielding required for protection against fallout.

Fortunately, both the neutrons and gamma rays produced by the fireball travel only short distances. Thus, while nuclear radiation of the delayed type present in fallout is most important from a survival standpoint, the immediate flash radiation is merely academic since an individual close enough and sufficiently exposed to be seriously affected would have already succumbed to thermal effects.

DELAYED EFFECTS

Serious as the immediate effects of a thermonuclear explosion may be, the delayed effects in the form of induced radiation at the site of detonation and the far-reaching fallout will result in a much higher number of casualties and loss of human life. Indeed, it is possible that over 90 per cent of casualties will be caused by fallout alone.

Frequently overlooked is the fact that at least a one-hour warning should be available if attack should come by manned bomber, and although an ICBM may arrive with little or no warning, precise accuracy between continents with such a weapon is difficult to achieve. It may easily be as much as 40 miles off target. With only this degree of accuracy an entire city might survive the immediate blast effects but *not* the lethal fallout.

Thus, even in a large city which may be a primary target, many hundreds of thousands may survive *if* shelters are available to protect from delayed radiation and the effect of possible secondary fires. On the other hand, it has been estimated that an attack *limited to military objectives alone* would kill 45 million Americans if we are not prepared to deal with fallout.

As in all exposure to radiation, the three factors determining total dosage are distance, shielding, and time. Unless we have adequate warning, the distance we are from the thermonuclear blast will be

FIGURE 3

PREVAILING WINDS DURING THE SUMMER

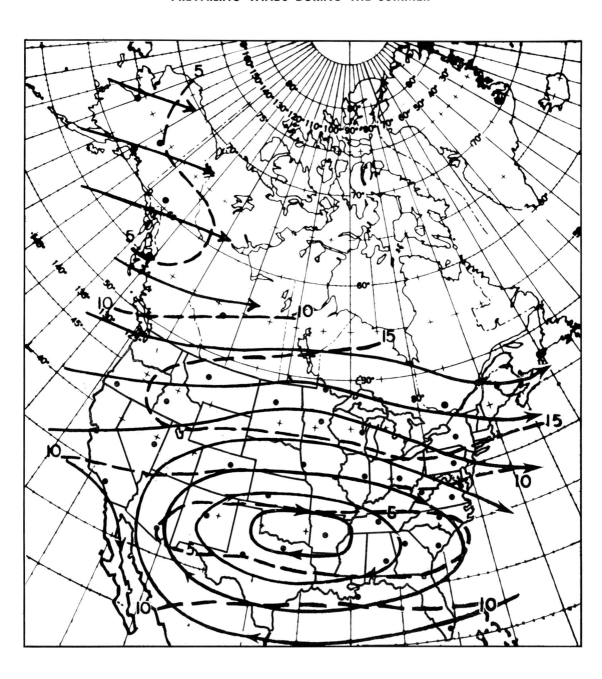

Prevailing winds at other seasons are usually west to east throughout the United States. However, during the summer months the prevailing winds in southern states are in other directions (U.S. Weather Bureau).

FIGURE 4

ISODOSE CONTOURS FOR A 20 MT SURFACE BURST PREDICTED
FOR THE WIND PATTERN OF MAY 12, 1956

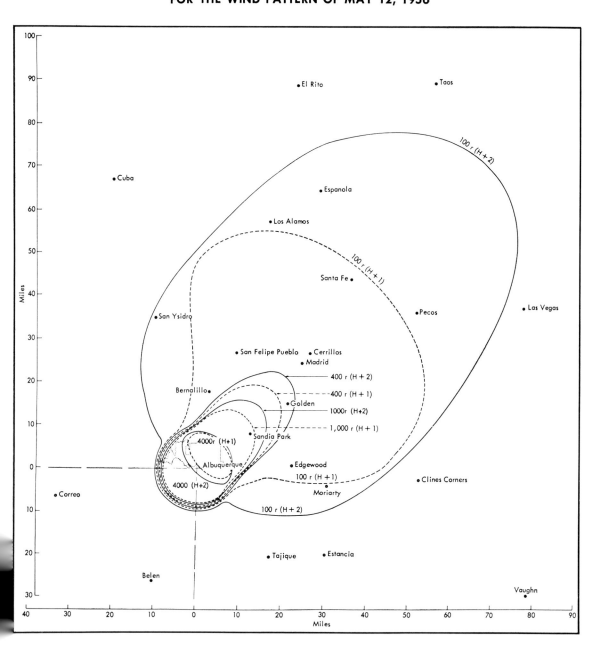

Accumulated doses received during the first and second hours (H+1 and H+2) following a 20 MT surface burst over Albuquerque, New Mexico, predicated on the wind pattern existing on May 12, 1956. Note that the schematic cigar-shaped patterns shown in Figures 1 and 2 may not develop under actual conditions.

beyond our control. We can, however, control the shielding we afford ourselves in the form of a shelter, and once in the shelter we can compute rather accurately the exposure we may have already suffered as well as that which we will receive during any outside mission undertaken at a later time (see pages 26 through 28).

How Much Fallout May Be Expected

The intensity and range of the fallout will depend upon many of the variables already mentioned. Since a surface blast in which the fireball touches the ground will produce the most massive fallout, we shall confine ourselves to discussing fallout from this type of blast. Here, large amounts of earth, dust, and debris, which become radioactive by neutron induction, are taken up into the fireball, where they are vaporized and become intimately mixed with fission products to form a tremendous number of particles, ranging from large lumps to fine dust, each of which is radioactive.

The larger pieces will not go up into the mushroom cloud, but will descend from the column, roughly in a circle around ground zero. (Usually the center of this column will be displaced somewhat from ground zero in the direction of the wind.) Thus, near the site of explosion, fallout will be most intense and, lacking adequate shelter, a lethal dose of radiation will be received within the first hour, even by many of those beyond the immediate effects of the explosion.

Figures 1 and 2 on pages 10 and 11 show the approximate extent of fallout at hours 1, 6, and 18, as well as the accumulated dosage that would have been received at those times, depending on wind direction. These calculations are based on a 15 m.p.h. wind.

Obviously, we cannot foretell the exact location of the target or how close to target the bomb might fall. Neither can we be assured of a 15 m.p.h. wind nor that it will be in the prevailing westerly direction.

Prevailing winds in the northern hemisphere are generally from a west to east direction, except for the summer in Gulf States (see Figure 3). However, the use of mean (prevailing) wind charts to predict the direction of fallout on any one day can be very misleading, as emphasized by the studies conducted by the Sandia Corporation, Albuquerque, New Mexico. On August 1, 1955, the effective wind would have carried the fallout produced by a 20 MT bomb directly west. On the same date in 1956, the fallout would have been carried northwest. On May 12, 1954, the fallout would have gone southeast. On the same date in 1956, the fallout would have been carried northeast.

Also the fallout may not be distributed in narrow bands as suggested by the schematic drawings in Figures 1 and 2. This is evident from calculation of the fallout from the hypothetical bomb of May 12, 1956, just referred to (see Figure 4).

The Sandia Corporation also computed the "maximized infinity isodose contours" around Albuquerque, showing the total accumulated exposure that would have been present following a 20 MT explosion on *any* one day over a period of five years. Isocontour lines thus plotted would of course represent highly unlikely possible exposures since they occurred under conditions present on only one day out of 1,825. Nevertheless, this study does emphasize the extent to which fallout *can* be disseminated from a single blast.

In this study, the isocontour of 100 r total exposure extended as far east as Detroit and Wheeling, West Virginia; 300 r extended east to the Oklahoma-Arkansas line and west to the Pacific Ocean beyond lower California. The 1,000 r contour extended east to Amarillo, a distance of 270 miles, and west 260 miles toward Phoenix.

The Time of Arrival of Fallout may be a matter of minutes for points close to ground zero, or hours for more distant

TABLE III

ESTIMATION OF DISTANCE FROM GROUND ZERO AND ARRIVAL OF
FALLOUT FROM INTERVAL BETWEEN FLASH AND SOUND

FLASH-SOUND INTERVAL (SECONDS)	DISTANCE (MILES)	PROBABLE TIME TO FALLOUT° (MINUTES)
Under 50	Under 10	10
60	12	12
90	18	18
120	24	24
200	40	40
300	60	60
500	100	100
750	150	150

°Individual in direct path of fallout, assuming winds in stratosphere to be 60 miles per hour — see also Figures 1, 2, and 4.

(Reproduced from "SURVIVAL IN A THERMONUCLEAR WAR — WHEN TIME IS SHORT," by Solomon Garb, M. D., *New York J. Med.* 60:4061-4064, 1960.)

points. Thus in Figure 2 it can be seen that an unshielded individual located directly downwind 18 miles from ground zero could have accumulated a lethal dose (1,000 r or more) within the first hour. One hundred miles away, 18 hours will elapse before a similar individual will have accumulated such a dose. Of course, these figures which were based on a 15 m.p.h. wind would be subject to great variation.

You can estimate your distance from ground zero and obtain a rough approximation of the earliest arrival of fallout by noting the direction of the flash in relation to wind direction and counting the seconds between flash and sound. Dividing the number of seconds in this flash-sound interval by 5 will give you the distance from ground zero in miles (see Table III).

When the fallout arrives, the exposure dose rate will be small, but it increases steadily as more and more fallout descends. In a few hours the fallout will be virtually (although not absolutely) complete. Then will begin a steady decrease in dose rate due to radioactive decay of fission products. This decay will be tenfold for every sevenfold elapse of time. Thus a rate of 1,000 r/hr. at the height of fallout will be reduced to 100 r/hr. in seven hours and to 10 r/hr. at seven times seven hours, or about two days.

PROTECTION PROVIDED BY SHELTER

Blast

An ideal shelter should provide protection against blast, heat, and fallout. Although no structure will withstand destruction within the radius of the fireball, reinforced concrete buildings are remarkably resistant to blast as indicated in Table II. Also, it can be seen from this table that properly designed underground

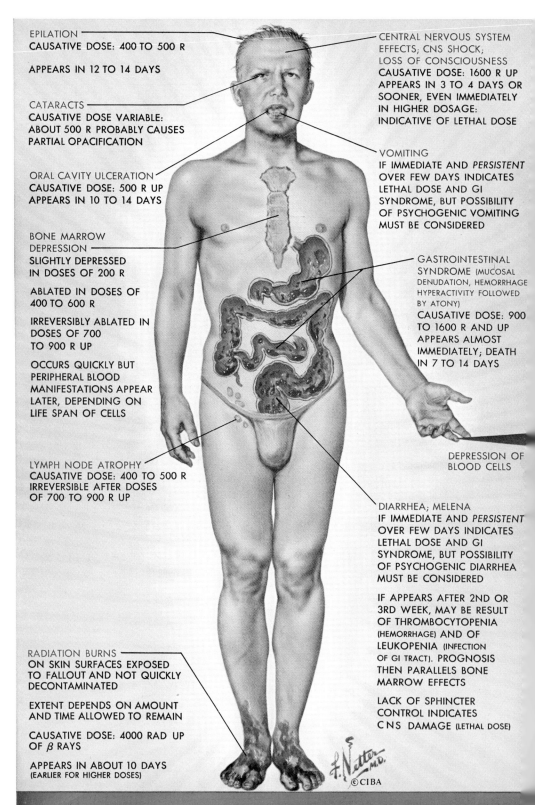

EPILATION
CAUSATIVE DOSE: 400 TO 500 R

APPEARS IN 12 TO 14 DAYS

CATARACTS
CAUSATIVE DOSE VARIABLE:
ABOUT 500 R PROBABLY CAUSES
PARTIAL OPACIFICATION

ORAL CAVITY ULCERATION
CAUSATIVE DOSE: 500 R UP
APPEARS IN 10 TO 14 DAYS

BONE MARROW
DEPRESSION
SLIGHTLY DEPRESSED
IN DOSES OF 200 R

ABLATED IN DOSES OF
400 TO 600 R

IRREVERSIBLY ABLATED IN
DOSES OF 700
TO 900 R UP

OCCURS QUICKLY BUT
PERIPHERAL BLOOD
MANIFESTATIONS APPEAR
LATER, DEPENDING ON
LIFE SPAN OF CELLS

LYMPH NODE ATROPHY
CAUSATIVE DOSE: 400 TO 500 R
IRREVERSIBLE AFTER DOSES
OF 700 TO 900 R UP

RADIATION BURNS
ON SKIN SURFACES EXPOSED
TO FALLOUT AND NOT QUICKLY
DECONTAMINATED

EXTENT DEPENDS ON AMOUNT
AND TIME ALLOWED TO REMAIN

CAUSATIVE DOSE: 4000 RAD UP
OF β RAYS

APPEARS IN ABOUT 10 DAYS
(EARLIER FOR HIGHER DOSES)

CENTRAL NERVOUS SYSTEM
EFFECTS; CNS SHOCK;
LOSS OF CONSCIOUSNESS
CAUSATIVE DOSE: 1600 R UP
APPEARS IN 3 TO 4 DAYS OR
SOONER, EVEN IMMEDIATELY
IN HIGHER DOSAGE:
INDICATIVE OF LETHAL DOSE

VOMITING
IF IMMEDIATE AND *PERSISTENT*
OVER FEW DAYS INDICATES
LETHAL DOSE AND GI
SYNDROME, BUT POSSIBILITY
OF PSYCHOGENIC VOMITING
MUST BE CONSIDERED

GASTROINTESTINAL
SYNDROME (MUCOSAL
DENUDATION, HEMORRHAGE
HYPERACTIVITY FOLLOWED
BY ATONY)
CAUSATIVE DOSE: 900
TO 1600 R AND UP
APPEARS ALMOST
IMMEDIATELY; DEATH
IN 7 TO 14 DAYS

DEPRESSION OF
BLOOD CELLS

DIARRHEA; MELENA
IF IMMEDIATE AND *PERSISTENT*
OVER FEW DAYS INDICATES
LETHAL DOSE AND GI
SYNDROME, BUT POSSIBILITY
OF PSYCHOGENIC DIARRHEA
MUST BE CONSIDERED

IF APPEARS AFTER 2ND OR
3RD WEEK, MAY BE RESULT
OF THROMBOCYTOPENIA
(HEMORRHAGE) AND OF
LEUKOPENIA (INFECTION
OF GI TRACT). PROGNOSIS
THEN PARALLELS BONE
MARROW EFFECTS

LACK OF SPHINCTER
CONTROL INDICATES
CNS DAMAGE (LETHAL DOSE)

F. Netter M.D.
©CIBA

EFFECTS OF ATOMIC RADIA

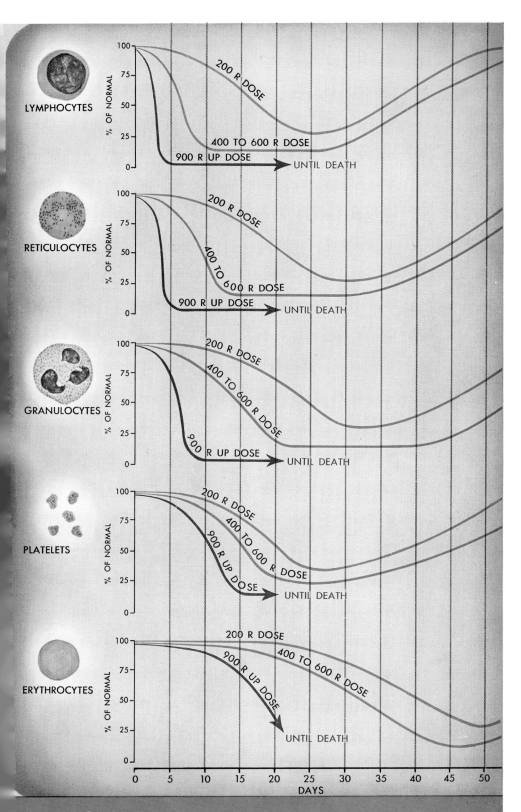

LYMPHOCYTES

100
75
50
25
0
% OF NORMAL

200 R DOSE

400 TO 600 R DOSE

900 R UP DOSE → UNTIL DEATH

RETICULOCYTES

100
75
50
25
0
% OF NORMAL

200 R DOSE

400 TO 600 R DOSE

900 R UP DOSE → UNTIL DEATH

GRANULOCYTES

100
75
50
25
0
% OF NORMAL

200 R DOSE

400 TO 600 R DOSE

900 R UP DOSE → UNTIL DEATH

PLATELETS

100
75
50
25
0
% OF NORMAL

200 R DOSE

400 TO 600 R DOSE

900 R UP DOSE → UNTIL DEATH

ERYTHROCYTES

100
75
50
25
0
% OF NORMAL

200 R DOSE

400 TO 600 R DOSE

900 R UP DOSE

UNTIL DEATH

0   5   10   15   20   25   30   35   40   45   50
DAYS

shelters offer even greater protection. These are available in such dimensions that they could easily be installed in many backyards of city dwellings as well as in suburban and rural areas. Shelters of this type must be equipped with air intake and exhaust pipes, suitably filtered with an air pump to assure a sufficient supply of oxygen. In addition, in areas subject to fire storms, a tank of oxygen would be required.

The protection against blast provided by a basement shelter will depend upon the construction of the building beneath which it lies. Within the area receiving 5 pounds per square inch of overpressure (Table I), a basement shelter can scarcely be depended upon to sustain the weight of a collapsed building. Therefore, basement shelters had best be relied upon mainly for protection against fallout.

Radiation

As in all forms of radiation, protection depends on distance, shielding, and time.

Distance: While we cannot control the distance we will be from the nuclear blast, we can as quickly as possible place ourselves at the greatest distance from fallout. For example, an inside corridor of an office building or apartment house would be safer than an exterior room; the basement would be still better. If only one side of a basement is underground, one had best lie against the wall nearest the earth and farthest from the exposed wall.

Shielding: It will be impossible to obtain *complete* shielding from all gamma rays. However, every inch of intervening material, even a pile of magazines, will absorb some of the rays.

In order to visualize the amount of shielding afforded by different structures and materials, "protection factors" are computed. If the protection factor is 2, one-half the rays will penetrate. If the protection factor is 10, only one gamma ray in 10 will penetrate.

The following are some approximate protection factors which will serve as a rough guide in computing the shielding efficiency of your own home or shelter. Structures:

Frame House		
First Floor		2
Basement		10
Multistory reinforced concrete building		
Lower floors away from windows		10
Basement (if surrounded by earth)		1,000+
Shelter below ground 3 ft. of earth		1,000+
Shelter below ground 5 ft. of earth		100,000+
Material: Concrete	8 inches	5
	12 inches	25
	16 inches	100
	22 inches	1,000
	28 inches	10,000
Earth	22 inches	100
	33 inches	1,000
	40 inches	10,000
Lead	1.9 inches	100
	2.5 inches	1,000

A basement shelter composed of solid concrete blocks 8 inches thick and covered with same thickness of concrete blocks would have a protection factor of approximately 100 (10 for its location, 5 for its inherent shielding plus an additional factor attributable to its distance from other basement walls, etc.).*

These protection factors are calculated against fallout. About double the thicknesses given are required against the more intense radiation of high energy gamma rays emitted directly from the fireball.

------

*Information on this and many other types of family shelters can be obtained from your local civil defense headquarters or from the Division of Protective Structures, Office of Civil Defense, Department of Defense, Washington 25, D. C., Attention: Family Shelters Branch.

Time: There is a direct relationship between total dose and time. If radiation is at the rate of 100 r/hr., 50 r will be received in one-half hour, and 200 r in two hours. If the radiation is at the rate of 4,000 r/hr., a fifteen-minute exposure would be fatal. Seven hours later, decay would have reduced the rate to 400 r/hr., and in a fifteen-minute exposure only 100 r would be acquired.

Rate of Decay

Fallout will "cool off" or decay rapidly. With passage of time a tenfold decrease in intensity may be expected with each sevenfold increase in time from the explosion. Thus:

One hour after explosion	1,000 r/hr.
Seven hours after explosion	100 r/hr.
About 2 days (7 hrs. × 7, or 49 hours)	10 r/hr.
About 2 weeks (49 hrs. × 7, or 343 hours)	1 r/hr.

Let us consider these figures in relation to expected fallout and permissible dosage in humans (see Biologic Effects, page 25).

It is conceivable that an area close to ground zero might receive a maximum fallout as high as 10,000 r/hr. Considering rate of decay, it could be assumed that a shelter having a protection factor of 1,000, providing it did not suffer destruction by the blast, could protect its occupants indefinitely from symptoms of radiation.

A shelter of the type advised for basements, having a protection factor of 100, if it withstood the blast, should protect against all symptoms if the maximum fallout were as much as 3,000 r/hr. (a fallout rate that would only be expected near ground zero or for a relatively short distance directly downwind therefrom). Such a shelter should permit survival at even higher dosages, if adequate treatment is given.

On the other hand, an ordinary base-

ment unshielded by top cover of concrete and adequate shielding over windows, and having a protection factor of 10, would probably protect against symptoms only in areas receiving 300 r/hr. or less of initial fallout. The first floor of a frame house would give but an insignificant 1:2 protection.

Since no one can foretell where a bomb may fall, it is clear from the above considerations that special shelter is an absolute necessity. Except for areas close to ground zero (and the immediate effects of blast, fire, and radiation), a basement shelter having a protection factor of 100 should be adequate. However, where ground is available (particularly near likely target areas), an underground shelter, able to withstand 10 p.s.i. of overpressure and thus able to escape much blast destruction, and having an efficiency of 1:1,000 or 1:10,000, would be far safer.

ESSENTIAL CONTENTS OF A SHELTER

Although it may not be necessary from the standpoint of radiation to remain continuously in the shelter for even as long as a week or two, it is highly probable that in thermonuclear war, production and distribution channels of food will be disrupted for a very long time. In addition, food stored above ground (including the 2 billion bushels of surplus grain) may be destroyed or seriously contaminated. Livestock may be killed. Fields may be unworkable. Therefore, where possible, it would be desirable to stock a food supply that will offer subsistence over a period of many months.

Food

Since space will be at a premium, food items should be selected which provide: (1) greatest number of calories per cubic foot, and (2) long shelf life. Examples of foods meeting these requirements are given in Table IV. Table V contains a

Table IV — FOODS WITH HIGH CALORIC VALUE AND LONG SHELF LIFE

Kind	Water (Per Cent)	Protein (Per Cent)	Important Vitamins and Minerals	Calories as Purchased (Per Cubic Foot)	Average Retail Price Per 1,000 Calories (Dollars)	Approximate Storage Life*
Sugars						
Granulated	0	0	0	90,000	0.07	1 year
Cubes or tablets	0	0	0	99,000	0.10	1 year
Honey (round 2½ pound can)	20	1	0	73,000	0.24	1 to 5 years
Oils & Fats						
Corn or cottonseed (round bottle)	0	0	0	132,000	0.09	1 to 5 years
Corn or cottonseed (rectangular gallon can)	0	0	0	196,000	0.08	1 to 5 years
Grains						
Wheat flour (unbaked)	12	11	Niacin Thiamine Riboflavin	54,000	0.06	6 months
Wheat (whole grain)	12	10	Niacin Thiamine Riboflavin	50,000	0.03	2 to 5 years
Rice (precooked)	7	9	Niacin Thiamine	38,000	0.28	6 months
Corn meal (cylindrical container)	12	9	Niacin	46,000	0.07	6 months
Corn meal (rectangular container)	12	9	Niacin	58,000	0.07	6 months
Corn (Whole kernel dried)	12	9	Niacin	48,000	0.02	2 to 5 years
Baked Goods						
New England brown bread (canned)	44	5	0	26,000	0.25	1 to 5 years
Cracker meal (rectangular container)	5	9	0	60,000	0.19	6 months to 1 year
Royal Lunch milk crackers (1 pound box)	5	7	0	27,000	0.20	6 months
Fig Newtons	13	3	0	41,000	0.30	6 months
Lorna Doone shortbread	3	7	0	42,000	0.33	6 months
Milk						
Evaporated (can)	74	7	Calcium	28,000	0.23	1 to 5 years
Sweetened condensed (can)	27	8	Calcium	86,000	0.18	1 to 5 years
Nonfat dry milk (not instant)	3	36	Calcium	41,000	0.19	6 months to 1 year
Dried Fruits						
Prunes, wax wrapped	24	2	0	44,000	0.29	1 year
Raisins	24	2	0	58,000	0.22	1 year
Dates, pitted	20	2	0	45,000	0.30	1 year
Figs	24	4	0	75,000	0.50	1 year
Meats (Canned)						
Corned beef	59	25	0	51,000	0.55	1 to 5 years
Roast beef	59	25	0	51,000	0.57	1 to 5 years
Ham (small can)	50	22	0	56,000	0.88	1 to 5 years
Corned beef hash (Armour)	65	9	0	40,000	0.41	1 to 5 years
Potted meat food product (Armour)	65	12	0	37,000	0.56	1 to 5 years
Beans						
Baked beans (can)	76	6	0	22,000	0.22	1 to 5 years
Pork and beans	70	6	0	25,000	0.22	1 to 5 years
Fish						
Sardines in oil	47	21	Niacin	58,000	0.38	1 to 5 years
Tuna in oil	52	24	Niacin	61,000	0.49	1 to 5 years
Salmon	65	20	Niacin	26,000	1.32	1 to 5 years
Spreads						
Peanut butter	2	26	Niacin	83,000	0.18	1 to 5 years
Jams, marmalades	28	0	0	68,000	0.31	1 to 5 years
Other						
Peanut Brittle (in compact bars)	2	8	Niacin	60,000	0.33	1 year

*Storage life based on careful packing in plastic to protect from moisture.

Tables IV and V have been reproduced from Survival in Thermonuclear War VIII, Basic Dietary Supplies and Equipment for Shelters, Garb, S.: New York J. Med. 60:3668, 1960, amplified by personal communication from Dr. Garb.

Table V

SUGGESTED SIX-MONTH FOOD SUPPLY FOR ONE PERSON IN SHELTER

Food	Net Weight (Pounds)	Cubic Feet (Approximate)	Calories	Estimated Retail Cost (Dollars)
Sugar	20	0.34	35,000	2.45
Corn oil	15 (2 gallons)	0.30	59,000	4.72
Flour	40	1.00	66,000	3.96
Corn meal	20	0.50	33,000	2.31
Cracker meal	10	0.32	19,000	3.61
Cookies (see Table IV)	20	0.50	19,000	4.92
Sweetened condensed milk	20	0.34	29,000	5.22
Dried fruits (see Table IV)	10	0.20	11,000	3.63
Meats (see Table IV)	20	0.41	18,000	12.00
Beans	50	1.27	28,000	6.16
Sardines and tuna fish	10	0.22	13,000	5.87
Peanut butter	8	0.25	21,000	3.74
Jams and marmalade	8	0.14	10,000	2.98
Peanut brittle	5	0.16	10,000	3.30
Canned vegetables, assorted	15	0.61	2,000	3.00
Canned citrus fruit juice	20	0.81	4,000	5.10
Totals	291	7.37	377,000	72.97

list of foods which will provide subsistence for an individual for a period of six months. In addition, one must remember that the body cannot subsist on calories alone. One gram of protein per kilogram of body weight is needed. Also required are essential amino acids that the body cannot manufacture itself. These are best found in meat, fish, and dairy products.

Canned goods will have a shelf life varying from one to five years. Packaged goods like granulated sugar and flour will keep reasonably well if wrapped in polyethylene to keep out excessive moisture. Packaged goods or even canned goods that are stored today should have the date written on the package so that after a suitable length of time, they can be utilized and replaced.

In addition to the food supply kept in the shelter, a secondary supply can be kept in a closet or trunk elsewhere, so that it will be available after leaving the shelter. For this purpose unopened cartons should be wrapped in a double layer of polyethylene and all openings sealed with tape to prevent entry of radioactive particles. Forty pounds of sugar, 4 gallons of corn oil, and 100 pounds of wheat flour thus stored will supply a person with sustenance for an additional six months at a cost of less than $25.

Water

The usual recommendation of 7 gallons per person for two weeks is sufficient to meet average intake requirements. However, much more will be needed to maintain fluid balance and insure cleanliness in case of radiation sickness. Moreover, the physician who must leave his shelter and enter a contaminated area should take steps to decontaminate himself on his return. This, too, will take water.

The minimum amount of water stored within the shelter should be 60 quarts (2 cubic feet) per person. Spacewise it is best that this be stored in 5- or 10-gallon containers.

Water is made unfit only by radioactive contaminants; *not* by radiation itself. Therefore, an additional supply of water for three months can be stored in a tank outside the shelter. This may be the usual basement water heater or an old hot water tank obtained from a junk yard and placed underground for protection against flying debris.

If the soil is sandy and the water table is within 20 feet of the floor of the shelter, an unlimited supply of water may be made available at reasonable cost by drilling a well and attaching an old-fashioned hand pump. However, water thus obtained would have to be monitored because the source might eventually become contaminated.

Vitamin Supplements

These are particularly necessary in the presence of radiation sickness and in the event food stored is inadequate in vitamin content.

Vitamin C: 1,000 tablets of 100 mg. each should be sufficient for three people for one year if taken at the rate of one a day. In addition, a like supply of multiple vitamin capsules containing A, B, and D should be obtained and stored.

Protein Supplements

Depending on the nature of other food stored, food supplements high in protein and concentrated to conserve space may be a desirable addition to the pantry, particularly if radiation sickness occurs.

Waste Disposal

A urinal may be made by sinking a 4-inch pipe 6 feet into the ground and filling it with gravel. A chemical toilet may be obtained but will require a 3-inch vent going outdoors and incorporating a Fiberglas filter. Plastic bags may be used for feces until disposal by burying is possible.

Medical Supplies

Since manufacture and channels of distribution of these items may also be disrupted, it obviously would be wise to lay in a supply of those items which will be most likely to be urgently needed. In-

cluded here will be sedatives, hypnotics, opiates, analgesics, antiseptics, antibiotics, antispasmodics, hypotensives, etc.

Patients suffering chronic diseases, such as diabetes, should be advised to lay in their own supplies of essential medicaments.

ESTIMATION OF RADIOACTIVITY

In case of failure of Conelrad or of your own radio, it may become necessary to do your own monitoring after 48 hours. In doing this, the graphs on pages 26 through 28 will help you determine initial radiation and other important facts.

A portable Geiger counter is useful to monitor the interior of the shelter, the food and the water supply. However, it is far too sensitive to be used to estimate outside fallout and cannot be used for monitoring in a high intensity background.

Least expensive, yet most convenient and highly useful, is the miniature ion chamber known as a dosimeter. This instrument is the size of a fountain pen. It can be used to monitor either inside or outside your shelter (monitoring both will give the efficiency coefficient of the shelter, which is a useful thing to know). For outside monitoring, it can be tied to a pole and pushed out a basement window or through the air exhaust pipe of an underground shelter, keeping it 3 feet above the ground. A reading taken for one minute or ten minutes will allow you to calculate the r/hr. dose.

Whereas a Geiger counter will cost in the neighborhood of $100, dosimeters are much less expensive. A special kit is available, containing two dosimeters and a recharger, which sells for something under $25.* One dosimeter acts as a rate meter

---

*EDITOR'S NOTE: A kit of this kind, manufactured by Bendix Corporation, is available through Nuclear Engineering, Inc., Naval Industrial Reserve Shipyards, Building 89, Kearny, New Jersey, or 65 Ray Street, Pleasanton, California.

to determine the radiation being received. Exposed for a period of either one minute or ten minutes, depending on intensity of radiation, the reading obtained is given in r/hr.

The other dosimeter is used to keep a continuing record of the total amount of radiation that has been received up to 600 r. The recharger, operating on a small flashlight battery, is provided to bring the reading of either dosimeter back to zero.

No one can foretell the date of a possible thermonuclear attack. Moreover, precise information as to the rate of exposure and accumulated dose is of utmost importance from the standpoint of additional risk to be assumed, or even individual survival. Therefore, the physician would be well advised to carry both types of dosimeter, fully charged, with him at all times.

ESTIMATION OF SAFE INTERVAL FOR LEAVING SHELTER

This is both a scientific and a philosophic problem. We will provide an estimate of the amount of radiation the body can withstand. The radiation in your area should be obtainable from Conelrad (or your own dosimeter — preferably after the first 48 hours). On succeeding pages we will give tables showing approximately how long you may stay out in order to receive the amount of radiation to which you feel justified in exposing yourself on a given day. So much for the science.

From a philosophic standpoint, the doctor must weigh his present and future value to his community against the urgency of the mission. In general, the fewer the doctors available and the younger the man (having an expectancy of more productive years), the more his potential value. Pending the development of organizations which will define specific tasks and assign them at specified times under a variety of circumstances, these will be questions that each must answer for himself.

In general, remember that an adequately equipped shelter is a sine qua non. Also remember that there is a direct relationship between total dose and time. If the exposure rate is 5 r/hr., a total dose of 10 r will be accumulated in 2 hours, so keep as exact a record as possible of all exposures. In using the graphs on pages 26, 27, and 28, remember that any present fallout may not be the last to which you are subjected. Also, some contamination may remain in the area for a very long time — so save up a margin of safety. In addition, it must be pointed out that these graphs may be misleading where overlapping fallout is received from several bombs dropped at different times.

If at all possible, remain in the shelter continuously for the first 48 hours. (In heavy fallout areas, unsheltered individuals will probably already have received a lethal dose.) Those who have received sublethal doses will probably not develop symptoms until *after* 48 hours.

BIOLOGIC EFFECTS OF FALLOUT
(Illustrated on pages 18 and 19)

Much has been written on the effect of radiation on various body tissues, on the carcinogenic effect, and the genetic changes that may be produced. Here we will focus our attention exclusively on the factors that affect survival.

The lethal dose of radiation is usually designated as LD_{50-30}. That is the dose that will kill 50 per cent of people within thirty days. For obvious reasons this has never been determined experimentally in humans. Extrapolating from animal experiments and results of the explosions in Japan, the figure of 450 r has been widely publicized. However, animals subject to radiation usually have been given no treatment. Therefore, my own estimate of the acute lethal dose (received within a

FIGURE 5

DETERMINATION OF DOSE RATES

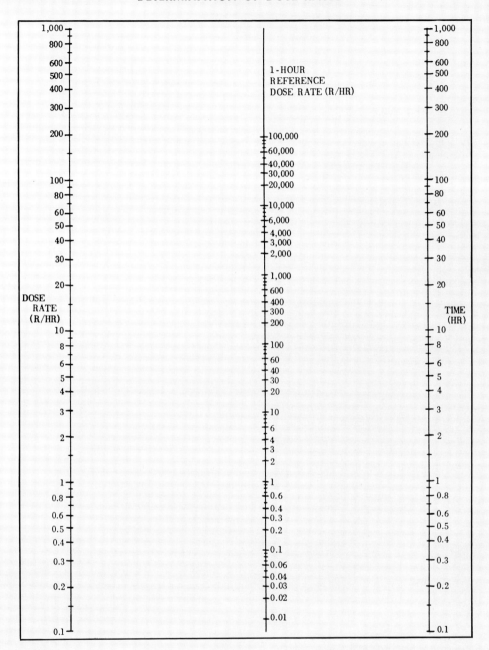

The left-hand line gives dose rates in r/hr. for any period after the explosion. The middle line gives the initial dose rate (either or both of these may have been received over Conelrad). The right-hand line gives the time in hours after the explosion. Knowing any two of these will enable determination of the other by placing a ruler or straight edge through two points and thus determining the third.

For example, if the local dose rate is 8 r/hr. 6 hours after the explosion, the *initial* dose rate may be obtained by placing the ruler on 8 r/hr. on the left-hand line and on 6 hours on the right-hand line. This will bisect the center line at 70 r/hr. which gives the initial rate of radiation.

Now to find out what the dosage will be at the end of 24 hours, simply lay the ruler on the initial rate of 70 r/hr. which was just determined (center line) and 24 hours (right line), and the answer is 1.4 r/hr.

To figure out how soon the radiation will be down to 1 r/hr., lay the ruler on 1 (left), 70 (middle), and the answer is 35 hours (right).

FIGURE 6

DETERMINATION OF DOSE RECEIVED DURING OUTSIDE MISSION

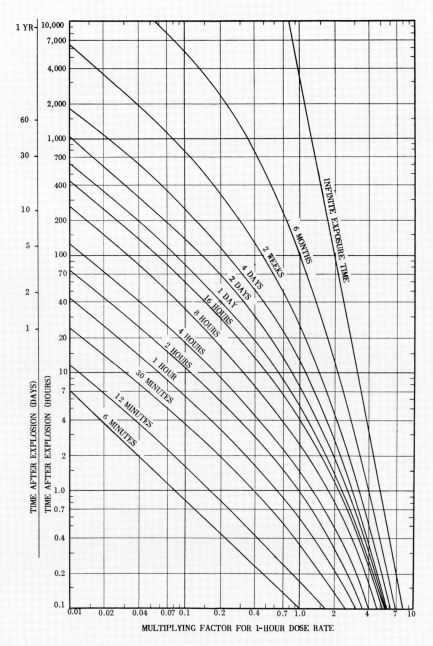

MULTIPLYING FACTOR FOR 1-HOUR DOSE RATE

Example: Given a dose rate of 6 r/hr. 4 hours after explosion. Calculate how much radiation will be received in 2 hours starting 6 hours after explosion.

First, calculate *initial* radiation rate from Fig. 5 (center line) as before. This time the answer is 32 r/hr. Place the ruler horizontally on the vertical scale at 6 hours. Referring to the horizontal scale at the bottom, it will be found that the ruler has bisected the 2-hour curve at 0.19. Multiplying this by the initial r/hr. just found to be 32, the answer will be 6.1 r, the amount of exposure suffered during the mission described.

When can a mission be started requiring 5 hours which will give a total exposure of 4 r under the above circumstances? Divide 4 (the total dose) by the initial radiation already found to be 32. The answer is 0.125. Locate this figure on the lower horizontal scale. Place the ruler vertically and it will be found to bisect the 5-hour (interpolated) curve at 19 hours on the vertical scale. This is the time after explosion that a 5-hour mission will give a total exposure of 4 r.

FIGURE 7

DOSE RECEIVED FROM RATE WHEN ENTERING CONTAMINATED AREA

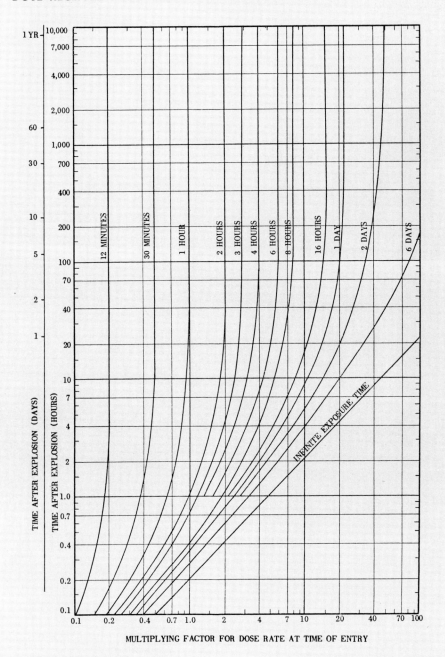

MULTIPLYING FACTOR FOR DOSE RATE AT TIME OF ENTRY

Suppose a contaminated area is entered 12 hours after explosion and the rate at that time is 5 r/hr. and it is desired to know how much radiation will be received in 2 hours: Lay the ruler horizontally on the vertical scale at 12 hours. This will bisect the 2-hour curve at a point corresponding with 1.9 on the lower horizontal scale. Multiplying this factor by 5 (the rate per hour), the answer will be 9.5 r, the total dose that will be received.

Now, under the same circumstances, to determine the length of stay outside that will result in a dosage of 10 r, divide 10 by 5 (the rate per hour). This gives you a factor of 2. Moving vertically upward from 2 on the lower horizontal scale, the ruler will intersect a horizontal line extending from 12 hours on the vertical scale at a point indicating a stay of about 2⅓ hours.

short time, as in a single day) in humans given adequate medical care would be in the neighborhood of 600 to 700 r.

If doses are divided, probably much more radiation can be sustained with survival. We base this opinion on our experience in total body irradiation of patients with incurable cancer. We have given such very ill patients 100 r doses two or three times a week, for two or three weeks, or a total dose of 600 r to 800 r, with no symptoms of radiation sickness. From this we would hazard the guess that one might probably receive divided doses of 100 r daily for two weeks, or a total of 1,400 r, and still survive.

Patients who have acquired an acute exposure of less than 300 r will probably need no special medical attention. Thus it can be seen that patients on whom treatment time can profitably be spent from the standpoint of saving life would be those estimated to have received between 300 r and 700 r as an acute dose. Some indication of the degree of exposure may be obtained from the known radiation present in the neighborhood and the history given by the patient. However, additional evidence can be obtained from the character of symptoms and their time of onset. These we will take up by systems affected.

Central Nervous System

An acute dose of 1,600 r or more will cause brain damage with edema. Loss of consciousness within three or four days may be expected, followed by certain death. The higher the dose the more rapid the onset of unconsciousness. Loss of sphincteric control may be an indication of central nervous system involvement and may indicate that a lethal dose has been received.

Gastrointestinal Tract

Radiation sickness with nausea, vomiting, and diarrhea will follow a dose of 400 to 450 r and higher. The bigger the dose the more quickly the nausea and vomiting will start. Indeed, where vomiting comes on immediately and persists for several days without interruption, the dose received was probably lethal. However, it is well to bear in mind that vomiting may be induced by psychogenic factors such as horrors experienced and the sight of others vomiting. This should be particularly suspected in suggestible neurotics.

Denudation of the Gastrointestinal Tract with hemorrhage will follow doses of 900 to 1,600 r and is lethal within one to two weeks. Early, the tract is hyperactive; later, atony sets in.

Bone Marrow

The clinical effect of radiation of the bone marrow lies in the reduction of various cellular elements of the blood, which is illustrated on page 19.

Depression of the bone marrow will follow doses as low as 200 r. However, with doses of 200-300 r, improvement may occur spontaneously without symptoms unless complications, such as pre-existing illness, pregnancy, trauma, and/or thermal burns, are also present. Doses of 400 to 600 r will result in *total ablation* of the bone marrow. However, subsequent restoration may occur spontaneously by proliferation of primordial cells, providing the patient can be carried over the acute depletion of cellular constituents of the blood. *Irreversible ablation* follows doses of 700 to 900 r.

The effect of radiation on the bone marrow appears quickly, but the results depend upon the life span of the individual blood cell which is the basis of symptoms, diagnosis, and prognosis.

Reticulocytes are one of the first affected. Indeed, the rate of fall of the reticulocyte count provides an excellent means of determining prognosis. However, from a practical standpoint this procedure is too time-consuming to be used in any major disaster.

Lymphocyte and granulocyte depletion, both in time of onset and in degree, also depend upon dosage received. Therefore, a simple white count may help in determining prognosis if the time element is taken into consideration. A white count that drops to 500 by the seventh day and fails to improve by the twenty-first day will invariably be followed by death. Symptomatically, depression of granulocytes makes its presence known by *ulcerations in the oral cavity*, appearing in ten to fourteen days with doses of 500 r and up. Those with depleted granulocytes (which may go as low as 500 with recovery) are subject to infection of all kinds, even through the puncture to obtain blood from a finger. Diarrhea with melena that comes on in the second or third week is usually due to leukopenia with thrombocytopenia.

Platelets are usually not depressed until the second or third week. This causes purpuric manifestations and the tendency to hemorrhage beginning about the end of the second week.

Red Blood Cells have a life span of approximately 120 days. Therefore, unless there is bleeding, anemia does not become a problem until the third or fourth week.

Lymph Nodes

These structures become atrophic and depleted of cells with doses of 400 to 500 r, a condition which is irreversible if 700 to 900 r have been received.

Epilation

Following an acute dose of 400 to 500 r, hair will usually be lost in bunches in about twelve to fourteen days.

Skin Burns Due to Radiation

If not washed off promptly, beta particles falling on the skin will cause skin burns to appear as early as the third or fourth day. Because of their lack of penetration, beta particles do not affect deeper structures. Alpha particles will cause damage only if inhaled or ingested.

TREATMENT

The treatment that may be effectively carried out will depend upon the availability of both private and public shelters for the civilian population and the thoroughness with which they are stocked with water for drinking and decontamination, medical supplies, and other materials essential for survival.

It is quite likely that most people within a 10-mile radius from detonation of a bomb of megaton power will be killed by blast and heat, unless they are fortunate enough to be in a blast-resistant structure or shelter, where they should stay for at least forty-eight hours. This area will probably be so "hot" from induced radiation and fallout that any efforts to reach survivors within this period would be fatal.

Farther out in the 10- to 20-mile radius and beyond, it may be possible to remove patients with traumatic injuries and thermal burns to shelter areas for treatment, provided sufficient time is available before expected arrival of fallout. Treatment of traumatic injuries and surface burns will follow usual methods of practice. However, one must keep in mind that these patients may later go through a period of bone marrow depression which may lower their natural resistance to the vanishing point. Therefore, excessive care should be taken to maintain sterile technique and to carry out thorough debridement of damaged tissue. In the case of burns, absolute surface cleanliness must be maintained. Antibiotics, which one might be tempted to use prophylactically under other conditions, should be reserved for those cases in whom their later use may be life-saving.

Burns may also be produced by beta

particles received in fallout. Therefore, patients who have been exposed should be thoroughly decontaminated by a shower with soap or detergent as quickly as possible, even before entering their own shelter or before being treated. This should be carried out even if the shower is in an unsheltered area since only a few minutes will be required. Burns of this type will require the same treatment as those caused by heat. However, healing time will probably be prolonged. Dosage to create skin burns is expressed in rads. A unit of absorbed dose, one rad is equivalent to 100 ergs/Gm.

Unfortunately, there is presently no specific treatment, nor are there any prophylactic measures that can be taken against *radiation sickness*, although this matter is under constant and intense investigation. However, meticulous nursing care with maintenance of scrupulous cleanliness, an adequate fluid intake, with a high-calorie, high-protein diet, rich in vitamins, may easily make the difference between life and death.

As previously stated, those who have received doses of 200-300 r will probably recover without special care or attention, provided they have been in relatively good health and no complications, such as trauma or thermal injury, are suffered. The most time must therefore be spent on those who have received between 300 and 700 r.

Since the central nervous system and gastrointestinal denudation syndromes are rather quickly lethal (within two weeks), the major problems are those associated with bone marrow depression or ablation (see page 19).

Bone Marrow Depression

Those individuals whose bone marrow is depressed, but not so severely that it cannot recover, must be afforded every opportunity to live long enough for this recovery to take place. Here the critical period will range from about ten days after exposure (*i.e.*, ten to fourteen days post-detonation, depending upon the time of arrival of fallout) to about thirty days after exposure.

If it were possible to store bone marrow from all of our citizens and then, after the two-week shelter stay, transfuse each exposed survivor with his own bone marrow (autogenous bone marrow), there is little doubt a tremendous number of lives could be saved. This, of course, would be a gigantic preparatory measure.

In addition, we do not have a method of preserving bone marrow over a long period of time. Therefore, we must assume there is no form of adequate therapy for individuals suffering from permanent bone marrow ablation due to gamma radiation from fallout (or any other type of ionizing radiation). Therefore, the treatment must be largely symptomatic.

In general, the suggestions which follow are those which any physician would automatically follow when caring for a weakened, debilitated individual.

Leukopenia

The first of the formal blood elements to fall, and perhaps disappear, are the leukocytes. This will result in a lowered resistance with susceptibility to infection. Thus the patient should be afforded the best nursing care possible, and be kept as clean as possible, with particular attention to the mouth, nares, anus, and vulva, all of which harbor saprophytes which are normally controlled by natural resistance. Meticulous care should be taken of all minor cuts and abrasions of skin and mucous membranes.

Antibiotics should not be used prophylactically but should be administered as generously as possible when signs of infection occur, because in these cases of radiation-induced leukopenia, the slightest infection is likely to become a full-blown septicemia in a very short time.

Choice of antibiotic will probably depend upon availability as well as clinical judgment. It is unlikely that bacteriologic sensitivity tests can be carried out.

These events will probably not occur for ten to fourteen days post-detonation, so there will probably be no reason for the doctor to leave his shelter earlier to care for this group of patients.

Thrombocytopenia

The next blood element to become depressed is the thrombocyte, or platelet. Thrombocytopenia may result in a hemorrhagic diathesis. Thus bleeding may occur from orifices as well as subcutaneously. Nose-pickers and people with poor dentition will likely bleed profusely from these areas. Again, nursing care and cleanliness are of paramount importance, or infection will be superimposed upon the bleeding sites and compound the treatment difficulties.

The best treatment for this type of bleeding is transfusion of *fresh* blood or platelet-rich plasma if available. There is no stored platelet product available at this time. Since banked whole blood does not contain platelets, it had better be reserved for traumatic cases and those suffering later persistent anemia.

Anemia

If the patient lives through the infection and bleeding phases, the later development of anemia will call for replacement of whole blood. In this instance, stored blood is adequate, for the replacement needed is of hemoglobin, not platelets.

Electrolyte and Water Balance

This is an extremely important supportive measure, and one with which most physicians are already conversant. The most practical way to maintain fluid and food intake is orally, of course. Patients with septicemia and/or hemorrhagic diathesis must be maintained on parenteral fluids containing required electrolytes as well as vitamins and nutrients. Again, the stockpiles of I.V. fluids and parenteral feedings must be hoarded and used only when absolutely necessary.

Gastrointestinal Symptoms

It has been previously mentioned that patients suffering from intractable *nausea and vomiting* from the early exposure and persisting through several days probably have suffered a lethal dose and present the gastrointestinal syndrome. These patients will probably die of this syndrome within two weeks. Medical care will not change the course.

Other patients may suffer from transient nausea and vomiting, some of which may be radiation-induced. Most such transient symptoms will be on a psychogenic basis and require only mild sedation and antiemetic drugs. However, in others, fluid replacement may become necessary.

Extreme, persistent, and early *bloody diarrhea* also signifies the gastrointestinal syndrome, and the prognosis is hopeless. Late (three to four weeks) bloody diarrhea may be caused by the thrombocytopenia. This latter type may be treated symptomatically, as any similar condition due to other etiologic agents, by fluids, sedation, cleanliness, and antidiarrheal drugs.

Nursing Care

This is the most important single phase of the treatment of radiation sickness. Various points of nursing care have already been mentioned and need not be repeated. In patients suffering from temporary bone marrow depression, emphasis must be placed on scrupulous cleanliness of body and clothing as well as linen. Skin, oral, and nasal hygiene must be maintained at high standards. Anal hygiene is extremely important. Saline mouth washes and gargles are adequate.

Careful cleansing of the skin prior to needle insertions or finger punctures must be emphasized. Rest and proper sedation are also important.

Speaking of sedation, it is quite probable that most adults who remain in a shelter for two weeks should be tranquilized if at all possible. The modern mother apparently cannot stand to have all the young children around her for a very long time, even under normal circumstances. Therefore, adequate sedation and tranquilization may change two weeks' restriction in a shelter from an impossible situation into one that is at least tolerable.

Home therapy and nursing management should be planned for in advance. Thus, antiseptics, antibiotics, sedatives, analgesics, antidiarrheal and antiemetic drugs, table salt, bicarbonate of soda, nose drops, cough syrup, etc., should be available in every shelter.

The mother will likely be the doctor as well as the nurse in most private shelters for about two weeks and should have instructions, as well as first aid equipment and drugs, to help her during this period.

EDITOR'S NOTE: Figures 1, 2, 5, 6, and 7, and much of the editorial content of this article have been derived from "The Effects of Nuclear Weapons" prepared by the United States Department of Defense, published by the United States Atomic Energy Commission, Samuel Glasstone, Editor. Copies may be obtained from the Superintendent of Documents, United States Government Printing Office, Washington 25, D. C. Price $2.00.

Figure 4 has been reproduced from CEX 58.8, "Comparative Nuclear Effects of Biomedical Interest," published by Lovelace Foundation of Medical Education and Research and the United States Atomic Energy Commission, Division of Biology and Medicine. Available from the Office of Technical Services, Department of Commerce, Washington 25, D. C. Price $1.00.

REMEMBER THESE WARNINGS

1. **A 3- TO 5-MINUTE STEADY TONE**
   TURN ON YOUR RADIO FOR DIRECTIONS.

2. **A 3-MINUTE WARBLING TONE OR SHORT BLASTS**
   TAKE COVER IMMEDIATELY.

3. **SUDDEN FLASH, FAR BRIGHTER THAN MID-DAY SUN**
   DON'T LOOK AT IT. DIVE UNDER FURNITURE, INTO DOORWAY, ONTO FLOOR OF YOUR CAR, UNDER A PARKED AUTO, OR EVEN INTO A GUTTER. STAY THERE FOR 5 MINUTES, OR UNTIL BLAST HAS PASSED. THEN FIND SHELTER FROM FALLOUT.

SECTION E

C I B A

DISEASES OF THE EYE
Dan M. Gordon, M.D.

DISEASES OF THE EYE

DAN M. GORDON, M.D.

Assistant Clinical Professor of Surgery (Ophthalmology)
Assistant Attending Staff
Cornell University Medical College — New York Hospital, New York.

At any moment of the day or night, the physician, regardless of his specialty, may be confronted with an ocular problem where accurate diagnosis and prompt treatment may save the vision or even save the eye.

Therefore, it may be of interest to review briefly the salient features of some of the common injuries and diseases which may affect this vital organ.

EXAMINATION

It is obviously impossible to examine the eye without ample illumination. In addition, particularly in corneal diseases, magnification is essential. Ideally, this is obtained by using a combination of lenses and prisms known as a loupe, which can be worn as a headband. In emergency, a common magnifying glass or even an extra pair of reading glasses will suffice.

Control of the eye for examination can be obtained by holding the upper lid firmly against the adjacent orbital margin and the lower lid forcibly against the lower bony margin, as illustrated in Plate III. This prevents blinking and stabilizes the globe.

Eversion of the upper lid must be carried out in order to examine the conjunctival lining of the upper lid. This is easily accomplished by pulling the lateral lash margin of the upper lid slowly and gently away from the eye and slightly downward and outward while the patient is looking down. Then with the other hand, the side of a cotton applicator (in emergencies a toothpick, thumb, or similar object may be employed) is gently pressed over the center of the lid, and at the same time the lid margin is turned rapidly outward and upward over the applicator, as illustrated in Plate III.

Any injury which may threaten vision is a potential malpractice suit or case of "compensationitis." Therefore, it is always wise to test the visual acuity and obtain a *written* history before prescribing treatment. It is amazing how often a simple foreign body in one eye will focus attention on an unnoticed or neglected presbyopia, and the patient will blame his need for glasses on the accident or the treat-

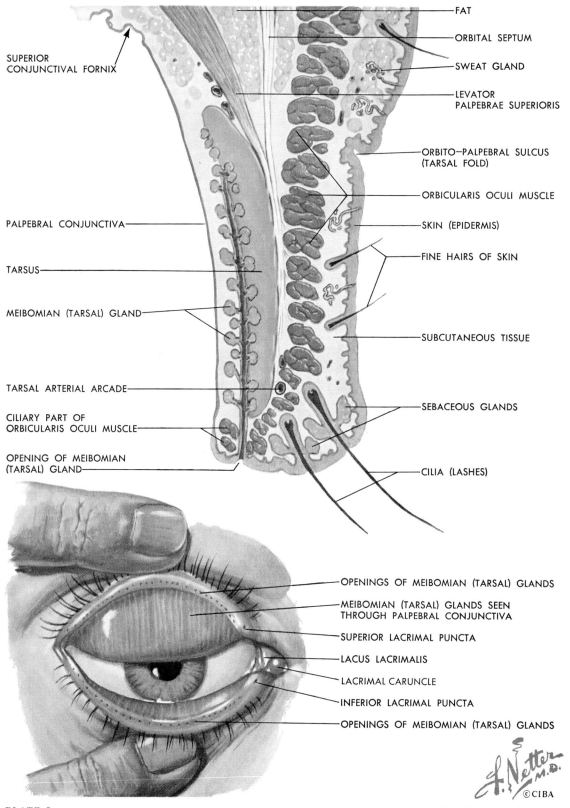

FAT

ORBITAL SEPTUM

SWEAT GLAND

LEVATOR
PALPEBRAE SUPERIORIS

ORBITO–PALPEBRAL SULCUS
(TARSAL FOLD)

ORBICULARIS OCULI MUSCLE

SKIN (EPIDERMIS)

FINE HAIRS OF SKIN

SUBCUTANEOUS TISSUE

SEBACEOUS GLANDS

CILIA (LASHES)

SUPERIOR
CONJUNCTIVAL FORNIX

PALPEBRAL CONJUNCTIVA

TARSUS

MEIBOMIAN (TARSAL) GLAND

TARSAL ARTERIAL ARCADE

CILIARY PART OF
ORBICULARIS OCULI MUSCLE

OPENING OF MEIBOMIAN
(TARSAL) GLAND

OPENINGS OF MEIBOMIAN (TARSAL) GLANDS

MEIBOMIAN (TARSAL) GLANDS SEEN
THROUGH PALPEBRAL CONJUNCTIVA

SUPERIOR LACRIMAL PUNCTA

LACUS LACRIMALIS

LACRIMAL CARUNCLE

INFERIOR LACRIMAL PUNCTA

OPENINGS OF MEIBOMIAN (TARSAL) GLANDS

F. Netter M.D.
©CIBA

PLATE I

ANATOMY OF THE LID

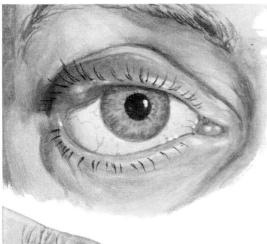

ACUTE
MEIBOMIANITIS

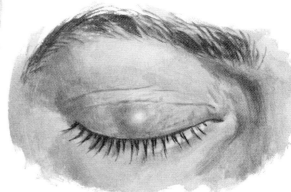

CHALAZION

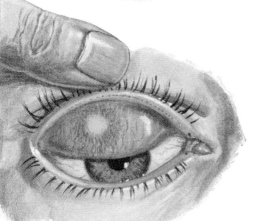

CHALAZION; LID EVERTED

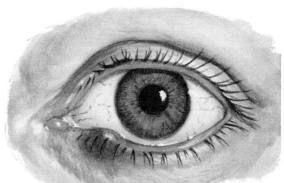

HORDEOLUM (STY) OF LOWER LID

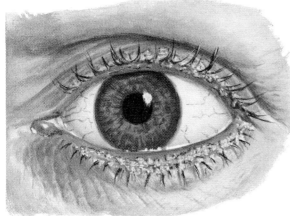

BLEPHARITIS

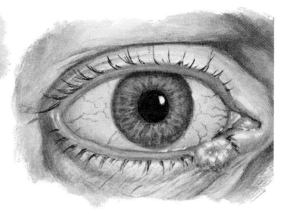

CARCINOMA OF LOWER LID

PLATE II

DISORDERS OF THE LID

ment. Therefore, whenever possible, vision should be determined and recorded before the eye is treated. Prognosis should not be discussed before the outcome is certain.

BLUNT INJURIES

When the eye is struck forcibly by a blunt object such as a ball or fist, a black eye (ecchymosis) may result. Absorption of the blood can usually be speeded by intramuscular injections of 1 ml. of trypsin daily, or by buccal streptokinase and streptodornase. If the floor of the orbit is fractured, diplopia usually results.

If intra-ocular injury has been produced, the most common findings are: (1) decrease in vision, (2) hemorrhage in the anterior chamber (hyphema), (3) tremor of the iris due to dislocated lens, (4) a black fundus reflex due to vitreous hemorrhage, and (5) retinal detachment.

Frequently, a traumatic hyphema is followed by absorption and then reoccurrence of the hemorrhage, plus secondary glaucoma. These require hospitalization with binocular bandaging plus specialized care.

THE EYELIDS

Plate I shows the anatomical details of the lid, most important of which from a practical standpoint is the location of the meibomian glands and the glands of Zeis or Moll.

Meibomianitis
(Also Called Meibomitis)

The meibomian glands are arranged in vertical columns forming yellowish streaks on the inside of the lid, forty in the upper lid, thirty in the lower lid. The ducts of these glands open on the lid margins, as depicted in Plate I.

These glands may be the seat of acute infection or *acute meibomianitis* (Plate II). The *treatment* consists of hot compresses and the frequent application of antimicrobial or steroid-antimicrobial combination drops — every one-half hour or every hour.

Chalazion

With or without antecedent acute meibomianitis, a cyst may form in a meibomian gland. This is known as a chalazion and is seen merely as a lump in an otherwise normal lid. The *treatment* of this condition is surgical excision or incision and drainage, preferably from the inner surface of the lid.

Hordeolum

This condition, commonly called a sty, is caused by an infection of one of the glands of Zeis, located around the follicles on the external lash margin, as shown in Plate I. Inflammation gives the appearance of a pimple or small boil pointing on the lash margin (Plate II). Here also the *treatment* is frequent hot compresses and the instillation of drops containing an antimicrobial. If this fails to abort the process, the sty must be incised with a sharp knife and the contents extruded. If the sty points at the base of a lash, removal of the involved lash may permit ample drainage. When stys tend to be recurrent, injections of staphylococcus toxoid are indicated.

Blepharitis

This condition is due to an infection of the lash margin which may be merely scaly like dandruff, or may be actually ulcerated. In the latter form, the affected lids often tend to become wholly or partially denuded of lashes. *Treatment* consists of the manual removal of the scales each night and morning by means of a moistened cotton applicator, followed by finger-tip application to all four lid margins of an antimicrobial or combination antimicrobial-steroid ointment. In the ulcerative form, staphylococcus desensitization may be required, and it may be necessary to cauterize the ulcers with 1 per cent silver nitrate. This latter procedure must be carried out with exceeding care because any of this solution getting into the eye will cause exquisite pain.

Allergy of the Lids

Because of their loose connective tissue, the lids tend to swell quite easily as a result of either systemic or local allergy. A systemic allergy usually affects both eyes. However, in some cases only a single lid may be involved. Local causes of lid allergy include such things as hair sprays, face powder, and particularly fingernail polish.

Treatment: This consists of the use of steroids topically applied, plus, in severe cases, one or two doses of a systemic steroid either by injection or orally. Cold applications for five minutes several times a day will help reduce the edema. Except in chronic cases an allergic work-up is rarely required. However, inquiry should always be made as to the recent use of hair sprays, etc. If cosmetics are suspected, the patient should be advised to switch to nonallergenic preparations.

Carcinoma of the Lid

Although relatively uncommon, this condition must always be kept in mind. The lesion is very slowly progressive, often being present for months or even years before the patient seeks medical advice. It is typically papular with a pearly sheen and a dimpled or ulcerated center, usually on the lower lid close to the lash margin, as shown in Plate II.

Treatment: Although these lesions may respond to radiation, full-width surgical excision is the treatment of choice. If less than one-third of the lid is involved, the operation is a relatively minor one. When a larger area of the lid is involved, a more formidable plastic procedure is required.

Chronic tearing or constant purulent conjunctival discharge points to obstruction of the lacrimal apparatus. The diagnosis and treatment of these conditions fall within the province of the specialist. Occasionally an obstruction will lead to a lacrimal sac abscess, with a painful swelling between the nose and lower eyelid. This requires antimicrobials and drainage.

THE EXTERNAL EYE

The two most common injuries affecting the external eye are chemical burns and foreign bodies. In either of these conditions the cardinal principle is *prompt* removal.

CHEMICAL BURNS

One should *never* wait to determine the proper neutralizing agent. Instead, the eye should be irrigated copiously and thoroughly at the earliest possible moment with water, milk, or any bland liquid from any available source. When no assistance is available, the eye can be controlled as previously explained, while water is poured in with the other hand. Also the upper and lower cul-de-sacs must be irrigated by pulling one lid and then the other away from the globe.

Acid burns tend to cause immediate, usually localized, and nonprogressive tissue necrosis. Therefore, the effect is usually immediate and complete. On the other hand, the action of alkalies, such as plaster and lime, is progressive so that particles must be diligently searched for and removed manually if necessary.

Later, adhesions may tend to form between denuded areas that have resulted from the burn. These can be prevented by instilling a bland ointment (such as boric acid ointment) between the lids,

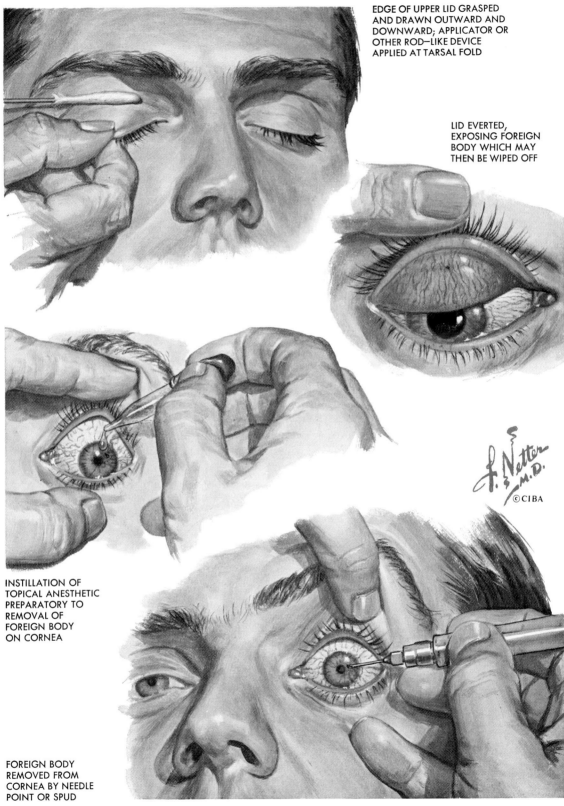

EDGE OF UPPER LID GRASPED AND DRAWN OUTWARD AND DOWNWARD; APPLICATOR OR OTHER ROD–LIKE DEVICE APPLIED AT TARSAL FOLD

LID EVERTED, EXPOSING FOREIGN BODY WHICH MAY THEN BE WIPED OFF

INSTILLATION OF TOPICAL ANESTHETIC PREPARATORY TO REMOVAL OF FOREIGN BODY ON CORNEA

FOREIGN BODY REMOVED FROM CORNEA BY NEEDLE POINT OR SPUD

PLATE III

FOREIGN BODIES

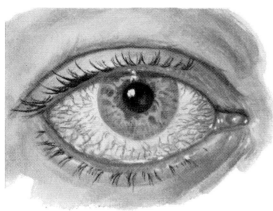

CONJUNCTIVITIS

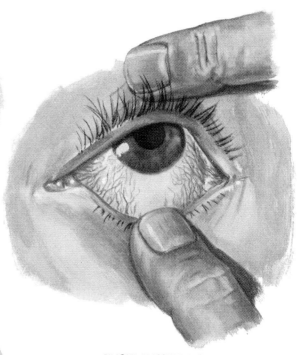

FINGER PRESSURE TEST

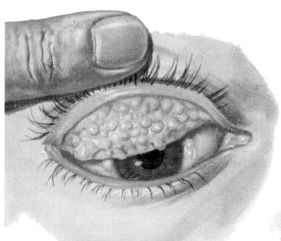

VERNAL CONJUNCTIVITIS

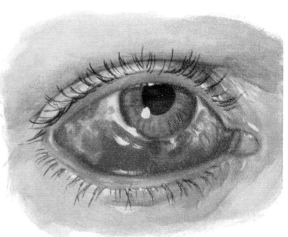

SUBCONJUNCTIVAL HEMORRHAGE

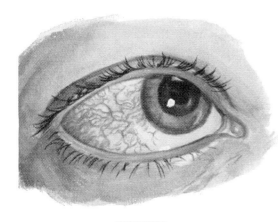

EPISCLERITIS

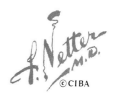

PLATE IV

CONJUNCTIVITIS; SUBCONJUNCTIVAL HEMORRHAGE; EPISCLERITIS

avoiding complete immobilization for long periods or, in severe cases, inserting a shape-retaining conformer made of dental wax or similar material.

Topical anesthesia may be used when the patient is first seen, but as infrequently as possible thereafter since such agents tend to delay healing. Antibiotic ointments also tend to interfere with healing and should be used only if infection is present or feared. Indeed, one should never put any medicament into the eye just for the sake of doing something!

FOREIGN BODIES

Foreign bodies adherent to conjunctiva are always found beneath the upper lid. Elsewhere they are carried into the corner of the eye by the tears. Usually after everting the upper lid, they can be visualized without difficulty and removed with a moistened applicator, or even the tip of a handkerchief. An exception may be a foreign body above the upper tarsal border, which may be difficult to see and wipe away unless the lid is doubly everted (turned again on itself).

A *foreign body on the cornea* is a different matter. While a conjunctival foreign body causes discomfort every time the lids blink, one on the cornea may cause no pain until it has produced an ulcer. If not over the pupil, there may be no impairment of vision except that produced by lacrimation. A sign that should arouse suspicion is the presence of localized redness on the adjacent sclera. Thus if the foreign body is at 9 o'clock, the area of injection will be localized to that particular area of the conjunctiva.

A corneal foreign body is difficult to visualize because of the dark background. Normally the cornea is smooth, glistening, and reflective like a mirror. Careful examination with good illumination will reveal a localized irregularity in this smooth surface. Where an ulcer has been formed, application of fluorescein will produce a greenish corneal stain (Plate V).

Because of the sensitivity of the cornea, a topical anesthetic should be applied before removal is attempted. Very early, the corneal foreign body can be removed by irrigation. However, it soon becomes imbedded so that it can be freed only by a semisharp metal instrument, known as an eye spud, or a hypodermic needle (Plate III). Whatever the instrument used, it should be sterile; otherwise an infected corneal ulcer may result.

There is no need to dilate the pupil or use any other medication if sterile technique has been followed. Under no circumstances should atropine be used because the prolonged dilatation of the pupil will partially incapacitate the patient for as long as two or three weeks!

A foreign body, if properly removed, will rarely leave a scar, unless it was so deeply imbedded as to involve Bowman's membrane. An exception is a metallic foreign body composed of either iron or steel. Here, even within an hour or so, *rust rings* will form which are very difficult to remove. If located over the pupil, they will interfere with vision, the degree depending upon their density and breadth.

Treatment: Removal of corneal rust rings requires equipment and technical skill usually possessed only by the specialist. By some they are curetted away with a cataract knife. Others use a dental drill. Our personal choice is the light application to the anesthetized eye of a 1 per cent solution of silver nitrate. This is applied only to the involved area with a tightly wound, fine-pointed, only slightly moistened applicator. The eye is then immediately lavaged with sterile saline or water. Anywhere from one-half hour to a day later, the area containing the rust ring can be lifted out on the point of a cataract knife. The eye is then bandaged for a day.

Penetrating Foreign Body: If protruding, such a foreign body should be removed immediately, provided this can be done without fear of breaking it off. If this is not possible, the eye should be anesthetized and both eyes covered with an occlusive dressing, so that they will be immobilized until specialized attention can be obtained.

Once the foreign body is removed, the cornea will usually heal spontaneously with simple patching, as will most simple corneal lacerations, unless the wound is large or gaping, in which case it must be sutured.

Loss of aqueous humor is unimportant of itself because it is rapidly replaced. However, where loss occurs in a rapid gush, the iris may become incarcerated in the wound. If this happens, a mydriatic may result in its release. If not, the protruding portion must be cut away. Otherwise the entire inner eye will become infected.

CONJUNCTIVITIS

This, the most common office ophthalmologic problem, is often called "pink eye" because of the injection of conjunctival vessels over the sclera. However, in some cases only the conjunctival surfaces of the lids are involved, the palpebral conjunctiva being beefy red, while the bulbar conjunctiva remains clear. Conjunctivitis may be due to allergy, infection, or some chemical or gaseous irritant.

Before treatment is instituted, one must rule out foreign body, carefully examine the cornea for disease (which would be more important than the conjunctivitis), and make sure there is no involvement of the inner eye.

Differentiation of Conjunctival Injection from Ciliary Injection: The conjunctival vessels reach toward the cornea from the periphery of the globe, while the ciliary vessels emerge from the inner eye at the corneoscleral junction (the limbus) and radiate outward. In conjunctivitis the

former vessels alone are injected. In disease of the inner eye, ciliary injection alone is present, or both sets of vessels may be engorged.

To differentiate between injection of these two vascular systems, press the lower lid firmly against the cornea and slowly draw it downward while maintaining the pressure, as shown in Plate IV. If the injection is conjunctival, a pallid area will remain next to the cornea, since the blood is coming from the periphery. On the other hand, if the area next to the cornea pales only momentarily as the lower lid is withdrawn and then quickly reddens again, the blood is coming from within the eye, indicating ciliary injection and inner eye disease.

Another method of differentiation is to instill a few drops of Privine 0.05 per cent. This will quickly blanch a conjunctival injection but not a ciliary injection.

Allergic Conjunctivitis

In this type of conjunctivitis, the palpebral conjunctiva will be found to be milky, pale, and edematous. Usually only the lower lid is involved. However, in *vernal conjunctivitis* the upper lid will be pale and milky and will have large cobblestone-like excrescences (Plate IV). In rare cases the limbal form of vernal conjunctivitis is seen, in which the conjunctiva is raised all around the limbus, but elsewhere it is clear. Although vernal conjunctivitis is said to be seasonal, in practice some patients will be found who are rarely free of symptoms.

This condition is best treated by the frequent use of topical steroids. Patients should be instructed to use the drops as necessary to obtain relief. This therapy may also be used when inflammation of the conjunctiva is caused by irritants.

Infective Conjunctivitis

In this condition the eye is red and bloodshot. Because of the effectiveness of

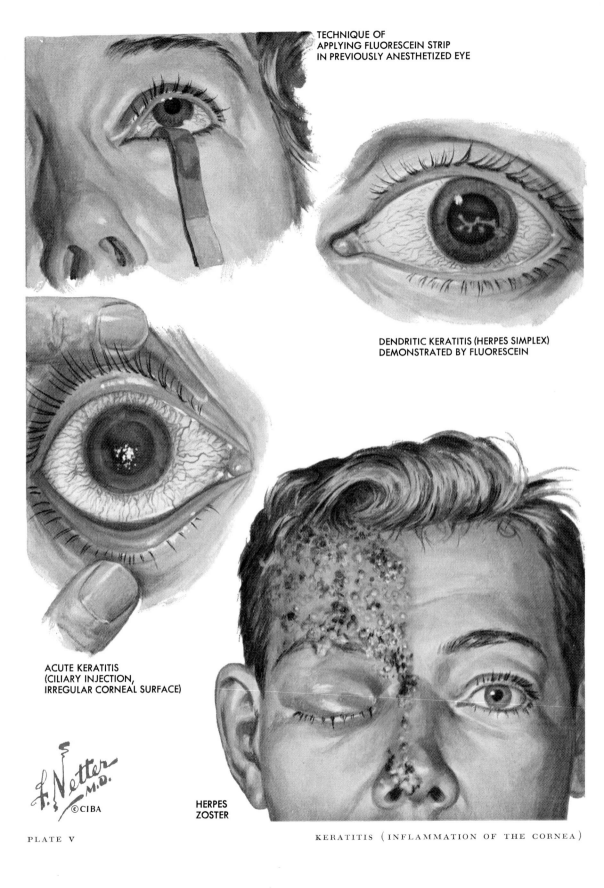

TECHNIQUE OF
APPLYING FLUORESCEIN STRIP
IN PREVIOUSLY ANESTHETIZED EYE

DENDRITIC KERATITIS (HERPES SIMPLEX)
DEMONSTRATED BY FLUORESCEIN

ACUTE KERATITIS
(CILIARY INJECTION,
IRREGULAR CORNEAL SURFACE)

HERPES
ZOSTER

PLATE V

KERATITIS (INFLAMMATION OF THE CORNEA)

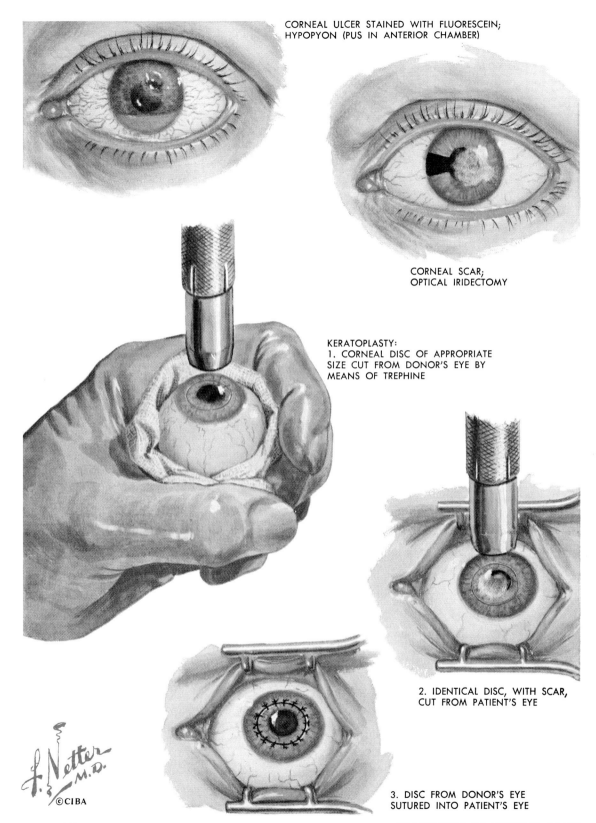

CORNEAL ULCER STAINED WITH FLUORESCEIN;
HYPOPYON (PUS IN ANTERIOR CHAMBER)

CORNEAL SCAR;
OPTICAL IRIDECTOMY

KERATOPLASTY:
1. CORNEAL DISC OF APPROPRIATE
SIZE CUT FROM DONOR'S EYE BY
MEANS OF TREPHINE

2. IDENTICAL DISC, WITH SCAR,
CUT FROM PATIENT'S EYE

3. DISC FROM DONOR'S EYE
SUTURED INTO PATIENT'S EYE

PLATE VI

TREATMENT OF CORNEAL SCARS

topical antimicrobials or steroid-antimicrobial preparations, it is rarely necessary to do a culture, unless there is no response to treatment after a fair trial of a week or so. Occasionally, there is a corneal complication with small marginal ulcers near the limbus, or junction between cornea and sclera. These respond to the same medications and need to be cultured only if they fail to respond.

Occlusive dressings are unnecessary in conjunctivitis. If there is discharge, it will remain pent up beneath the lids and will macerate the cornea.

SUBCONJUNCTIVAL HEMORRHAGE

A painless, homogenous, red area, which is easily differentiated from injection, is usually limited to one quadrant (Plate IV). It appears suddenly and will be reabsorbed spontaneously within about two weeks. Cold compresses may be applied for the first few days. Afterwards, hot compresses may be used in the hope of hastening reabsorption.

EPISCLERITIS

This is an inflammation of the loose connective tissue between the sclera and the conjunctiva. A red or slightly purplish area, over which the overlying conjunctiva can be moved, may be localized or diffuse (Plate IV). It is distinguished from conjunctivitis by tenderness to pressure exerted upon the overlying lid and by the fact that it is usually localized to one quadrant, while conjunctivitis tends to be diffuse. It may be a forerunner of iritis.

An unusual form of conjunctivitis, the angular conjunctivitis of Morax-Axenfeld, may cause some confusion in diagnosis because it is quadrantic, more commonly occurring in the outer angle of the eye. However, angular conjunctivitis, like other forms of conjunctivitis, will blanch out entirely on application of Privine 0.05 per cent, whereas the injection of episcleritis will not. Episcleritis usually responds to frequently applied topical steroids.

SCLERITIS

This uncommon condition is found in people with rheumatoid arthritis or a "rheumatic tendency." The engorged deep blood vessels tend to be purplish. Yellow, gelatinous nodules may form, or ulceration may result in perforation and loss of the globe. Since this condition is usually refractory to treatment, it had best be referred to a specialist.

KERATITIS
(Inflammation of the Cornea)

Keratitis is always a serious condition. The eye is painful, there will be ciliary injection, and probably conjunctival injection as well. Part or all of the cornea will appear rough, and the light reflections coming from it will be rough or irregular (Plate V).

Herpes Simplex

In the eye, this virus infection causes the so-called dendritic keratitis or branch-like ulceration of the cornea, the end of each branch terminating in a little round knob (Plate V). It is probably the most common form of keratitis seen today and often occurs in patients who have had a cold sore on the lips or face.

Typical of this condition is a partial or complete loss of corneal sensation. Thus if the cornea of the affected eye is found relatively anesthetic as compared with the other eye by drawing a hair or a wisp of cotton across it, the diagnosis is dendritic keratitis unless proved otherwise.

Diagnosis: The diagnosis is confirmed by *fluorescein*, which is best applied as a moistened sterile strip of impregnated paper placed inside the lower lid while the patient is looking up and left in place for a few moments (Plate V). This results in a greenish discoloration of the denuded epithelium, easily visible with good focal illumination and magnification.

Treatment: The traditional treatment consisted of the manual or chemical removal of all of the diseased epithelium. This was accomplished by scraping with a sterile cataract knife, or the application of tincture of iodine followed by 4 per cent cocaine and irrigation.

Recently there has become available a new medication which appears to be specific. It is 5-iodo-2′-deoxyuridine. This is known as IDU* and is applied one drop every hour during the daytime and every two hours at night. This can be used as initial treatment or following the traditional scraping if desired. Little or no scarring should result from this treatment.

Previous to the introduction of IDU, steroids were contraindicated in dendritic keratitis. However, now they may be added to the IDU regimen. If steroids are given from the first day of application, the reaction is minimized and, again, little or no scarring will result.

Herpes Zoster

This is usually readily diagnosed because of the hemifacial distribution of the typical lesions extending down to the tip of the nose (Plate V). When the eye is affected, it produces a keratitis which may be very severe and is accompanied always by a concomitant severe iritis. In this condition the corticosteroids are of value, 3 to 4.5 mg. of dexamethasone† being given daily in divided doses.

Another form of keratitis is the *indolent ulcer produced by fungi.* This is a dirty gray, very slowly progressive ulceration of the cornea, which comes on weeks or

---

*At the time of publication this drug had not yet become commercially available.

†Dexamethasone is available as Gammacorten.

months after an original injury. It is rarely seen except in states where such organisms are prevalent, such as California, Missouri, southern Illinois, and Texas. For diagnosis, culture must be made on special media, or in some cases the fungus can be seen in a smear. Here, sodium sulfacetamide by iontophoresis, or the topical application of thimerosal 1:1,000, amphotericin B, or sodium sulfacetamide 30 per cent are useful in the relative order mentioned.

Corneal Ulcer

A corneal ulcer is a localized necrosis of corneal epithelium usually caused by an infection following trauma to the cornea, or spread of infection from the conjunctiva or an infected lacrimal sac.

Limbal corneal ulcers, or ulcers at the edge of the cornea where it joins the sclera, are usually found in association with conjunctivitis. These are benign and respond to steroid-antimicrobial combinations.

The more serious corneal ulcers usually occur away from the limbus. As a rule, they are easily seen with proper illumination and magnification and stain readily with fluorescein. There is frequently an associated iritis.

Severe progressive corneal ulcers, known as serpent ulcers, will show a collection of pus in the bottom of the anterior chamber. This is known as *hypopyon* (Plate VI).

Because of the seriousness of this situation, antimicrobials should be administered systemically and topically in large doses while awaiting the results of culture.

CORNEAL SCARS

A corneal scar causes trouble only if it is over the pupil and especially over the center of the pupil. If only the periphery of the pupil area is involved, little difficulty in vision is to be anticipated.

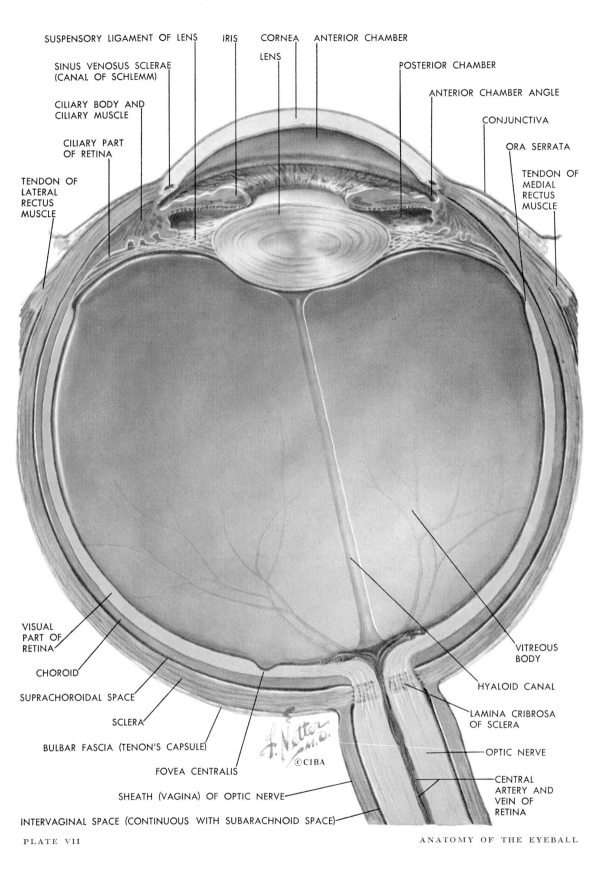

SUSPENSORY LIGAMENT OF LENS   IRIS   CORNEA   ANTERIOR CHAMBER

SINUS VENOSUS SCLERAE
(CANAL OF SCHLEMM)   LENS

CILIARY BODY AND
CILIARY MUSCLE

CILIARY PART
OF RETINA

POSTERIOR CHAMBER

ANTERIOR CHAMBER ANGLE

CONJUNCTIVA

ORA SERRATA

TENDON OF
MEDIAL
RECTUS
MUSCLE

TENDON OF
LATERAL
RECTUS
MUSCLE

VISUAL
PART OF
RETINA

CHOROID

SUPRACHOROIDAL SPACE

SCLERA

BULBAR FASCIA (TENON'S CAPSULE)

FOVEA CENTRALIS

VITREOUS
BODY

HYALOID CANAL

LAMINA CRIBROSA
OF SCLERA

OPTIC NERVE

CENTRAL
ARTERY AND
VEIN OF
RETINA

SHEATH (VAGINA) OF OPTIC NERVE

INTERVAGINAL SPACE (CONTINUOUS WITH SUBARACHNOID SPACE)

F. Netter M.D.
©CIBA

PLATE VII   ANATOMY OF THE EYEBALL

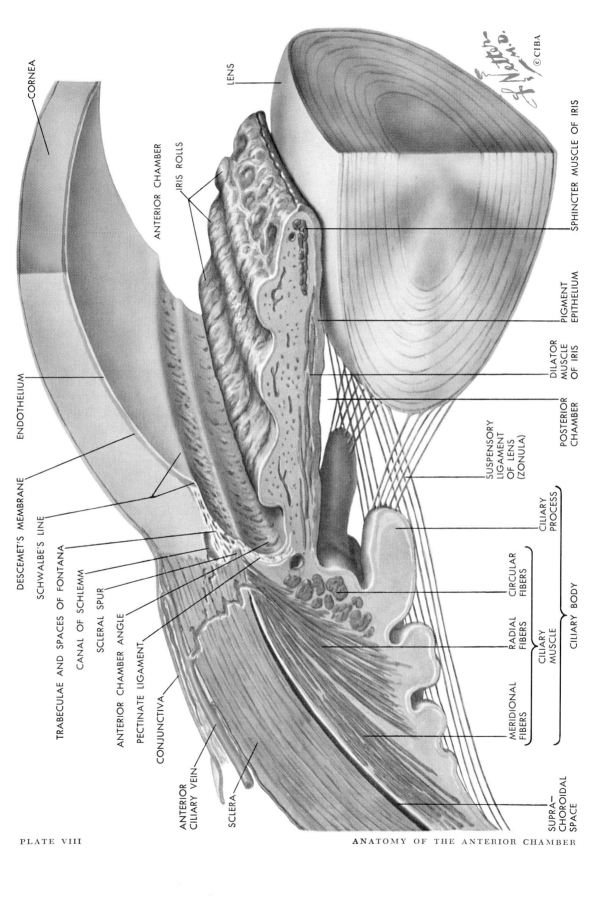

CORNEA

LENS

ANTERIOR CHAMBER

IRIS ROLLS

SPHINCTER MUSCLE OF IRIS

ENDOTHELIUM

PIGMENT EPITHELIUM

DILATOR MUSCLE OF IRIS

POSTERIOR CHAMBER

DESCEMET'S MEMBRANE

SCHWALBE'S LINE

TRABECULAE AND SPACES OF FONTANA

CANAL OF SCHLEMM

SCLERAL SPUR

ANTERIOR CHAMBER ANGLE

PECTINATE LIGAMENT

CONJUNCTIVA

ANTERIOR CILIARY VEIN

SCLERA

SUSPENSORY LIGAMENT OF LENS (ZONULA)

CILIARY PROCESS

CIRCULAR FIBERS

RADIAL FIBERS

MERIDIONAL FIBERS

CILIARY MUSCLE

CILIARY BODY

SUPRA-CHOROIDAL SPACE

©CIBA

PLATE VIII

ANATOMY OF THE ANTERIOR CHAMBER

Surgical Treatment

This consists of either optical iridectomy or keratoplasty (the so-called corneal transplant). In the former, a portion of the iris is removed (Plate VI). This procedure is only of value if a clear area is found toward the periphery of the cornea and vision is improved by dilating that segment of the iris which lies behind it.

Keratoplasty: When the scar is only superficial, or where for technical reasons it is desired to create a better bed for a subsequent complete corneal graft, only the outer layers of the cornea are replaced with donor cornea of similar thickness. For full-thickness corneal graft, the donor eye must be injected with saline so that the cornea will have the same convexity as that of the patient's eye. A trephine with identical setting removes cornea from donor eye and the patient's eye as shown in Plate VI. The transplanted cornea is sutured in place by about 16 sutures, each pair of sutures being diagonally opposite each other.

THE INTERNAL EYE

The two diseases of the internal eye which cause pain and are most easily confused are: iritis or inflammation of the iris, and glaucoma, in which intra-ocular pressure is elevated. (Pain is also caused by optic or retrobulbar neuritis, but here sudden loss of vision is a distinguishing feature.)

Iritis must be differentiated from glaucoma because much of the treatment is diametrically opposed. In treating iritis, the pupil may be dilated. This would be dangerous in glaucoma. The reverse is true of the use of miotics to constrict the pupils. They are indicated in glaucoma; they may or may not do harm in iritis.

Both of these conditions must be differentiated from conjunctivitis which also causes redness of the eye. Lack of treatment of conjunctivitis will only prolong the discomfort, whereas in iritis and glaucoma lack of treatment may result in permanent damage (see Table 1 opposite).

IRITIS (IRIDOCYCLITIS)

Inflammation of the iris may be acute, recurrent, or chronic. When the ciliary body (Plate VIII) is involved, as it usually is, the condition is known as *iridocyclitis.* (The uveal tract includes the iris, ciliary body, and choroid. Therefore, a synonym of iridocyclitis is *anterior uveitis.*)

The main symptoms are pain and blurring of vision. The pain, due to spasm of the ciliary body, is localized in the temporal region of the same side. Blurring of vision may be due to several factors: loss of ability to focus due to spasm of the ciliary body, fibrin in the anterior chamber, edema of the cornea, or edema of the retina if the posterior eye becomes involved.

On examination there is often unilateral edema of the upper lid, constriction of the pupil which may be irregular due to adhesions, and ciliary injection which must be differentiated from conjunctival injection (see page 123). The typical appearance is shown in Plate IX.

Having noted these signs and symptoms, the intra-ocular pressure of the two eyes should be compared to rule out glaucoma. A rough estimate can be made by placing the index fingers against the upper lid while the patient is looking down. Alternate pressure, first with the right and then with the left index finger, may show that the affected eye is as soft as the unaffected one if the patient has iritis. In glaucoma, the affected eye will be tense and even stony hard to the touch. Of course, a more accurate determination can and should be made by a tonometer (see page 134). In considering the differential diagnosis, it is well to remember that occasionally iritis is accompanied by secondary glaucoma.

TABLE 1

DIFFERENTIAL DIAGNOSIS OF THREE FREQUENTLY ENCOUNTERED OCULAR ABNORMALITIES

SIGN OR SYMPTOM	ACUTE CONJUNCTIVITIS	ACUTE IRITIS	ACUTE GLAUCOMA
Injection	Conjunctival (superficial)	Ciliary (deep)	Intense conjunctival and ciliary
Pain	Sandy sensation	Moderate	Severe
Vision	Normal	Impaired	Severely impaired
Pupil	Normal	Small	Dilated
Discharge	Watery to purulent	None	None
Anterior chamber	Normal	Normal	Shallow
Media	Clear	Corneal deposits Hazy aqueous	Steamy cornea
Iris	Normal	Muddy markings	Congested
Intra-ocular pressure	Normal	Usually normal	Elevated

Iris Bombé

In iridocyclitis, the formation of adhesions, or synechiae, between the posterior surface of the iris and the lens may progress until a complete uninterrupted ring has formed about the pupil. When this happens, the aqueous humor formed in the posterior chamber behind the iris cannot pass into the anterior chamber, and the iris balloons forward like a doughnut around the pupil (Plate IX).

This produces a secondary glaucoma, and vision will be destroyed unless an artificial pupil is created, which will permit free flow of aqueous humor from the posterior to the anterior chamber.

Treatment of Iritis

Topical steroids are valuable in iritis, and in acute glaucoma they may be of some value in preventing adhesions in the anterior chamber, if instilled about every hour, or initially even more often.

Carbonic anhydrase inhibitors are often helpful in acute glaucoma and will do no harm in acute iritis. Therefore, any of these agents may be used if there is doubt as to the diagnosis. If there is *no* doubt about the diagnosis, the pupil should be dilated, using any short-acting mydriatic such as cyclopentolate hydrochloride. This dilates the pupil and helps prevent adhesions (synechiae) between the iris and either the cornea or the lens.

GLAUCOMA

In glaucoma, aqueous humor accumulates within the eye, creating an increase in intra-ocular pressure. It may be acute or chronic, primary or secondary to another condition such as intra-ocular tumor or uveitis (iritis, choroiditis).

ACUTE GLAUCOMA

This is always due to an acute obstruction of the anterior chamber angle, or angle between the root of the iris and cornea, through which the aqueous humor drains back into the circulation (Plate VIII). Rarely is this obstruction relieved spontaneously. If unrelieved, the vision will be lost.

Symptoms

Tension in any hollow viscus causes excruciating pain. Acute glaucoma is no exception, creating as it does the most

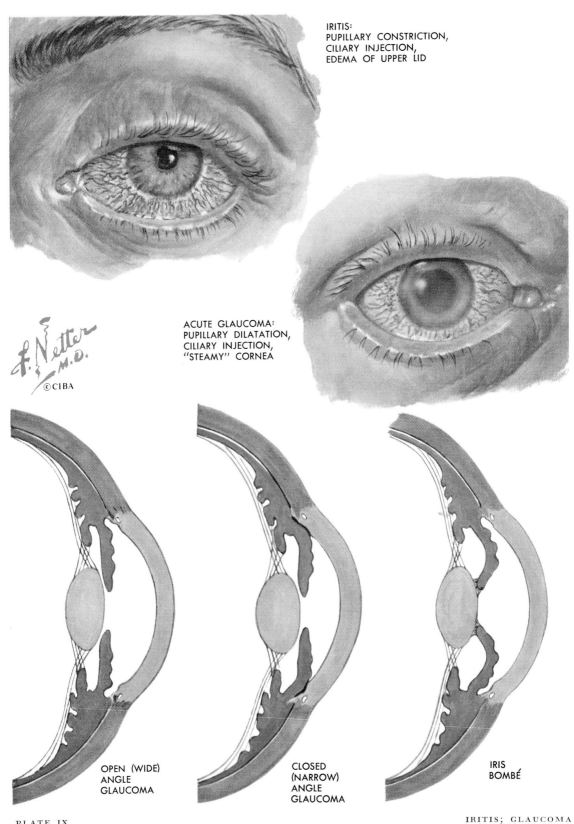

IRITIS:
PUPILLARY CONSTRICTION,
CILIARY INJECTION,
EDEMA OF UPPER LID

ACUTE GLAUCOMA:
PUPILLARY DILATATION,
CILIARY INJECTION,
"STEAMY" CORNEA

OPEN (WIDE)
ANGLE
GLAUCOMA

CLOSED
(NARROW)
ANGLE
GLAUCOMA

IRIS
BOMBÉ

PLATE IX

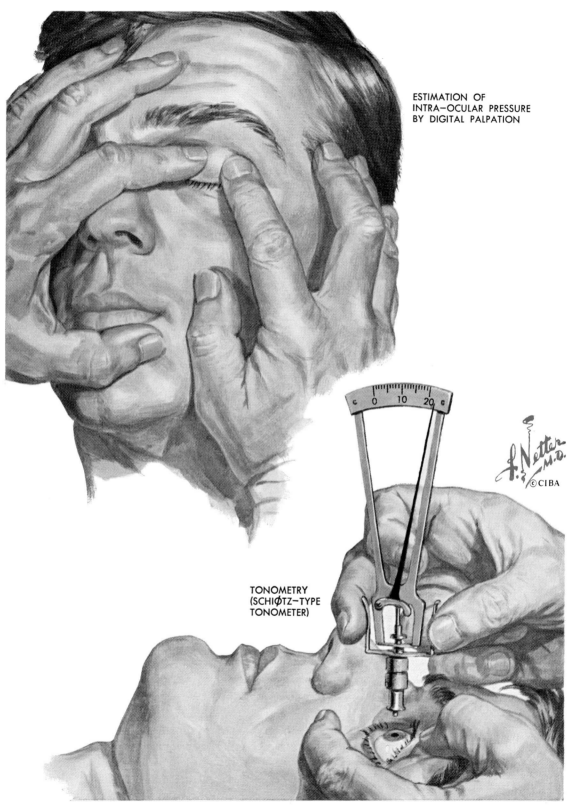

ESTIMATION OF
INTRA–OCULAR PRESSURE
BY DIGITAL PALPATION

TONOMETRY
(SCHIØTZ–TYPE
TONOMETER)

PLATE X   ESTIMATION OF INTRA-OCULAR PRESSURE

agonizing discomfort. Vomiting is often present, so that a gastrointestinal disease may be erroneously suspected. Halos or rainbows around lights, a symptom also produced by sclerosis of the nucleus of the lens and sometimes by tears or mucus on the eye, are often seen in chronic glaucoma and are caused by corneal edema. In acute glaucoma they may not be noticed because of loss of visual acuity.

Signs

The eye is reddened by ciliary injection (which must be differentiated from conjunctival injection, see page 123), the pupil is dilated, the anterior chamber is shallow, and the cornea is steamy with irregular light reflexes (Plate IX).

As previously mentioned, alternate pressure on the globe by the index fingers as shown in Plate X will reveal a hardness, even a stony hardness, of the affected eye as compared with the normal eye.

Tonometry: Obviously a more accurate determination of intra-ocular pressure can be obtained by direct measurement. This is carried out as follows: The patient lies down. Both eyes are anesthetized (both should be tested). Then as the patient looks directly upward at his own index finger or some other object, the lids are separated (see Plate X), the foot of the Schiøtz tonometer is set lightly but firmly on the center of the cornea, and a reading is promptly taken while the shaft of the tonometer is held absolutely vertical.

The lower the reading on the scale, the higher the intra-ocular pressure. The tonometer is equipped with a built-in 5.5-mg. weight. With this weight, a reading of 4 is considered the upper limit of normal. A reading of 3 is probably pathologic. A reading of less than 3 must be considered pathologic unless proved otherwise. Any reading of 3 or less should be correlated with the reading obtained using a heavier weight (a card for such correlation accompanies the instrument).

Low or questionable readings indicate referral to an ophthalmologist, or if this is impossible, the patient must be closely followed. While the vision-destroying capacity of glaucoma must never be forgotten, it is almost equally important that a definite diagnosis of chronic glaucoma not be made on the basis of a single reading. Rather, if asymptomatic, the patient should be told that his pressure is high and that careful follow-up and additional confirmatory tests should be carried out.

Gonioscopy: The gonioscope is a combination of a contact lens and mirror which allows the observer to look directly into the angle of the anterior chamber. He is thus able to determine whether the angle is normally open or closed (Plate XI).

Treatment

The treatment of acute glaucoma consists of the use of double or quadruple doses of a carbonic anhydrase inhibitor orally, such as acetazolamide, ethoxzolamide, or dichlorphenamide. If effective, intra-ocular tension will be considerably reduced within one and one-half hours.

Simultaneously, the patient is given miotics, such as 2 to 4 per cent pilocarpine, which may be alternated with 0.25 per cent eserine applied topically every 15 minutes until the pupil is constricted. If the intra-ocular tension is not reduced within 90 minutes, the patient should be given acetazolamide intravenously. Often this will reduce the tension when the oral medication has failed and will produce an effect within 15 to 30 minutes. If these measures fail, the patient should be given urea intravenously in a dosage of 1 Gm./kg. of body weight. This will reduce pressure in practically every patient, not only in the hard eye but also in the normal one.

If these measures have produced no relief, an iridectomy, preferably a peripheral iridectomy, should be carried out without delay. This will usually control the patient's symptoms and, in addition, prevent further attacks (see page 138).

If the acute attack responds to the medical therapy outlined, the patient should be advised to have a peripheral iridectomy to prevent further attacks. Preferably this surgery should not be carried out until the eye has become pale and quiescent.

In these patients, the tension is often elevated in the opposite eye as well. In any event, that eye must be regarded as potentially glaucomatous. Where a moderate elevation is found, or where patients reside long distances from medical help, a prophylactic peripheral iridectomy of the other eye may be desirable.

Occasionally, acute glaucoma may be simulated by a *glaucoma-cyclitic crisis* which, however, is usually not as severe. This is a very uncommon form of iridocyclitis, which is accompanied by an attack of acute glaucoma due to edema of the choroid body. Here, the anterior chamber angle is found to be open when examined by gonioscope, and the slit lamp will reveal signs of anterior uveitis, including deposits on the corneal endothelium. There may be little other evidence of iritis until the following day, however. This condition should not be operated upon since it usually responds quite well to carbonic anhydrase inhibitors and topical or systemic steroids.

CHRONIC GLAUCOMA

The chronic forms of glaucoma are divided into those with an open or wide anterior chamber angle and those in which the angle is closed or narrow.

Open (Wide) Angle Glaucoma
(Plate IX)

This condition is due to some failure in the facility of outflow of aqueous humor possibly due to a defect in the trabeculae of the anterior chamber. It is a chronic, slowly progressive disease, rarely associated with acute attacks or with definitive symptoms. The patient may complain of vague headaches, he may be continually wiping his glasses, or his glasses may require frequent changing.

Since there are no distinguishing symptoms and the intra-ocular pressure may not be greatly elevated, diagnosis may be impossible unless the patient is examined with a tonometer, with repeated testing in suspicious cases. Indeed, it has been suggested that tonometry be a part of every routine physical examination in order to pick up patients of this sort before damage to vision results.

Course: Eventually, if untreated and possibly even if treated, excavation of the optic nerve will occur (with loss of visual field and vision).

Treatment: This type of chronic glaucoma responds very well to miotics, starting with 0.5 per cent pilocarpine or 0.75 per cent carbachol, and increasing the dosage to 1 or 2 per cent pilocarpine or 1½ per cent carbachol. Both drugs, when they fail to control the condition adequately, can be supplemented by epinephrine bitartrate or borate. (These latter drugs should *not* be used in closed angle glaucoma.) Eserine ointment can be applied at night, and/or carbonic anhydrase inhibitors can be given. With early diagnosis and adequate medical care, few of these patients should come to surgery.

Closed (Narrow) Angle Glaucoma
(Plate IX)

This type of chronic glaucoma occurs in intermittent attacks during which the angle closes. In many patients the attacks will be of brief duration and clear up spontaneously. However, each attack tends to produce adhesions in the angle of the anterior chamber, and eventually the angle will be either partially or completely obliterated, so that surgery becomes an absolute necessity.

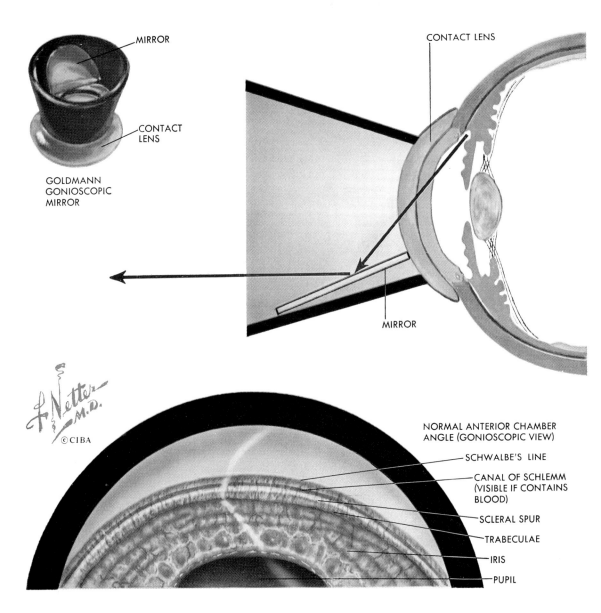

MIRROR

CONTACT
LENS

GOLDMANN
GONIOSCOPIC
MIRROR

CONTACT LENS

MIRROR

NORMAL ANTERIOR CHAMBER
ANGLE (GONIOSCOPIC VIEW)

SCHWALBE'S LINE

CANAL OF SCHLEMM
(VISIBLE IF CONTAINS
BLOOD)

SCLERAL SPUR

TRABECULAE

IRIS

PUPIL

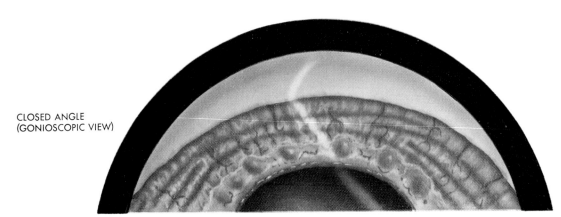

CLOSED ANGLE
(GONIOSCOPIC VIEW)

PLATE XI   GONIOSCOPY

PERIPHERAL IRIDECTOMY

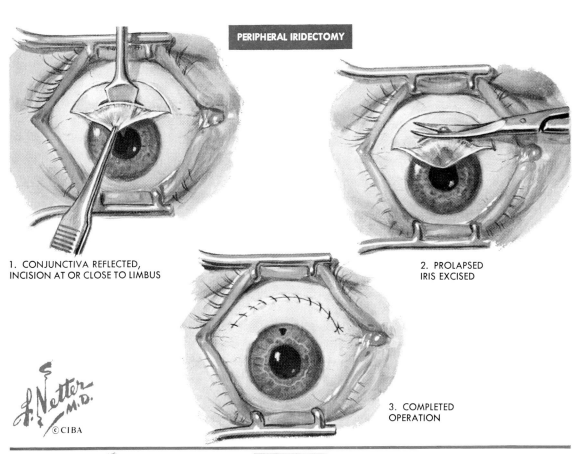

1. CONJUNCTIVA REFLECTED,
INCISION AT OR CLOSE TO LIMBUS

2. PROLAPSED
IRIS EXCISED

3. COMPLETED
OPERATION

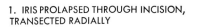

IRIDENCLEISIS

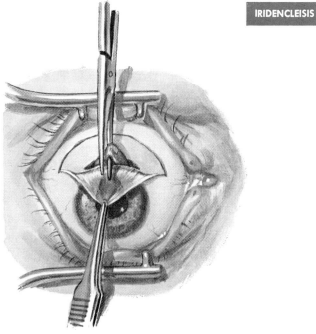

1. IRIS PROLAPSED THROUGH INCISION,
TRANSECTED RADIALLY

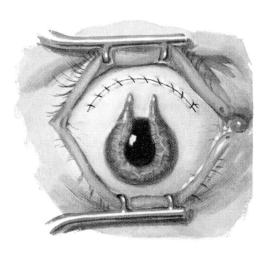

2. COMPLETED OPERATION

PLATE XII

SURGICAL TREATMENT OF GLAUCOMA

In this type of chronic glaucoma, surgery is the treatment of choice. When done early, a peripheral iridectomy will usually be adequate to prevent further attacks. This operation is much neater cosmetically and just as effective as the old full iridectomy. One advantage of peripheral iridectomy is that it does not prevent more extensive surgery later, if that should prove necessary.

OPERATIVE PROCEDURES FOR GLAUCOMA

Peripheral Iridectomy

This is the surgical procedure of choice in any form of closed, or narrow angle, glaucoma. Unless a good many adhesions (synechiae) have formed in the anterior chamber as a result of previous attacks, this operation can practically always be depended upon to prevent future episodes of acute glaucoma.

This operation gives a better cosmetic result than a full iridectomy. Moreover, even when the pupil is dilated, the opening that has been created will permit an adequate outflow of aqueous humor.

The steps of peripheral iridectomy are illustrated in Plate XII. They can perhaps be better visualized by also referring to the cross section in Plate VIII.

The conjunctiva is incised and reflected as shown, and an incision made through the limbus (or the sclera, 1 mm. behind the limbus) into the anterior chamber at the root of the iris. The root of the iris is then prolapsed through this incision by pressure on the lip of the sclera. Both layers of the prolapsed iris are then excised close to the ciliary body. The corneoscleral incision is then closed with a single suture. The result is an opening through which aqueous humor can escape at the anterior angle.

The Scheie Procedure

This is a procedure of choice in open, or wide angle, glaucoma. It differs from the peripheral iridectomy in only two respects. The conjunctival flap must be approximately 8 mm. in height to permit formation of a filtering bleb. In addition, the opening at the limbus is made with a cautery instead of a knife.

The result is that in addition to a peripheral iridectomy, a new filtering scar forms an opening between the inner and outer eye, thus enabling aqueous humor to escape into the space beneath Tenon's capsule, forming a bleb on the surface of the globe.

Iridencleisis

This operation, like the Scheie procedure, provides for filtration of aqueous humor from the inner eye to the space beneath Tenon's capsule.

As shown in Plate XII, it differs from peripheral iridectomy in that the root of the iris is transected radially, and the two tongues of iris are brought out through the incision to lie upon the sclera and provide external drainage.

CATARACT

The multilayered lens is composed of a nucleus, surrounded by a cortex consisting of a number of layers like an onion, all enclosed in a capsule.

The nucleus begins to dry at birth and with increasing age tends to shrink and harden. Indeed, everyone past the age of 40 has some degree of nuclear sclerosis. This is rarely important, however, until it becomes moderately advanced, when it produces an artificial myopia.

Gradually progressive opacities can occur in the cortex and in the subcapsular area, as well as in the nucleus (Plate XIII). The term "complicating" is usually appended to posterior subcapsular cataracts because opacities in this area are often produced by some other disease such as uveitis or retinal detachment.

At one time, operation was discouraged

until the cataract became "ripe," that is, until a complete breakdown of cortical material caused the lens to appear white. Today, however, we operate as soon as the patient no longer has useful vision to carry out his usual work or duties.

An intracapsular extraction is illustrated in Plate XIII. Incisions are made as shown, the iris incised or a piece excised, a suction device known as an erysiphake or a capsule forceps inserted, and the lens removed through the openings provided. To facilitate removal, particularly in younger people, a trypsin enzyme, alpha chymotrypsin, may be used to dissolve the zonula which holds the lens in place.

The extracapsular operation is more difficult, is not uniformly successful the first time as is an intracapsular extraction, and is used today only in infants and children or when the lens capsule ruptures accidentally. In this operation the nucleus is rather easy to remove, but the cortical material being tenacious and gummy must be removed piecemeal, aided by repeated washings. If a good opening is not created through the remaining capsular and cortical material, repeated surgery is necessary.

SUDDEN PAINLESS LOSS OF VISION

Sudden loss of vision without pain is practically always due to an *occlusion of the central retinal artery* or an *occlusion of the central retinal vein* (Plate XIV). Vision may or may not be affected if only a branch vessel is involved. Although often considered "sudden," *retinal detachment* (Plate XIV) usually takes place more slowly — hours or days.

Arterial Occlusion

If the occlusion is arterial, the retina is usually edematous and nonhemorrhagic. The macula, since it is not ophthalmoscopically involved in the retinal edema, will appear as a cherry red spot in con-

trast to the edematous retina around it. The arteries are narrowed or absent. At times one sees a broken column of blood, the so-called segmentation (trucking), especially in the veins. This phenomenon is also seen in dying patients (*The Eye in Death*, CLINICAL SYMPOSIA, Vol. 13, No. 2).

Treatment: Rapid decompression of the eye will sometimes relieve the arterial occlusion. This is accomplished by paracentesis of the anterior chamber through a keratome incision. This closes immediately when the keratome is removed but can be reopened by pressure within a day or so. At the same time, a whiff of amyl nitrite can be given or Priscoline injected intravenously.

Another method of rapidly decompressing the eye is the retrobulbar injection of procaine, followed by massage of the eyeball through closed lids. This will usually reduce the pressure within a matter of two or three minutes. Still another method, which has a less rapid effect, is the intravenous injection of urea (1 Gm./kg.).

Venous Occlusion

When the central retinal vein is occluded, a hemorrhagic retinitis is produced with blood and transudate covering the entire retina (Plate XIV). If the occlusion is only of a single branch, the blood is confined to the quadrant served by that branch. However, some blood will gravitate from the superior branch to the macular area, thus obscuring the vision. The *treatment* of venous occlusion is the immediate institution of anticoagulant therapy. Fibrinolytic therapy for vascular occlusion is still experimental, although some successes have been reported.

Retinal Detachment

Another cause of sudden loss of vision, although usually requiring several hours to a few days to develop, is retinal detach-

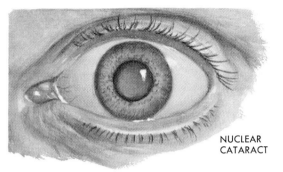

NUCLEAR
CATARACT

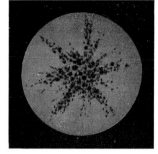

POSTERIOR
SUBCAPSULAR
(COMPLICATING)
CATARACT:
OPHTHALMOSCOPIC
VIEW

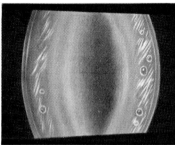

CORTICONUCLEAR
CATARACT:
DIRECT FOCAL
ILLUMINATION
WITH SLIT LAMP
MICROSCOPE

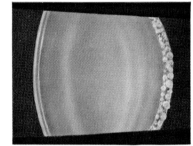

POSTERIOR
SUBCAPSULAR
(COMPLICATING)
CATARACT:
DIRECT FOCAL
ILLUMINATION
WITH SLIT LAMP
MICROSCOPE

CATARACT
EXTRACTION
(INTRACAPSULAR)

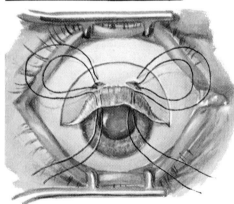

1. CONJUNCTIVA REFLECTED; MCLEAN–TYPE
CORNEOSCLERAL SUTURES PLACED

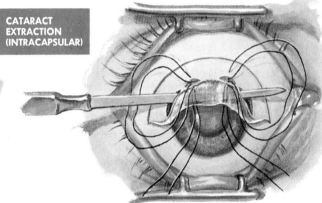

2. CATARACT KNIFE INTRODUCED,
INCISING LIMBUS BETWEEN SUTURES

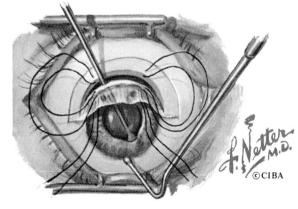

3. LENS GRASPED WITH ERYSIPHAKE AFTER
IRIDOTOMY (OR IRIDECTOMY); ZONULAR
ATTACHMENT BROKEN BY PRESSURE OF HOOK

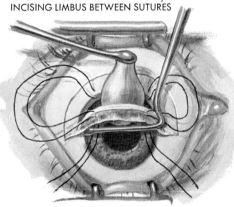

4. LENS EXTRACTED BY ERYSIPHAKE,
AIDED BY EXTERNAL PRESSURE OF HOOK

PLATE XIII

CATARACT

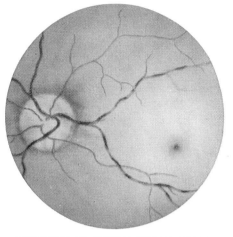

OCCLUSION OF CENTRAL RETINAL ARTERY

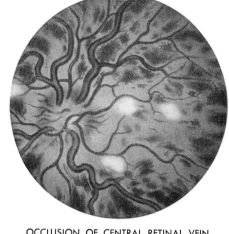

OCCLUSION OF CENTRAL RETINAL VEIN

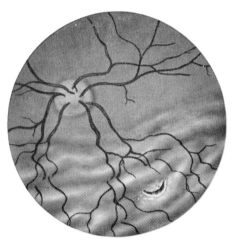

DETACHMENT OF RETINA (WITH TEAR)

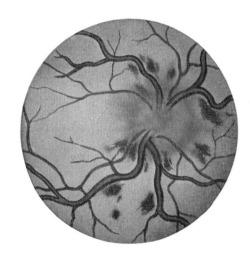

OPTIC NEURITIS

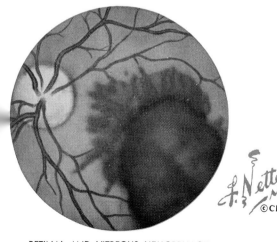

RETINAL AND VITREOUS HEMORRHAGE

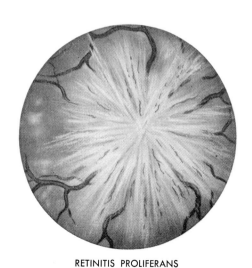

RETINITIS PROLIFERANS

PLATE XIV

LESIONS OF RETINA AND OPTIC NERVE

ment. Here there may or may not be a history of injury. The patient is often myopic.

Symptoms: The patient will first notice stars or scintillating flashes out of one corner of the eye, followed several hours later by a curtain moving across the eye, and later a progressive and marked loss of vision.

Treatment: The commonest treatment is diathermic reattachment. Here a thermal choroiditis is produced which will result in adhesions between the choroid and retina. This is often combined with various forms of shortening, or buckling, the sclera in such a way as to bring the choroid into better contact with the detached retina.

Another more recent innovation is the use of photocoagulation, in which light of high intensity is focused upon the retina to produce a localized burn, creating an adhesion to the underlying choroid. It is of value only in flat detachments, or prophylactically in treating certain retinal tears.

Retinal and Vitreous Hemorrhage

The vitreous body contains no blood vessels. However, in case of a huge retinal hemorrhage, blood will soak into the vitreous, completely obscuring retinal details and destroying the vision until absorbed or removed (Plate XIV).

Retinitis Proliferans

This condition is always secondary to one or more severe hemorrhages most commonly seen in diabetics. In an effort to absorb the hemorrhagic material, new vessels and fibroblastic tissue are formed. This condition is hopeless from the standpoint of treatment. Indeed, subsequent contraction of the fibrous tissue often results in retinal detachment.

SUDDEN LOSS OF VISION WITH PAIN ON MOVEMENT OF THE EYE

Optic neuritis and *retrobulbar neuritis* may be responsible for sudden loss of vision. In contrast to the conditions previously mentioned, these are both distinguished by the fact that movements of the eye cause pain, due to the posterior insertion of some of the extrinsic muscles to the sheath of the optic nerve.

In optic neuritis the examiner sees a red, engorged edematous nerve head (Plate XIV). In retrobulbar neuritis the fundus appears essentially normal, or as the saying goes, "Neither the patient nor the ophthalmologist can see anything!" Both of these conditions respond very beautifully, as a rule, to steroid treatment given by either the oral or parenteral routes in rather large doses.

CLINICAL SYMPOSIA REPRINTS

EDITOR'S NOTE: So great has been the popularity of CLINICAL SYMPOSIA that it has become impossible to fill all requests for back issues or extra copies of current issues. Therefore, a new policy was adopted with the last issue devoted to "The Cellular Elements of the Blood." An unusually large supply of reprints without ads has been printed for subsequent distribution. These will be available at $1.00 per copy, to defray extra printing and handling charges. (Ordered in quantities of 25 to 49, the cost will be 75 cents per copy; 50 to 99, 60 cents per copy; and 100 or over, 45 cents per copy.)

Issues which are still on hand, such as *Pulmonary Emphysema* and *Survival in Nuclear Warfare*, will continue to be distributed gratis.

SECTION F

C I B A

THE ADRENAL GLAND

PETER H. FORSHAM, M.A., M.D.

Professor of Medicine and Pediatrics; Chief, Endocrinology and Metabolism;
Director, Metabolic Research Unit, University of California School of Medicine,
San Francisco, California.
Active Physician, University of California Hospitals, San Francisco.

The adrenal glands are flattened, cap-like structures covering the superior pole of each kidney at the level of the first lumbar vertebra. Normally, each adrenal weighs between 5 and 7 grams. In males they are about 30 per cent heavier than in females. The adrenal gland and kidney lie within a tough, fibrous, fascial compartment composed of Gerota's fascia. The gland is composed of an inner core, the medulla, and an outer shell, the cortex, the latter comprising about 80 per cent of the entire weight of the gland.

The *medulla* is dark red or brown in color and composed largely of cells called chromaffin cells, because they stain brown with chromic acid. This portion of the gland is derived from ectodermal stem cells which migrate down from the neural crest. Therefore, these chromaffin cells may be found not only in the adrenal medulla, but wherever sympathetic nerve tissue is found, particularly in the sympathetic nerve ganglia and plexuses and in the organ of Zuckerkandl at the bifurcation of the aorta.

The catecholamines manufactured by these cells as a result of sympathetic nerve stimulation are important in the reaction to acute, transient stress.

The *cortex* which surrounds the medulla is composed of large, lipid-laden epithelial cells, giving this portion of the gland its yellowish appearance. The cortex is divided into three layers or zones. The outer, zona glomerulosa, is the narrowest. Here the cells produce mostly mineralocorticoids and are little affected by corticotropin.

Beneath this zone are the much wider zona fasciculata and the zona reticularis, lying next to the medulla. These inner layers form glucocorticoids, 17-ketosteroids, and estrogens predominantly, and are dependent on corticotropin for growth and secretory stimulation.

In the inactive state, lipid-laden "vacuolated" cells predominate. During periods of increased secretory activity, these cells take on a "compact" appearance because of the discharge of stored lipid and cholesterol, the latter having been changed into steroid hormones.

Blood Supply

The adrenals are richly supplied with arterial blood through branches arising from the phrenic artery above, the aorta laterally, the renal artery below, and often from the intercostals as well. Additional branches may be received from the ovarian or internal spermatic artery on the left. On entering the gland, the vessels break up into sinusoids devoid of endothelial lining, which run through the cortex, ending in large, venous lacunae in the medulla, from which blood is collected into one large venous trunk and a number of smaller ones, ending in the renal vein.

Nerve Supply

The nerve supply is derived from the celiac and renal plexuses. Entering the lower and middle parts of the capsule,

3

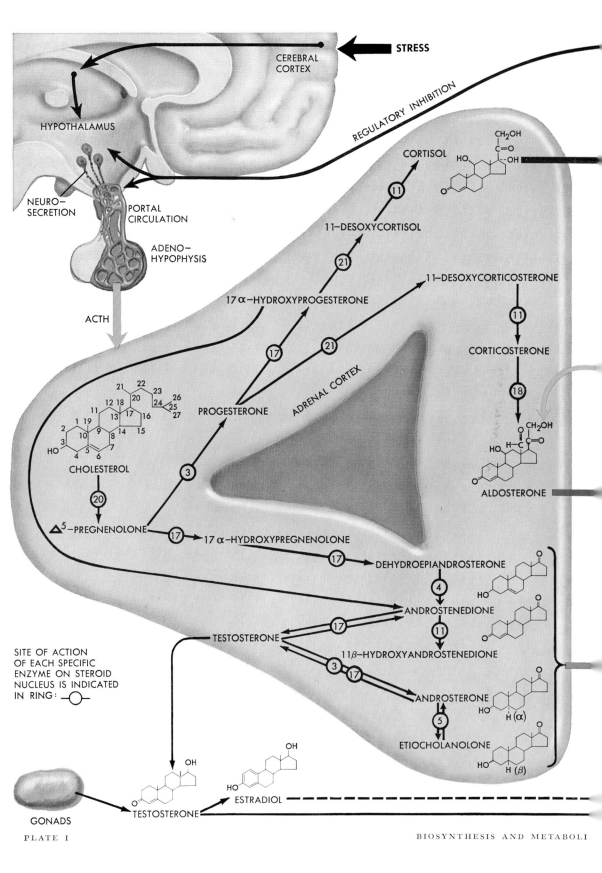

PLATE I

BIOSYNTHESIS AND METABOLI

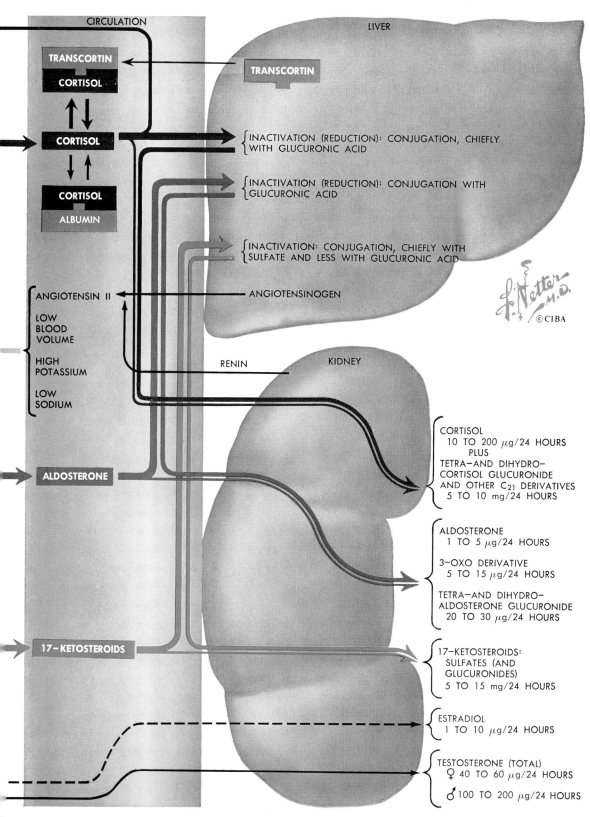

CIRCULATION

TRANSCORTIN

CORTISOL

TRANSCORTIN

LIVER

CORTISOL

{ INACTIVATION (REDUCTION): CONJUGATION, CHIEFLY
WITH GLUCURONIC ACID

CORTISOL

ALBUMIN

{ INACTIVATION (REDUCTION): CONJUGATION WITH
GLUCURONIC ACID

{ INACTIVATION: CONJUGATION, CHIEFLY WITH
SULFATE AND LESS WITH GLUCURONIC ACID

ANGIOTENSIN II

LOW
BLOOD
VOLUME

HIGH
POTASSIUM

LOW
SODIUM

ANGIOTENSINOGEN

RENIN

KIDNEY

ALDOSTERONE

CORTISOL
10 TO 200 μg/24 HOURS
PLUS
TETRA—AND DIHYDRO-
CORTISOL GLUCURONIDE
AND OTHER C$_{21}$ DERIVATIVES
5 TO 10 mg/24 HOURS

ALDOSTERONE
1 TO 5 μg/24 HOURS

3—OXO DERIVATIVE
5 TO 15 μg/24 HOURS

TETRA—AND DIHYDRO-
ALDOSTERONE GLUCURONIDE
20 TO 30 μg/24 HOURS

17- KETOSTEROIDS

{ 17—KETOSTEROIDS:
SULFATES (AND
GLUCURONIDES)
5 TO 15 mg/24 HOURS

{ ESTRADIOL
1 TO 10 μg/24 HOURS

{ TESTOSTERONE (TOTAL)
♀ 40 TO 60 μg/24 HOURS

♂ 100 TO 200 μg/24 HOURS

ADRENAL CORTICOIDS

©CIBA

they traverse the cortex and end around the cells of the medulla, where there are many small ganglia.

The steroid hormones produced by the adrenal cortex may be grouped broadly into corticoids, adrenal androgens (17-ketosteroids), aldosterone, estrogens, and progesteroids. Some of these hormones are highly potent biologically, while others are relatively inactive. In contrast to the adrenal medulla which is stimulated by sympathetic nerves, the activity of this portion of the gland is apparently wholly under the regulation of humoral mechanisms, no secretory nerve endings ever having been demonstrated here.

Structure, growth, and secretory activity (except for aldosterone) are entirely regulated by the anterior pituitary hormone, corticotropin. This hormone is produced and released from certain basophils as well as some large chromophobe cells in the anterior pituitary gland or adenohypophysis.

As indicated by the arrows in Plate I, stressful stimuli reaching the cerebral cortex release the inhibition of the reticular formation or of the limbic system upon hypothalamic centers in and around the tubero-infundibular nucleus and the median eminence. Large neurons then secrete corticotropin-releasing factor (CRF), a polypeptide hormone mediator. Pitressin (ADH), as well as other synthetic short-chain peptides, also has a corticotropin-releasing effect.

Of the various hormones released as a result of corticotropin secretion, only cortisol (hydrocortisone) has a feedback inhibitory effect. The higher the level of cortisol, the lower the secretion of corticotropin and vice versa. This "servoregulation" maintains the level of circulating plasma cortisol within relatively narrow limits unless there is a stressful situation, which will induce an increase in ACTH, irrespective of the level of circulating cortisol.

There is a diurnal variation in the levels of both corticotropin and cortisol. Soon after midnight, levels of 17-hydroxycorticoids in the blood rise, rapidly reaching a maximum about 6 a.m., after which there is a gradual decline to the lowest level reached between early evening and midnight. Under basal conditions the adrenals secrete 70 per cent of their 17-hydroxycorticoids between midnight and 6 a.m., the other 30 per cent during the remainder of the day.

Changes in urinary levels reflect plasma levels with a brief lag. Thus, if three 8-hour collections are made starting at 7 a.m., one finds most of the 17-hydroxycorticoids in the first 8 hours, least in the next 8 hours (3 p.m. to 11 p.m.). The 11 p.m. to 7 a.m. specimen contains an intermediate amount.

This diurnal rhythm is abolished in most cases of Cushing's syndrome due to bilateral adrenal hyperplasia or tumor and also by destruction of the pretectorial or temporal lobe as well as other central nervous system lesions.

As indicated in Plate I, all adrenal steroid hormones are derived from cholesterol, which is present in abundance in the gland in the inactive state. The basic cyclopentanophenanthrene ring of cholesterol is modified by enzymes (hydroxylases) which introduce hydroxy groups into specific positions of the ring, each of which is numbered, as shown in Plate I and also in Figure 1. Other enzymes (dehydrogenases) may remove hydrogen from an OH group, while others (oxidases) remove hydrogen from a CH group, each at specific positions.

More than 50 different steroids have so far been isolated from the adrenal cortex.

6

Of these, only a few are normally secreted into the blood stream. The rest are intracellular intermediates. The compounds isolated normally from the adrenal vein may be divided into glucocorticoids, the mineralocorticoids, weak androgens, progesteroids, and estrogens.

The *glucocorticoids* are distinguished by an alpha-ketol group and an 11-hydroxyl group. These include cortisol, bearing a 17-hydroxyl group, of which 15 to 20 mg. are secreted each day in adults under basal conditions, and corticosterone, of which 2 to 5 mg. are secreted daily.

The *mineralocorticoids* include aldosterone, 75 to 125 micrograms of which are secreted daily, and 11-desoxycorticosterone, normally found only in traces.

The weak *androgens* produced by the adrenal are known as *17-ketosteroids* or 17-oxosteroids because each has an atom of oxygen in the 17 position. Also, testosterone, a 17-hydroxy derivative, has recently been isolated from normal human adrenal tissue in vitro. Of the 17-ketosteroids, about 75 per cent is in the form of dehydroepiandrosterone (DEA), a weak androgen about 1/20th the potency of testosterone. It is secreted in quantities of about 25 to 30 mg. daily, an amount which exceeds that of cortisol. DEA secretion is depressed by cortisol but stimulated 2-fold by ACTH. The biologic synthesis of all of these hormones is indicated in Plate I and Figure 1. In addition, the adrenal secretes approximately 0.4 to 0.8 mg. daily of progesterone and small amounts of estradiol derived from testosterone and estrone derived from androstenedione.

METABOLISM OF ADRENAL STEROIDS

Metabolism of Glucocorticoids

Cortisol represents over 80 per cent of the total 17-hydroxycorticoids, or Porter-Silber chromogens, found in the blood stream. About one-half circulates in the form of the original molecule. The remainder circulates as the reduced, inactive tetrahydro- derivative, conjugated at C-3 with glucuronic acid, and to a much smaller extent with sulfate.

The biologically active, unconjugated cortisol in the plasma is bound to some extent by albumin and also to an alpha-globulin derived mainly from the liver. This latter substance is called *transcortin* or corticosterone-binding globulin (CBG). The CBG mechanism assures a ready source of available circulating hormone, while protecting it from inactivation and conjugation in the liver. In addition, CBG solubilizes cortisol which of itself has only limited solubility. The binding mechanism affects the unconjugated metabolites very little and the conjugated material not at all.

The production of CBG is increased markedly by estrogen therapy. In the later stages of pregnancy, the titer of CBG-bound cortisol may be increased 3-fold. Yet there are no manifestations of hyperadrenocorticism since most of the active hormone is not available to the tissue. Conversely, a lowering of transcortin occurs in various conditions which are characterized by abnormalities of serum proteins. These include cirrhosis, nephrosis, and multiple myeloma. In these diseases the relative excess of unchanged cortisol rapidly suppresses ACTH secretion so that hyperadrenocorticism does not usually develop.

The half-life of free cortisol in the plasma, determined with C-14 labeled cortisol in tracer amounts, is normally about 2 hours. This period is markedly increased by liver dysfunction and decreased by thyrotoxicosis. This results from changes in the catabolism of cortisol in the liver, which reduces cortisol to tetra- and dihydrocortisol, which is quickly solubilized by conjugation with glucuronic acid, preparing it for rapid urinary clearance.

7

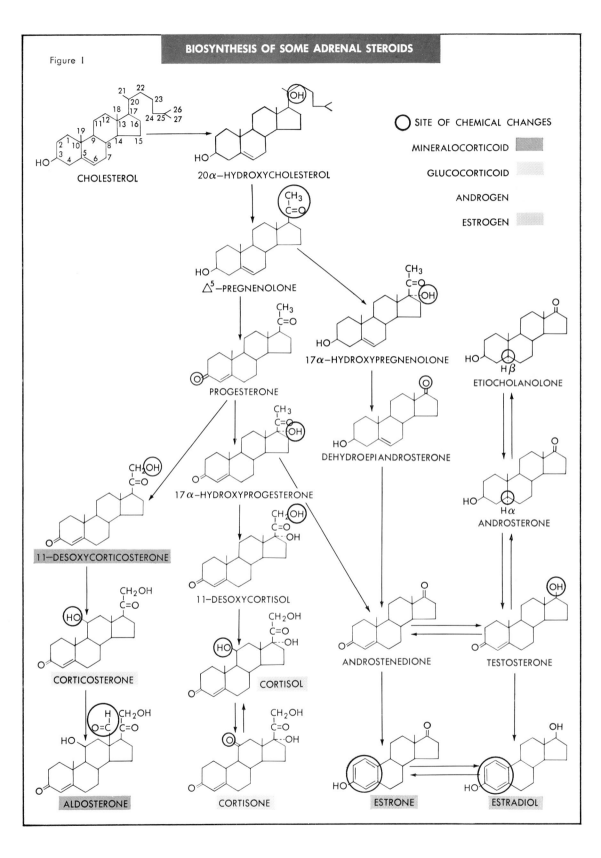

BIOSYNTHESIS OF SOME ADRENAL STEROIDS

Figure 1

CHOLESTEROL

20α–HYDROXYCHOLESTEROL

○ SITE OF CHEMICAL CHANGES

MINERALOCORTICOID

GLUCOCORTICOID

ANDROGEN

ESTROGEN

Δ⁵–PREGNENOLONE

17α–HYDROXYPREGNENOLONE

ETIOCHOLANOLONE

PROGESTERONE

DEHYDROEPIANDROSTERONE

ANDROSTERONE

17α–HYDROXYPROGESTERONE

11–DESOXYCORTICOSTERONE

11–DESOXYCORTISOL

CORTICOSTERONE

CORTISOL

ANDROSTENEDIONE

TESTOSTERONE

ALDOSTERONE

CORTISONE

ESTRONE

ESTRADIOL

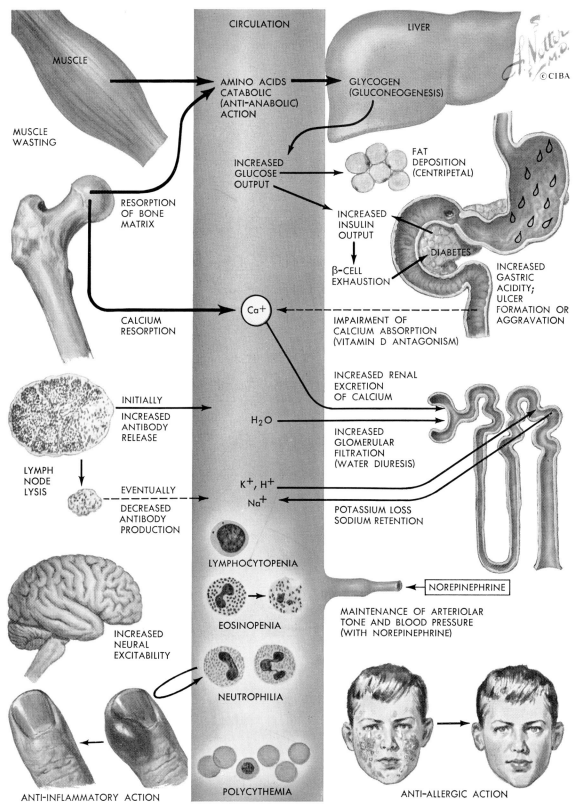

CIRCULATION

LIVER

MUSCLE

MUSCLE WASTING

AMINO ACIDS CATABOLIC (ANTI-ANABOLIC) ACTION

GLYCOGEN (GLUCONEOGENESIS)

RESORPTION OF BONE MATRIX

INCREASED GLUCOSE OUTPUT

FAT DEPOSITION (CENTRIPETAL)

INCREASED INSULIN OUTPUT

DIABETES

β-CELL EXHAUSTION

INCREASED GASTRIC ACIDITY; ULCER FORMATION OR AGGRAVATION

CALCIUM RESORPTION

Ca^+

IMPAIRMENT OF CALCIUM ABSORPTION (VITAMIN D ANTAGONISM)

INCREASED RENAL EXCRETION OF CALCIUM

H_2O

INITIALLY INCREASED ANTIBODY RELEASE

INCREASED GLOMERULAR FILTRATION (WATER DIURESIS)

LYMPH NODE LYSIS

EVENTUALLY DECREASED ANTIBODY PRODUCTION

K^+, H^+

Na^+

POTASSIUM LOSS SODIUM RETENTION

LYMPHOCYTOPENIA

EOSINOPENIA

NOREPINEPHRINE

INCREASED NEURAL EXCITABILITY

MAINTENANCE OF ARTERIOLAR TONE AND BLOOD PRESSURE (WITH NOREPINEPHRINE)

NEUTROPHILIA

ANTI-INFLAMMATORY ACTION

POLYCYTHEMIA

ANTI-ALLERGIC ACTION

PLATE II

ACTION OF CORTISOL

The degradation of cortisone into inactive metabolites is quite similar to that of cortisol. Since hydrocortisone (cortisol) and cortisone are freely interchangeable by enzymic action in the adrenal and the liver (Figure 1), a considerable amount of tetrahydrocortisone and cortisone may be found in the urine, particularly so in the hyperthyroid state.

Metabolism of 17-Ketosteroids

As shown in both Plate I and Figure 1, the dehydroepiandrosterone (known in the past as dehydro-isoandrosterone) is a precursor of a number of adrenal 17-ketosteroids, including etiocholanolone and androsterone. It has been shown to be present largely as the water soluble sulfate in the adrenal cortex itself. It is apparently carried to enzyme sites in this form, and in the presence of sulfatase at these enzyme sites, it is hydrolyzed and then transformed as shown in Plate I. In addition to the production of 17-ketosteroids, the adrenal, like the testes and to a smaller extent the ovaries, produces testosterone. This is the most potent of the androgens, being approximately 20 to 30 times as potent as any of the 17-ketosteroids. The biosynthesis of testosterone in the adrenal is shown in Figure 1. In females, up to 40 to 60 micrograms of free testosterone are found daily in the urine. These are mostly of adrenal origin. In young males, as much as 100 micrograms are excreted daily, and fully twice as much may be recovered when the glucuronides in the urine are first hydrolyzed.

The 17-ketosteroids, such as dehydroepiandrosterone, are conjugated at the C-3 position mainly by sulfate, whereas etiocholanolone and androsterone are found mainly as glucuronides in the urine. Both are solubilized forms which are rapidly excreted. The daily excretion of 17-ketosteroids amounts normally to 10 mg. ± 5 mg. in females, 12 to 15 mg. ± 5 mg. in males.

Metabolism of Aldosterone

This hormone follows the same metabolic pattern as cortisol, consisting of intrahepatic reduction and biologic inactivation, and conjugation of the tetrahydro- derivative with glucuronate at the C-3 hydroxyl group. Twenty to 30 micrograms of this conjugate are excreted daily. In addition, 5 to 15 micrograms of the 3-oxo glucuronic acid conjugate are excreted daily. A much smaller fraction of aldosterone, between 1 and 5 micrograms, appears in the urine in the free form.

ACTION OF GLUCOCORTICOIDS

By far the most abundant and active glucocorticoids in man are cortisol and cortisone. The various physiologic actions of these hormones are diagrammatically illustrated in Plate II.

As the term "glucocorticoid" implies, one of the most important actions of these hormones is gluconeogenesis.

Gluconeogenesis

This is fundamentally a catabolic process in which there is deamination of amino acids making up the protein, with nitrogen loss and increased formation of glucose, with a rise in both liver glycogen and blood sugar. The rise in the glucose level of the blood may temporarily be counterbalanced by an increase in insulin output, which may or may not be sufficient to prevent glycosuria. In the end, however, if cortisol is present in excess (Cushing's syndrome) or administered for prolonged periods, the beta cells of the pancreas may become exhausted, and a true *steroid diabetes* (metadiabetes) ensues.

The abnormal breakdown of protein results in *muscle weakness and wasting* and *loss of bone matrix*. Loss of bone matrix results in *resorption of calcium* content and increased excretion of calcium in the

10

TABLE 1.

RELATIVE ANTI-INFLAMMATORY POTENCY AND SODIUM-RETAINING EFFECT OF VARIOUS CORTICOIDS USED IN THERAPY

COMPOUND	RELATIVE POTENCY COMPARED TO CORTISOL	RELATIVE SODIUM-RETAINING ACTIVITY
Cortisol	1	+ +
Cortisone Acetate	0.8	+ +
Prednisolone	4	+
Prednisone	3.5	+
Triamcinolone	5	0
6-Methylprednisolone	5	0
Haldranolone	10	0
Betamethasone	25	0
Dexamethasone*	30	0
9 α-fluorohydrocortisone	15	+ + + + +

*Available commercially as Gammacorten®.

urine. In addition, calcium absorption from the gut is impaired because of cortisol antagonism to vitamin D. In Cushing's syndrome and prolonged corticoid therapy, the result is osteoporosis, and spontaneous fractures may occur.

In children receiving corticoid therapy, the epiphysial plate is thinned, cartilage development is impeded, formation of new bone is blocked at the level of the matrix, and osteoblasts are scarce. Consequently, there is temporary growth arrest.

Effect on Fat Metabolism

As in the case of glucose, total fat is increased at the expense of protein. This is deposited in a characteristic distribution limited to the head and trunk, with the moon face, "buffalo hump," supraclavicular fat pads, and pendulous abdomen seen in Cushing's syndrome. Chronic excess of cortisol leads to hyperlipemia and hypercholesterolemia.

Effect on Water Metabolism

Both cortisol and cortisone enhance water diuresis. This is probably due mostly to increased glomerular filtration and to a lesser extent to antagonism of the antidiuretic hormone's effect on water reabsorption at the tubular level. In the absence of cortisol and cortisone, a water load is not disposed of for 12 hours or more, a fact utilized in the socalled water test for adrenocortical insufficiency. The dehydration of Addison's disease is, of course, secondary to salt loss, rather than a result of any primary changes in the movement of water.

Effect on Ion Exchange in the Kidney

These hormones have a relatively minor effect on sodium reabsorption in the kidney. Nevertheless, they do have some slight effect in increasing the reabsorption of sodium, with consequent loss of potassium and hydrogen ions given in exchange

11

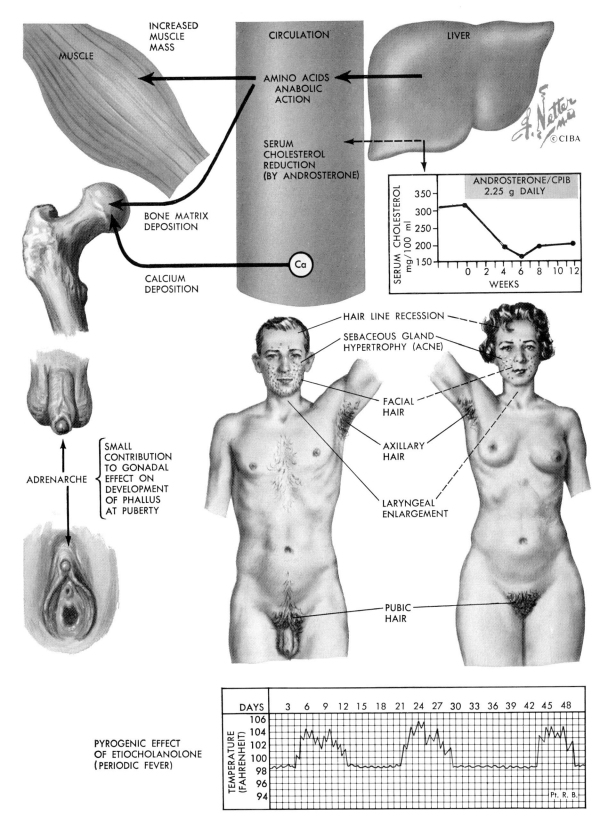

MUSCLE

INCREASED
MUSCLE
MASS

CIRCULATION

LIVER

AMINO ACIDS
ANABOLIC
ACTION

SERUM
CHOLESTEROL
REDUCTION
(BY ANDROSTERONE)

ANDROSTERONE/CPIB
2.25 g DAILY

SERUM CHOLESTEROL
mg/100 ml

350
300
250
200
150

0 2 4 6 8 10 12
WEEKS

BONE MATRIX
DEPOSITION

CALCIUM
DEPOSITION

Ca

HAIR LINE RECESSION

SEBACEOUS GLAND
HYPERTROPHY (ACNE)

FACIAL
HAIR

AXILLARY
HAIR

LARYNGEAL
ENLARGEMENT

ADRENARCHE

SMALL
CONTRIBUTION
TO GONADAL
EFFECT ON
DEVELOPMENT
OF PHALLUS
AT PUBERTY

PUBIC
HAIR

PYROGENIC EFFECT
OF ETIOCHOLANOLONE
(PERIODIC FEVER)

DAYS   3   6   9 12 15 18 21 24 27 30 33 36 39 42 45 48

TEMPERATURE
(FAHRENHEIT)

106
104
102
100
98
96
94

Pt. R. B.

PLATE III

ACTION OF ADRENAL ANDROGENS

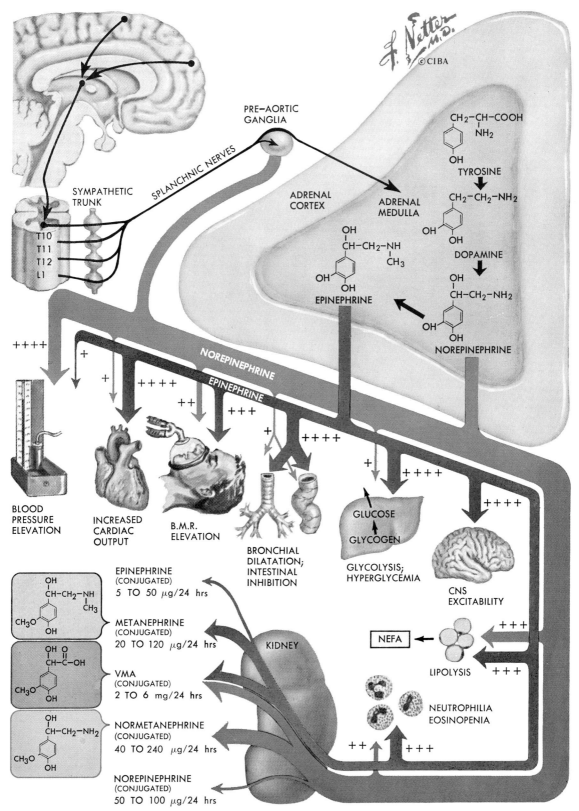

PRE–AORTIC
GANGLIA

SYMPATHETIC
TRUNK

SPLANCHNIC NERVES

T10
T11
T12
L1

ADRENAL
CORTEX

ADRENAL
MEDULLA

$CH_2-CH-COOH$
NH_2
OH
TYROSINE

$CH_2-CH_2-NH_2$
OH
OH
DOPAMINE

OH
$CH-CH_2-NH_2$
OH
OH
NOREPINEPHRINE

OH
$CH-CH_2-NH$
CH_3
OH
OH
EPINEPHRINE

++++
+
+
++++
EPINEPHRINE
++
+++
NOREPINEPHRINE
+
++++
+
++++
++++

BLOOD
PRESSURE
ELEVATION

INCREASED
CARDIAC
OUTPUT

B.M.R.
ELEVATION

BRONCHIAL
DILATATION;
INTESTINAL
INHIBITION

GLUCOSE
GLYCOGEN

GLYCOLYSIS;
HYPERGLYCEMIA

CNS
EXCITABILITY

+++
NEFA
LIPOLYSIS   +++

OH
$CH-CH_2-NH$
CH_3
CH_3O
OH

EPINEPHRINE
(CONJUGATED)
5 TO 50 μg/24 hrs

METANEPHRINE
(CONJUGATED)
20 TO 120 μg/24 hrs

KIDNEY

OH O
$CH-C-OH$
CH_3O
OH

VMA
(CONJUGATED)
2 TO 6 mg/24 hrs

OH
$CH-CH_2-NH_2$
CH_3O
OH

NORMETANEPHRINE
(CONJUGATED)
40 TO 240 μg/24 hrs

NEUTROPHILIA
EOSINOPENIA

++
+++

NOREPINEPHRINE
(CONJUGATED)
50 TO 100 μg/24 hrs

PLATE IV

SYNTHESIS, METABOLISM, AND ACTION OF CATECHOLAMINES

in the distal tubule. However, most of the modern synthetic corticoids, such as dexamethasone,* are devoid of any sodium retaining effect (see Table 1).

Immunologic Effects

Initially, antibodies may be increased by lysis of lymph nodes and plasma cells. However, this effect is quite transient and requires large doses. Resistance to infection is eventually reduced by loss of antibody-forming tissues. Glucocorticoids also protect target tissue against the ill effects of antigen-antibody complexes, doing this even at moderate dose levels.

Central Nervous System Effects

Apparently the central nervous system requires a near-optimal level of cortisol, because psychiatric disturbances are common both when there is either a deficiency or an excess of this hormone. As many as 40 per cent of patients with Cushing's syndrome show some major psychotic abnormalities. Indeed, one of Dr. Cushing's first cases was found in an insane asylum.

In adrenocortical insufficiency, a slowing of the electrical discharges in the electroencephalogram, reversible with cortisol, has been clearly shown. In excess, the threshold of electrical excitation of the brain is lowered by this hormone — a phenomenon that accounts for the increased tendency of epileptic seizures in patients treated with cortisol.

Hematologic Effects

Because of the lysis of lymphoid tissue already mentioned, circulating lymphocytes are reduced by glucocorticoids with or without a 17-hydroxyl group. Thus in Cushing's syndrome, the lymphocytes usually make up less than 15 per cent of the total leukocytes. Indeed, an intramuscular injection of corticotropin will

---

*Available commercially as Gammacorten®.

reduce circulating lymphocytes as much as 45 per cent in 4 hours. Eosinophils are depressed by cortisol and cortisone and also by aldosterone. This effect is not due to suppression of bone marrow but to increased sequestration in lungs and spleen and increased destruction in the blood. The basophils suffer a similar fate. However, the over-all white count is significantly raised, reaching 12,000 to 15,000 following corticoid administration for any length of time. In the presence of infection the count may reach 20,000 to 30,000. This is in part due to increased formation as indicated by an increased number of young forms and also to a sharp decrease in diapedesis around foci of infection. Erythrocytes are increased, leading to polycythemia. Thrombocytes also are increased in number.

Potentiation of Vasopressors

On occasion a hypotensive state unresponsive to pressor agents, such as norepinephrine, will yield promptly to a large dose (100 mg. or more) of cortisol or an equivalent synthetic corticoid given intramuscularly. An immediate rise in blood pressure follows in spite of a preceding normal level of 17-hydroxycorticoids. Apparently a sensitization of the vessel wall to the catecholamine is responsible.

Anti-inflammatory and Anti-allergic Action

These actions of the glucocorticoids form the basis of their widespread clinical use. Inflammatory responses are decreased, fibrosis is prevented, and subsequent degeneration is minimized. Thus these hormones tend to abolish the manifestations of disease without antagonizing the causative agent directly. Yet, when administered early, they help to prevent death during the acute phases of inflammatory or allergic disease. They also inhibit subsequent reparative and fibrotic changes to some extent.

This then is the rationale underlying their therapeutic use: the early preventive use of high doses or the late establishment of a maintenance regimen with a moderate, near physiologic dosage when the disease continues to smolder. When used in this way, they have proved lifesaving in some, life-maintaining in many.

Specific recommendations for therapy are beyond our present scope; however, a few words of a general nature may be desirable.

Therapeutic Use of Corticoids

In the therapeutic use of corticoids and corticotropin, clinical response is the only criterion on which to base dosage, constantly weighing the improvement that may be produced with the side effects which will be discussed below.

High dosage of 60 to 1,000 mg. of cortisol or 2 to 30 mg. of dexamethasone* is required where *mesenchymal suppression* is desired. Doses of this magnitude may be administered for less than 1 week in the following conditions:

Aspiration pneumonitis

Lye and other burns of the esophagus

Acute serum disease, e.g., penicillin reaction, bee sting

Acute secondary glaucoma

Acute vascular collapse unresponsive to pressor agents.

Dosage of the order mentioned above may be required for prolonged periods in the following conditions:

Pemphigus

Lupus crises

Nephrosis unresponsive to intermittent therapy

Chronic pulmonary fibrosis no longer responding to moderate dosage

Acute phase of rheumatic fever early in the course

Overwhelming polyarteritis including trichinosis

Waterhouse-Friderichsen syndrome

Subacute lymphatic leukemia

Thrombotic thrombocytopenic purpura.

Moderate dosage in the range of 30 to 60 mg. of cortisol or 1 to 2 mg. of dexamethasone* may be given in a number of conditions including:

Allergic Conditions: bronchial asthma; severe hay fever; allergic rhinitis; angioneurotic edema; atopic dermatitis; neurodermatitis; allergic eczema.

Blood Dyscrasias: idiopathic thrombocytopenic purpura; allergic purpura; acquired hemolytic anemia.

Eye Diseases: acute uveitis; choroiditis; optic neuritis; sympathetic ophthalmia; macular degeneration.

Collagen Diseases: disseminated lupus erythematosus; dermatomyositis; only exceptionally and in small dosage in scleroderma and rheumatoid arthritis; erythema nodosum; nonsupportive panniculitis.

Gastrointestinal Diseases: ileitis; ulcerative colitis.

Infectious Diseases: in conjunction with specific antibiotics, but only for *selected* cases of pulmonary, urogenital, or bone tuberculosis, and in tuberculous meningitis.

Miscellaneous Conditions: Bell's palsy; nasal polyps; sarcoidosis; nephrosis; pulmonary emphysema; acute gouty arthritis only in patients sensitive to colchicine; androgenital syndrome; adrenal insufficiency; supportive therapy in terminal cases of leukemia, Hodgkin's disease, carcinoma.

One must bear constantly in mind that when treating chronic disease one should start with the smallest possible dose, gradually increasing it, but never aspiring to more than 60 per cent clinical improvement. To expect more is to court the inevitable appearance of serious side effects.

Of course, in life-threatening situations one may be forced to start with a maximal dose equivalent to 200 mg. of cortisol or 7 mg. of dexamethasone.* This should not be maintained longer than 10 days and then reduced gradually. In general, dose

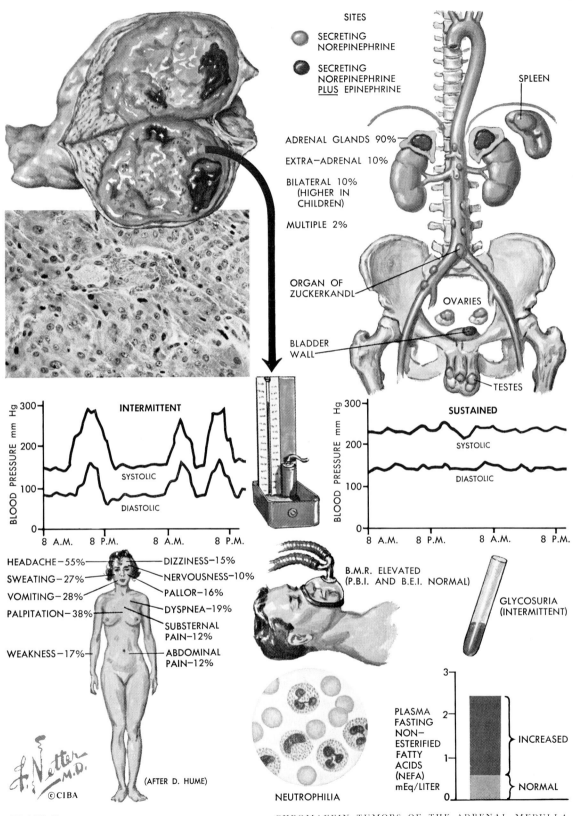

SITES

SECRETING NOREPINEPHRINE

SECRETING NOREPINEPHRINE PLUS EPINEPHRINE

SPLEEN

ADRENAL GLANDS 90%

EXTRA–ADRENAL 10%

BILATERAL 10% (HIGHER IN CHILDREN)

MULTIPLE 2%

ORGAN OF ZUCKERKANDL

OVARIES

BLADDER WALL

TESTES

INTERMITTENT

BLOOD PRESSURE mm Hg

300

200

100

0

SYSTOLIC

DIASTOLIC

8 A.M. 8 P.M. 8 A.M. 8 P.M.

SUSTAINED

BLOOD PRESSURE mm Hg

300

200

100

0

SYSTOLIC

DIASTOLIC

8 A.M. 8 P.M. 8 A.M. 8 P.M.

HEADACHE–55%

SWEATING–27%

VOMITING–28%

PALPITATION–38%

WEAKNESS–17%

DIZZINESS–15%

NERVOUSNESS–10%

PALLOR–16%

DYSPNEA–19%

SUBSTERNAL PAIN–12%

ABDOMINAL PAIN–12%

(AFTER D. HUME)

B.M.R. ELEVATED (P.B.I. AND B.E.I. NORMAL)

GLYCOSURIA (INTERMITTENT)

NEUTROPHILIA

PLASMA FASTING NON–ESTERIFIED FATTY ACIDS (NEFA) mEq/LITER

3

2

1

0

INCREASED

NORMAL

F. Netter M.D.
©CIBA

PLATE V

CHROMAFFIN TUMORS OF THE ADRENAL MEDULLA

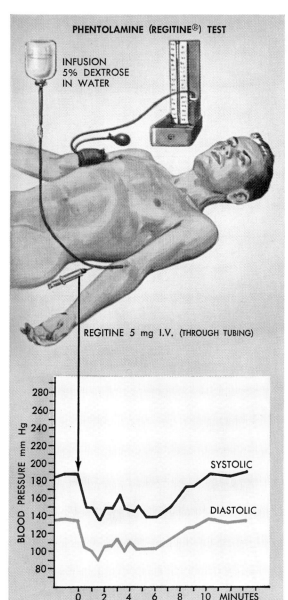

PHENTOLAMINE (REGITINE®) TEST

INFUSION 5% DEXTROSE IN WATER

REGITINE 5 mg I.V. (THROUGH TUBING)

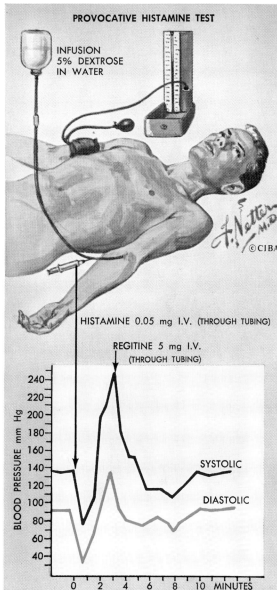

PROVOCATIVE HISTAMINE TEST

INFUSION 5% DEXTROSE IN WATER

HISTAMINE 0.05 mg I.V. (THROUGH TUBING)

REGITINE 5 mg I.V. (THROUGH TUBING)

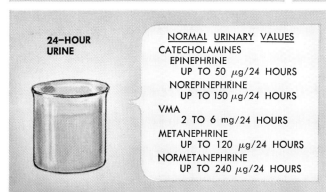

24-HOUR URINE

NORMAL URINARY VALUES

CATECHOLAMINES
EPINEPHRINE
UP TO 50 μg/24 HOURS
NOREPINEPHRINE
UP TO 150 μg/24 HOURS
VMA
2 TO 6 mg/24 HOURS
METANEPHRINE
UP TO 120 μg/24 HOURS
NORMETANEPHRINE
UP TO 240 μg/24 HOURS

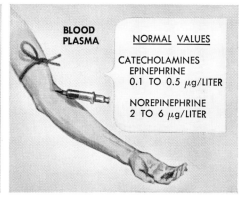

BLOOD PLASMA

NORMAL VALUES

CATECHOLAMINES
EPINEPHRINE
0.1 TO 0.5 μg/LITER

NOREPINEPHRINE
2 TO 6 μg/LITER

PLATE VI   TESTS FOR PHEOCHROMOCYTOMA

"from the bottom up" in long-range therapy; "from the top down" only when handling acute, self-limited conditions.

Side Effects

(1) *Weight gain and edema.* Weight gain may be decreased by a high protein, low caloric diet. Salt and water retention, leading to edema, is no longer important with the latest synthetic corticoids which are devoid of sodium-retaining effect (see Table 1, page 11).

(2) *Hypochloremic-hypokalemic alkalosis.* This is rarely of disturbing magnitude. It may be completely prevented by giving supplemental potassium.

(3) *Negative nitrogen balance.* May be partly decreased by an anabolic agent such as methandrostenolone (Dianabol).

(4) *Thrombophlebitis and coronary occlusion* tends to occur when the dose of corticosteroid is reduced or especially when treatment is stopped suddenly. This is prevented by good hydration, exercise, and anticoagulant therapy on slightest suspicion.

(5) *Bleeding tendencies and ecchymoses,* found increasingly with the use of more potent derivatives, are due to loss of vascular elastic tissue rather than blood dyscrasia and call for avoidance of any superficial trauma.

(6) *Increased gastric acidity* and *ulcer formation* may be minimized by antacids and anticholinergics.

(7) *Glycosuria* should be controlled by tolbutamide or insulin when fasting blood sugar is above 130, especially where there is a family history of diabetes.

(8) *Sleeplessness* can be minimized by giving the last dose of corticosteroid at 6 p.m. Sedatives or tranquilizers are helpful.

(9) *Psychosis.* Danger signals are inability to concentrate, weird dreams, and nightmares and are an indication to decrease the dose gradually. However, one must not stop suddenly since this may be catastrophic in terms of the original disease.

(10) *Superinfection.* This is a dreaded complication, to be minimized by extreme cleanliness, aseptic techniques, and appropriate and preferably bactericidal agents as opposed to bacteriostatic ones.

ACTION OF 17-KETOSTEROIDS

The 17-ketosteroids produced by the adrenal include dehydroepiandrosterone, etiocholanolone, and androsterone, all weak androgens which are excreted as sulfates, glucuronidates, and 11-oxy derivatives in an amount of 5 to 15 mg. daily. In addition, the adrenal is an important source of testosterone in both males and females.

The action of these androgens may be divided into their anabolic effect on protein synthesis and breakdown and their effect on secondary sex characteristics.

Anabolic Effect

Nitrogen balance studies have repeatedly proved that androgens retain nitrogen due to increased synthesis of protein from amino acids. This leads to increased muscle strength and development (Plate III). Also a greater degree of assurance and aggressiveness has been attributed to the anabolic influence of androgens. These effects can perhaps best be visualized by contrasting the bull and steer in both muscular development and mental outlook.

Since protein is an important constituent of bone matrix, the anabolic effect improves bone development and increases the utilization of calcium.

Androgenic Effects

Androgens are stimulating to male sex characteristics — inhibiting to female sex characteristics. However, they stimulate growth of pubic hair in both sexes. Androgens in the male promote growth of phallus and prostate, cause a deepening of voice, growth of facial and axillary hair, and in some men baldness (a sex-linked characteristic).

In normal subjects, the relatively low androgenic potency of adrenal 17-keto-steroids contributes mainly an anabolic effect, adding little to normal development of sex characteristics. However, in the abnormal amounts present in the adrenogenital syndrome, conspicuous alterations in sex characteristics are encountered in the female.

Pyrogenic Effect

Etiocholanolone and related compounds produce hyperpyrexia on intravenous administration — and have been found in excessive amounts in certain patients with unexplained periodic fevers.

Cholesterol-Lowering Effect of Androsterone

Unlike testosterone, androsterone has been found to lower serum cholesterol when given by mouth as a solubilized (CPIB) derivative.

THE ADRENAL MEDULLA

The adrenal medulla supplies the catecholamines, epinephrine and norepinephrine, which are so essential to successful "fight or flight." One of the important effects of these humoral substances is the temporary elevation of blood pressure which they so characteristically produce.

Thus they share a function possessed by one of the cortical hormones, aldosterone, which in a different fashion helps maintain a normal level of blood pressure. This interrelationship is of considerable practical importance because hypertension may be caused by abnormally high levels of either catecholamines or aldosterone. Because of the importance of this differential point, the medulla will be discussed before the remaining cortical hormone, aldosterone, is considered.

Physiology

The polyhedral chromaffin cells of the medulla are arranged in networks of anastomosing chords. They respond primarily to splanchnic nerve stimulation. Thus they are designed to respond to emergency situations.

As indicated in Plate IV, these cells receive sympathetic stimuli from T-10 through L-1 via pre-aortic ganglia. Thus stimulated by acetylcholine, the chromaffin cells produce the catecholamines, norepinephrine and epinephrine. Certain cells produce only norepinephrine, others only epinephrine. Indeed, the fetal adrenal contains only norepinephrine, epinephrine appearing some time after birth.

Insulin hypoglycemia will deplete the epinephrine-secreting cells, sparing the norepinephrine cells, while on the other hand reserpine in low doses causes the loss of norepinephrine only. Section of the splanchnic nerves abolishes the secretory response of the adrenal medulla.

Biosynthesis of Catecholamines

This process starts with phenylalanine, which is oxidized to tyrosine enzymatically. Tyrosine in turn is transformed into dihydroxyphenylalanine (DOPA) by the enzyme, tyrosinase. This is then transformed into dopamine (hydroxytyramine), which is then converted by an alphahydroxylase to norepinephrine, and thence by an N-methylating enzyme to epinephrine as shown in Plate IV. The average combined norepinephrine-epinephrine content of the normal human adrenal medulla is 2 to 4 mg. per gram of tissue, of which only 20 to 30 per cent is norepinephrine, whereas this latter hormone predominates in all extramedullary catecholamine-secreting tissues.

Metabolism of Medullary Hormones

Both epinephrine and norepinephrine are inactivated rapidly in the blood stream. Following intravenous infusion, less than 4 per cent is recovered as such in the urine. Both are normally metabolized by a combination of oxidative deamination (20 per cent) and ortho-methylation (80 per cent).

Catechol methyltransferase is present in all tissues in which the catecholamines exert an effect, with the exception of plasma and skeletal muscle. The metabolic end products excreted in the urine are shown in Plate IV. It will be noted that both epinephrine and norepinephrine yield metabolites in considerable quantity, being excreted as metanephrine, normetanephrine, and vinyl mandelic acid (VMA).

Pharmacophysiology

Epinephrine and norepinephrine differ considerably in the degree of their pharmacologic and physiologic actions as indicated in Plate IV. At one end of the scale, norepinephrine has far greater effect on blood pressure than does epinephrine. On the other hand, epinephrine stimulates the central nervous system, accelerates the heart, and dilates the bronchi far more than does norepinephrine. Also, hyperglycemia produced by activation of the liver enzyme, phosphorylase, for the degradation of glycogen to glucose is primarily affected by epinephrine.

Both have equal effect in the liberation of nonesterified fatty acids (NEFA) from the neutral lipids of fat depots, thus raising the NEFA levels in the plasma above the normal 0.4 ± 2 mEq. per liter.

PHEOCHROMOCYTOMA

This is a chromaffin tissue tumor, 90 per cent of which occur in the adrenal gland itself. In about 10 per cent of all cases tumors are found bilaterally, a figure that is higher in children, lower in adults. The extra-adrenal locations of pheochromocytoma (10 per cent of cases)

are indicated in Plate V. In about 14 per cent of cases, the tumor is large enough to be palpated. In most locations these tumors secrete only norepinephrine; in tumors of the adrenal medulla and rare tumors implanted in the wall of the bladder, both norepinephrine and epinephrine are secreted.

In autopsies performed at the Mayo Clinic the incidence of pheochromocytoma was 1 per 1,000. Both higher and lower figures have been reported elsewhere. Thus, it is a rare cause of hypertension, but being a curable one it deserves consideration and appropriate diagnostic testing in suspected cases.

Clinical Picture

As indicated in Plate V, elevation of blood pressure may be intermittent or sustained. Occasionally it is absent. Although paroxysmal hypertension is often considered characteristic, only 20 to 50 per cent of adults show this type of hypertension, and in over 50 per cent of adults and 90 per cent or more of children, a sustained rather than an intermittent hypertension is found. The frequency of symptoms in adults suffering the paroxysmal type of hypertension is shown in Plate V.

In children, the sweating and visual complaints are more common, constipation is frequently present, and about 10 per cent have puffy, red, cyanotic hands, a symptom not usually found in adults.

Attacks of *paroxysmal hypertension* come on suddenly, last for minutes or hours and are usually brought on by some emotional or postural trigger mechanism such as a sudden change in posture or urination. Following the attack, which ends with sweating, there is extreme fatigue and prostration.

The *sustained* type of *hypertension* is hard to distinguish clinically from essential or malignant hypertension, except for the signs of epinephrine excess such as prodromal anxiety, tremor, difficulty in focusing, and dilatation of the pupils.

A pheochromocytoma should be suspected in patients having a continuous hypertension, atypical paroxysmal attacks of hypertension, unexplained hypertensive reactions during induction of anesthesia, unexplained shock during anesthesia in the absence of demonstrable hemorrhage, hypertension with signs of hyperthyroidism, including an elevated basal metabolic rate but normal cholesterol and normal protein-bound iodine values, intermittent glycosuria, or acute anxiety attacks.

Diagnosis

In preliminary work-up a neutrophilia with a "shift to the left," hyperglycemia, an elevated postprandial, nonesterified fatty acid level in the plasma, or elevated basal metabolic rate may be found.

Regitine Test: This test, illustrated in Plate VI, is of value during a hypertensive phase and is carried out as follows: After the patient has been lying down for at least 10 minutes, an intravenous infusion of 5 per cent dextrose in water is started. When the patient is in the basal state, blood pressure readings are taken every minute and recorded for 5 consecutive readings. Then, so as not to disturb the patient, 5 mg. Regitine (phentolamine) is given intravenously through the tubing over a period of 1 minute. A reduction of blood pressure exceeding 35 mm. Hg systolic and 25 mm. Hg diastolic, lasting for 3 to 5 minutes, strongly suggests pheochromocytoma. A less marked hypotensive effect may be found in normal subjects, most of whom will however show a rise in blood pressure.

Patients should not receive any sedatives, antihypertensives, or narcotics for at least 3 days prior to the Regitine test. Reserpine should be discontinued several weeks or even longer before the test is carried out. Such medication may produce false-positive reactions, which always occur in uremic patients. However, in severely hypertensive patients who cannot be taken off their hypotensive medications, the test can still be performed. In these cases, if there is no significant hypotensive response, pheochromocytoma is clearly ruled out. False-negative tests may occur if the hypertension due to pheochromocytoma has become fixed as a result of secondary vascular changes.

The Provocative Histamine Test: This is used only during a lull in paroxysmal hypertension or in the sustained type of hypertension. It must be employed with great care, 5 mg. of Regitine (phentolamine) being immediately available to counteract any excessive rise in blood pressure.

The histamine test is carried out as follows: Histamine is given over a 1- to 2-minute period in maximum intravenous dosage of 0.05 mg. in 10 ml. of saline. A significant rise in blood pressure, occurring within 2 minutes after the injection, is suggestive of pheochromocytoma. False-positive results do occur, but in normal subjects or those with essential hypertension, a flush or a headache is usually accompanied by a slight fall in blood pressure. Rapid intravenous injection of 5 mg. of Regitine (phentolamine) will depress any alarming rise in blood pressure produced by the histamine.

Determination of Catecholamines

Determinations of catecholamines in urine and blood offer the most direct and conclusive test for overactivity of the adrenal medulla. Normal values for these determinations are given in Plate VI.

The determination of the metanephrines and particularly VMA is preferable to that of the catecholamines because of the far greater quantities available and the much better stability of VMA, even in acidified urines. Plasma catecholamines, though chemically unstable, provide sensitive measurements of secretory activity.

21

ALDOSTERONE

EDWARD G. BIGLIERI, M.D.

Assistant Professor of Medicine,
University of California School of Medicine;
Chief, Endocrine-Metabolic Division,
San Francisco General Hospital.

Of all the hormones produced by the adrenal cortex, one of the most important to survival of the organism is aldosterone. With deprivation of this hormone, salt (sodium) is lost, blood volume shrinks, and blood pressure falls. In excess, as in primary hyperaldosteronism, sodium is retained, blood volume increases, and blood pressure rises. Thus primary hyperaldosteronism is an important cause of hypertension. Like pheochromocytoma (see page 20), from which it must be differentiated, the hypertension caused by this condition is curable, providing diagnosis is made before irreversible vascular changes have occurred.

REGULATION OF ALDOSTERONE

Because of the importance of this hormone to the organism's survival, it is fortunate that its regulation does not depend entirely upon one source, the pituitary gland. While the secretion of adrenocorticotropin (ACTH) by the pituitary is wholly responsible for the regulation of cortisol secretion, it affects the production of aldosterone to only a comparatively minor extent.

Ablation of the pituitary practically abolishes cortisol secretion, but it reduces aldosterone by only 60 to 80 per cent. Administration of ACTH increases aldosterone levels 2- or 3-fold for a short period, but a fall in blood volume raises levels 30-fold, and deprivation of sodium will increase aldosterone more than 10-fold (see Plate X). The aldosterone response to sodium deprivation can be reduced by concurrent potassium depletion and augmented by potassium administration. Therefore, it has been suggested that a rise in the plasma potassium level might be a stimulus for aldosterone release.

Obviously, other aldosterone-stimulating mechanisms are far more important than the anterior pituitary. Perhaps, like the kidney, the zona granulosa acts with a certain degree of autonomy. Also, aldosterone stimulation has been attributed in part to the pineal gland or surrounding brain tissue where a humoral substance, glomerulotropin, may perhaps be produced (Plate VII).

Neither ablation of the pituitary nor removal of the pineal gland and surrounding tissue prevents the increase of aldosterone that follows a reduction in blood volume or sodium depletion. However, when the kidney also is removed the

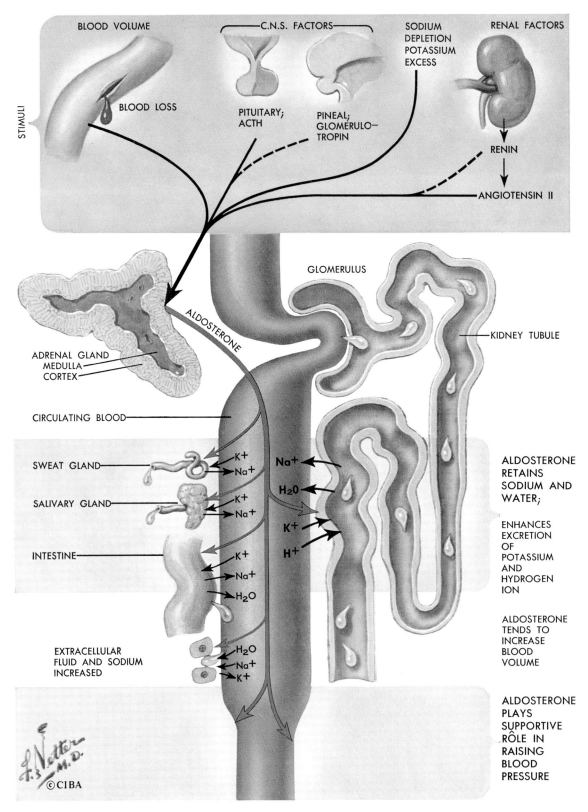

STIMULI

BLOOD VOLUME

C.N.S. FACTORS

SODIUM
DEPLETION
POTASSIUM
EXCESS

RENAL FACTORS

BLOOD LOSS

PITUITARY;
ACTH

PINEAL;
GLOMERULO—
TROPIN

RENIN

ANGIOTENSIN II

GLOMERULUS

ALDOSTERONE

ADRENAL GLAND
MEDULLA
CORTEX

KIDNEY TUBULE

CIRCULATING BLOOD

SWEAT GLAND

K+
Na+

Na+

H₂O

SALIVARY GLAND

K+
Na+

K+

H+

INTESTINE

K+
Na+
H₂O

ALDOSTERONE
RETAINS
SODIUM AND
WATER;

ENHANCES
EXCRETION
OF
POTASSIUM
AND
HYDROGEN
ION

ALDOSTERONE
TENDS TO
INCREASE
BLOOD
VOLUME

EXTRACELLULAR
FLUID AND SODIUM
INCREASED

H₂O
Na+
K+

ALDOSTERONE
PLAYS
SUPPORTIVE
RÔLE IN
RAISING
BLOOD
PRESSURE

©CIBA

PLATE VII

PHYSIOLOGY OF ALDOSTERONE

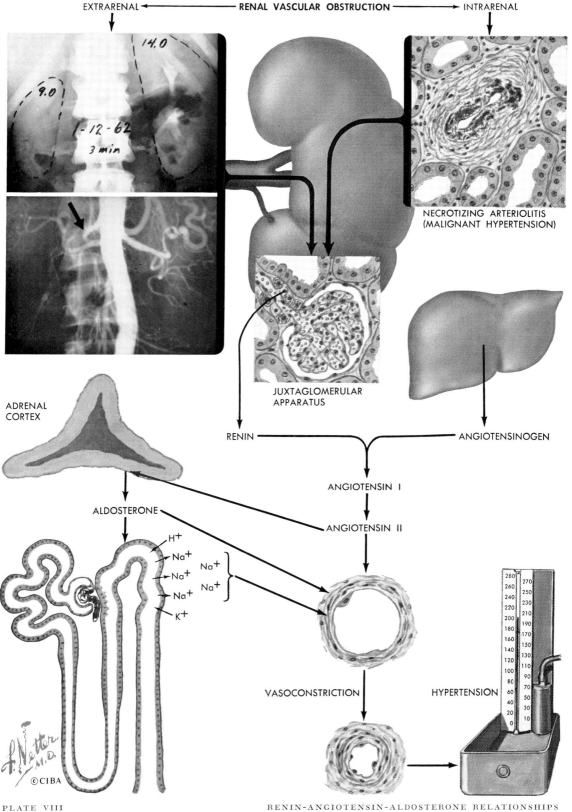

EXTRARENAL ◄———— **RENAL VASCULAR OBSTRUCTION** ————► INTRARENAL

14.0

9.0

1-12-62
3 min

NECROTIZING ARTERIOLITIS
(MALIGNANT HYPERTENSION)

JUXTAGLOMERULAR
APPARATUS

ADRENAL
CORTEX

RENIN ————————————— ANGIOTENSINOGEN

ANGIOTENSIN I

ALDOSTERONE

ANGIOTENSIN II

H+
Na+
Na+   Na+
Na+
Na+   Na+
Na+
K+

VASOCONSTRICTION   HYPERTENSION

PLATE VIII

RENIN-ANGIOTENSIN-ALDOSTERONE RELATIONSHIPS

aldosterone-stimulating effect of hemorrhage is lost. This directs attention to the
kidney.

Renin-Angiotensin Mechanism

The effect of the kidney in stimulating
aldosterone, as presently visualized, is
illustrated in Plate VIII. Between the
afferent renal arteriole and the macula
densa of the distal tubule is located a collection of cells known as juxtaglomerular
cells. These cells are ideally located to act
as stretch receptors, monitoring the pressure of blood entering the glomerulus.

The intra-arteriolar pressure exerted on
the juxtaglomerular cells may be decreased
by intra-renal or extra-renal vascular lesions. Within the kidney the necrotizing
arteriolitis of malignant hypertension is
the characteristic lesion. Outside the kidney a thickening of the subendothelial
layers of one of the renal arteries with
superimposed atheromatous deposit may
reduce intra-arteriolar pressure on the
juxtaglomerular cells. Also, of course, a
similar effect can be produced by more
diffuse lesions involving smaller intra-
renal vessels.

Any of the vascular changes just
described may cause an increase in the
secretion of renin by the juxtaglomerular
apparatus, an increase that can be correlated with the granularity of the individual cells.

Renin changes angiotensinogen, produced by the liver, to angiotensin I. In
the plasma, the latter is converted further
to angiotensin II,* one of the most potent
vasopressors. Beside its effect on smooth
muscle of the arterioles, angiotensin II
strongly stimulates aldosterone secretion.
Aldosterone itself has a hypertensive
effect. This may be due to an increase in
sodium in the walls of arterioles, directly

---

*A substance identical in action and practically
identical in structure has been synthesized and
is commercially available under the trade name
Hypertensin-CIBA® (angiotensin amide).

decreasing their lumen or increasing their
sensitivity to vasopressor agents. In this
way the combined effects of angiotensin
II and aldosterone produce vasoconstriction with increase in blood pressure.

Rate of Aldosterone Secretion

Under conditions of normal sodium
intake, the normal subject secretes from
100 to 200 micrograms per day. Sodium
deprivation may increase the secretory
rate to 1,000 micrograms per day. The
level of aldosterone in the peripheral
blood is approximately 0.01 micrograms/
100 ml. Its disappearance time from the
plasma is rapid, requiring only 20 to 30
minutes.

Catabolism of Aldosterone

Very little of this hormone is bound to
corticosteroid-binding globulin (transcortin), most being bound loosely to albumin.
Only a small amount, 1 to 5 micrograms,
is excreted as the 3-oxo derivative and
20 to 30 micrograms as the tetrahydro-
metabolites devoid of biological activity.

ACTION OF ALDOSTERONE

Aldosterone is the electrolyte regulating hormone of the adrenal cortex. Herein
lies its major contribution to the survival
of the organism — the maintenance of
electrolyte equilibrium. Secondary to this
is the maintenance of blood volume and
blood pressure.

The chief action of this hormone is the
conservation of sodium, which it accom-
plishes mainly in the distal tubule of
the kidney. (Although 86 per cent of the
sodium present in the glomerular filtrate is reabsorbed in the proximal tubule,
the fine adjustments to maintain equilibrium are carried out in the distal
tubule, and these are largely regulated by
aldosterone.)

Most of the excess acid resulting from
body metabolism is excreted as carbon

dioxide from the lungs. However, it remains for the kidney to conserve sodium in order to maintain the 7.4 pH of the various blood buffers: $NAHCO_3/HHCO_3$, $NAHPO_4/NAH_2PO_4$, etc. This is accomplished in the distal tubule by returning sodium ions present in the glomerular filtrate to the blood in exchange for ions of hydrogen and potassium (Plates VII and IX).

The rate of this exchange is largely regulated by aldosterone; the greater the secretion of aldosterone, the more sodium that is reabsorbed and the more hydrogen or potassium that is excreted in the urine.

Also under the influence of aldosterone, the sweat and saliva contain less sodium and more potassium (a ratio of diagnostic importance). In addition, sodium and water absorption from the intestine may be increased and more potassium lost in the stool.

With the retention of sodium there must be a retention of water with increase in plasma volume and extracellular fluid. This may tend to increase blood pressure. However, in the regulation of blood pressure, aldosterone probably does not depend entirely upon its influence on the excretion or retention of electrolytes and water. It probably also has a direct effect upon the vasculature, as previously mentioned, and illustrated in Plate VIII. This latter effect on vascular tonus it probably shares with the medullary catecholamines (see Plate IV).

A deficiency of aldosterone, as in Addison's disease, results in a very low blood pressure. An excess, as in primary hyperaldosteronism, leads to high blood pressure.

PRIMARY HYPERALDOSTERONISM

This condition, also known as Conn's syndrome, is comparatively rare. Like pheochromocytoma (see page 20) it is usually curable. Therefore, appropriate diagnostic tests should be carried out in every hypertensive patient to differentiate this condition from renovascular hypertension (also often curable), pheochromocytoma, and various other causes of hypertension, particularly if refractory to treatment.

The cause is nearly always a small adenoma, whose cells resemble those of the zona glomerulosa, the zona fasciculata, or both. The contiguous adrenal tissue is usually of normal size and histology. To date all but one tumor has been benign.

Signs and Symptoms

From the action of aldosterone already described, the signs and symptoms are easily explained (see Plate IX).

Hypertension: This is present in nearly all patients. The mechanism is really unknown but may be related to salt retention, hypervolemia, and direct effect of aldosterone on vessel walls. The hypertension is usually benign, with elevation of both systolic and diastolic pressures. Impairment of reflex circulatory regulation is often manifested by a fall of blood pressure on standing and the fact that the pulse rate is usually slow and relatively fixed, not tending to vary with changes in posture and activity.

Hypokalemia: Low serum potassium with an abnormally high excretion of this ion in the urine are practically always found at least once in 2 or 3 consecutive determinations, *if* the patient is on a normal salt intake of 5 to 8 Gm. of sodium chloride per day. If salt is restricted, potassium may be retained because too few sodium ions are available for exchange. Indeed, both serum potassium and the ECG abnormalities caused by hypokalemia can return to normal on salt restriction alone!

Chief clinical results of hypokalemia are fatigue and loss of stamina. Paresthesias are common, and occasionally ascending paralysis may be encountered. ECG

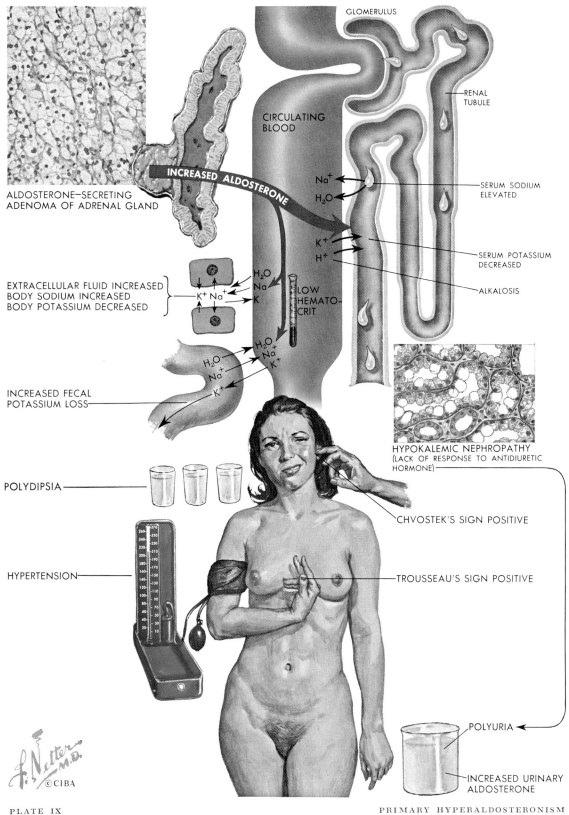

GLOMERULUS

ALDOSTERONE–SECRETING
ADENOMA OF ADRENAL GLAND

CIRCULATING
BLOOD

INCREASED ALDOSTERONE

RENAL
TUBULE

Na^+
H_2O

SERUM SODIUM
ELEVATED

K^+
H^+

SERUM POTASSIUM
DECREASED

ALKALOSIS

EXTRACELLULAR FLUID INCREASED
BODY SODIUM INCREASED
BODY POTASSIUM DECREASED

H_2O
Na
K^+ Na^+
K

LOW
HEMATO-
CRIT

INCREASED FECAL
POTASSIUM LOSS

H_2O
Na^+
Na^+
K^+
K^+

HYPOKALEMIC NEPHROPATHY
(LACK OF RESPONSE TO ANTIDIURETIC
HORMONE)

POLYDIPSIA

CHVOSTEK'S SIGN POSITIVE

HYPERTENSION

TROUSSEAU'S SIGN POSITIVE

POLYURIA

INCREASED URINARY
ALDOSTERONE

PLATE IX

PRIMARY HYPERALDOSTERONISM

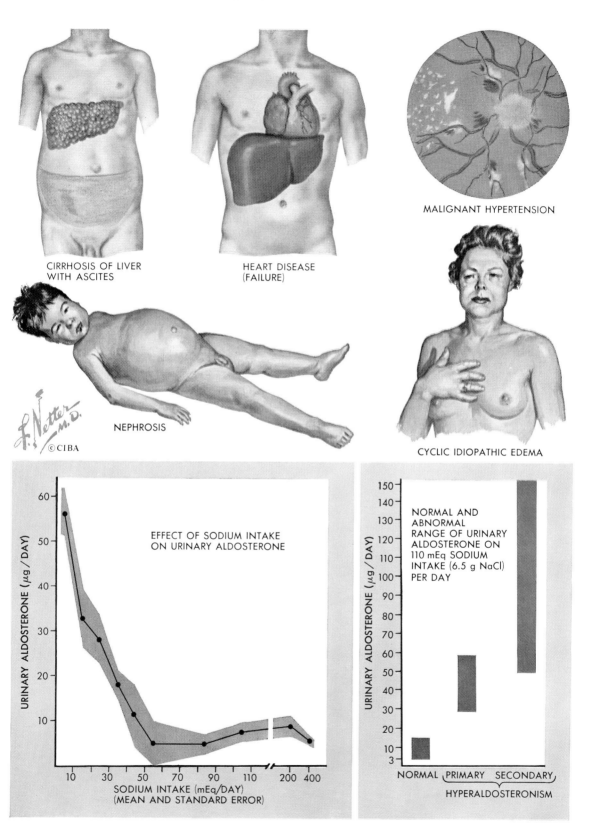

CIRRHOSIS OF LIVER
WITH ASCITES

HEART DISEASE
(FAILURE)

MALIGNANT HYPERTENSION

NEPHROSIS

CYCLIC IDIOPATHIC EDEMA

EFFECT OF SODIUM INTAKE
ON URINARY ALDOSTERONE

URINARY ALDOSTERONE (µg / DAY)

SODIUM INTAKE (mEq/DAY)
(MEAN AND STANDARD ERROR)

NORMAL AND
ABNORMAL
RANGE OF URINARY
ALDOSTERONE ON
110 mEq SODIUM
INTAKE (6.5 g NaCl)
PER DAY

URINARY ALDOSTERONE (µg / DAY)

NORMAL PRIMARY SECONDARY

HYPERALDOSTERONISM

PLATE X

SECONDARY HYPERALDOSTERONISM

changes characteristic of hypokalemia should arouse immediate suspicion if found in a hypertensive subject.

Hypokalemia produces functional changes or even structural vacuolization in the renal tubule — a hypokalemic nephropathy. The result is a loss of urine concentration, even after dehydration or antidiuretic hormone administration. There is then polydipsia, polyuria, and often a marked nocturia.

The administration of spironolactone which competes with aldosterone at the distal tubule will assist in retention of potassium but does little to the hypertension. This agent may prove helpful in diagnosis since 1 gram of spironolactone given by mouth daily for 3 days brings serum potassium toward normal temporarily. Five to 7 days after cessation of the drug, serum potassium again falls to hypokalemic levels, since tumor secretion is not reduced, but frequently is increased.

Alkalosis: Excessive reabsorption of sodium causes abnormal loss of hydrogen ions in the exchange. This may result in alkalosis, with positive Chvostek and Trousseau signs (Plate IX).

Hypernatremia: The increase in sodium absorption leads to increased concentration of salt in the plasma, along with increase in plasma volume and usually a low hematocrit. The apparently paradoxical absence of edema in these cases, in spite of sodium retention, has been attributed to an increase in glomerular filtration rate. This increases the sodium load offered the exchange mechanism, thus limiting the net amount of sodium reabsorbed.

Diagnosis

The triad of hypertension, hypokalemia, and polyuria should arouse immediate suspicion. Indeed, hypernatremic, hypokalemic alkalosis with increased plasma volume and excessive urinary potassium loss are almost diagnostic.

The definitive diagnosis of primary hyperaldosteronism is established by measuring the rate of secretion of aldosterone or the daily excretion of one of its metabolites, making sure the patient is on a normal salt intake. The various diagnostic points we have mentioned are summarized in Table 2.

Treatment

At present, treatment of primary hyperaldosteronism is always surgical. Operation should be deferred, however, until body potassium stores have to some extent been replenished, giving 4 to 12 Gm. of potassium daily for a week while sodium intake is restricted.

Extirpation of the adenoma may be expected to provide cure if no irreparable vascular damage has been produced by the hypertension. Improvement or cure is seen in over 80 per cent of these cases. The administration of spironolactone may help correct electrolyte imbalance but does little for the hypertension.

SECONDARY HYPERALDOSTERONISM

Aldosterone is increased secondarily in a number of conditions, in none of which the adrenal cortex is primarily at fault. Rather, aldosterone is increased by one of the extrapituitary regulating mechanisms already enumerated, and its increase is, in fact, an attempt to "normalize" an existing pathologic state.

Secondary hyperaldosteronism occurs in certain edematous states as well as in renovascular and malignant hypertension (Plate X).

Edematous States

Nephrosis: The nephroses are all characterized by massive proteinuria, which causes a reduction of blood proteins. As a result, the colloidal osmotic pressure, which tends to hold water within the capillaries, is reduced. This in turn increases

TABLE 2.

HYPERTENSION ASSOCIATED WITH PRIMARY
AND SECONDARY HYPERALDOSTERONISM
Similarities and Differences

TESTS	PRIMARY HYPERALDOSTERONISM	MALIGNANT HYPERTENSION	RENOVASCULAR HYPERTENSION
Spironolactone Test	Positive	Positive	Positive
Blood Pressure	Moderately or severely elevated	Elevation severe and progressive	Rapid onset of severe elevation
Aldosterone Secretion	Always elevated	Usually elevated	Occasionally elevated
Serum Potassium Concentration	Often severely decreased	Normal, or slight decrease	Normal, or occasionally decreased
Urinary Potassium	Usually increased	Normal	Normal, or increased
Serum Sodium Concentration	Usually increased	Normal, or decreased	Normal, or decreased
Blood Volume	Usually increased	Normal, or decreased	Normal, or decreased
Circulatory Reflexes	Impaired	Normal	Normal
Chief Diagnostic Findings	Hypokalemia Hypernatremia Hypervolemia	Progressive course leading to Keith-Wagener IV eyegrounds	Abnormal intravenous pyelogram, renal arteriogram, Howard test

transudation of fluid from the capillaries into the extracellular space, producing edema. Because of increased transudation, the plasma volume is reduced — one of the most potent stimulants to aldosterone secretion.

The higher level of aldosterone in this condition is an attempt to correct the situation by increasing the reabsorption of sodium and water, thus returning the blood volume to normal. Often, however, a vicious cycle is created, correctable mainly by reducing the proteinuria and other therapeutic measures utilized in nephrosis.

In contradistinction to primary hyperaldosteronism, serum electrolytes are within physiologic limits unless diuretics have been used within a week before the test. There is no potassium depletion. The normalcy of electrolytes in secondary hyperaldosteronism has been attributed to an intense proximal reabsorption of sodium, diminishing its availability to the exchange mechanism we have discussed under primary hyperaldosteronism.

Hepatic Cirrhosis: This condition is also characterized by low blood proteins, due in this case to a deficiency in their manufacture. There is also loss of fluid from the vascular compartment, due to impedance of portal return and ascites. As in the case of nephrosis, aldosterone secretion is increased with the same objective, often leading to the same vicious cycle.

As in the nephroses, the serum electrolytes are usually within normal limits. However, levels of both potassium and sodium may be reduced because of dietary lack of potassium.

Congestive Heart Failure: Here the loss of water from the vascular compartment is probably largely due to increased venous pressure, preventing return of water at the venule end of the capillary. Again the result may be a reduced blood volume in some critical area with the same chain of events already described. In this case, however, an additional stimulant to aldosterone production may be activation of the juxtaglomerular apparatus by decreased renal blood flow.

As in other edematous states, serum electrolytes are usually within normal limits.

Cyclic Idiopathic Edema: The cause of this condition is often an excessive secretion of pituitary antidiuretic hormone under the influence of psychic stimuli. Aldosterone secretion is increased in some cases, but not in all. The reason is unknown. When increased, aldosterone levels are often unresponsive to methods usually effective in their reduction. Serum electrolytes are usually normal.

Malignant Hypertension and Renovascular Hypertension with Secondary Hyperaldosteronism

Aldosterone secretion is invariably elevated in malignant hypertension and occasionally elevated secondarily to a unilateral stenosis of a renal artery, doubtless due to overactivity of the juxtaglomerular cells.

Renovascular hypertension should be suspected if there is a 2 cm. difference in kidney size on intravenous pyelogram (Plate VIII, upper left). An arteriogram (Plate VIII) may reveal the exact site of the lesion. In *malignant hypertension*, however, one may be dealing with diffuse lesions involving smaller intra-renal vessels which are not demonstrable (except by renal biopsy). The diagnosis of pheochromocytoma as a cause of endocrine hypertension has been previously described, see page 20 and Plate VI.

In contrast to the secondary hyperaldosteronism caused by edematous states, where electrolytes are essentially normal, these hypertensive disorders may have certain electrolyte abnormalities resembling those of primary hyperaldosteronism, namely, hypokalemia and alkalosis. The hypokalemia, however, is frequently not as severe as in primary hyperaldosteronism.

These similarities, as well as certain contrasting findings, helpful in differentiating hypertension due to primary hyperaldosteronism from renovascular and malignant hypertension, are listed in Table 2.

In secondary hyperaldosteronism caused by renovascular or malignant hypertension, the serum sodium concentration is normal or low, in sharp contrast to the usually high concentration found in primary hyperaldosteronism. Moreover, blood volume, instead of being increased, is reduced, probably because of intense vasoconstriction, a phenomenon readily observed in the eyegrounds which show Keith-Wagener III and IV. This is an important diagnostic point because in primary hyperaldosteronism eyeground changes are usually benign in nature. A further useful point may well be the presence of normal circulatory reflexes in these conditions and their impairment in primary hyperaldosteronism as described on page 27.

Treatment

The differentiation of secondary hyperaldosteronism from the primary variety is most important from the standpoint of definitive treatment. In secondary hyperaldosteronism, reduction of increased aldosterone levels can at best be regarded as adjunctive or supplementary to the treatment of the primary disease. Where increase in aldosterone is secondary to hypertensive states, vigorous antihypertensive therapy is required. Any renal vascular obstruction that is discovered should be attacked surgically.

SECTION G

C I B A

ABNORMALITIES OF THE ADRENAL CORTEX
Peter H. Forsham, M.A., M.D.

ABNORMALITIES OF THE ADRENAL CORTEX

PETER H. FORSHAM, M.A., M.D.

Professor of Medicine and Pediatrics; Chief, Endocrinology and Metabolism;
Director, Metabolic Research Unit, University of California School of Medicine,
San Francisco, California.
Active Physician, University of California Hospitals, San Francisco.

Illustrations by FRANK H. NETTER, M.D.

The chief steroids secreted by the adrenal cortex may be divided into the glucocorticoids (11- and 11-17-hydroxycorticoids, chiefly cortisol), adrenal androgens (17-ketosteroids and, in small amounts, testosterone), estrogen, and mineralocorticoids, mainly aldosterone.

Secretion of the adrenal corticoids is regulated exclusively by corticotropin (ACTH), produced by the anterior pituitary. One exception to this, however, is aldosterone, which has a multiplicity of regulatory mechanisms. Abnormalities of secretion specifically confined to this latter hormone have been described elsewhere.*

Here we will discuss those conditions in which there is a generalized abnormality of the adrenal cortex leading to an excess, an imbalance, or a deficiency of adrenal corticoids. These abnormalities may be secondary to a disorder of the anterior pituitary or inherent in the adrenal cortex itself.

ADRENOCORTICAL INSUFFICIENCY

An insufficiency of hormones produced by the adrenal cortex may be acute or chronic, primary or secondary. Because of their different sites of production and

mechanisms of secretory stimulation, glucocorticoids, mineralocorticoids, and androgenic hormones may be affected selectively. For example, a selective lack of 17-ketosteroids is the rule normally in prepuberal children up to the age of 8 or 10, but is not seen in adults. In androgenic, adrenocortical hyperplasia, a deficiency of cortisol accompanies an excess of 17-ketosteroids. In secondary (pituitary ACTH type) adrenal insufficiency, aldosterone secretion is well preserved, only cortisol and 17-ketosteroid secretion being reduced. Rare cases of exclusive hypoaldosteronism have been described.

ACUTE ADRENOCORTICAL INSUFFICIENCY (ADRENAL CRISIS)

This may follow destruction of the adrenal cortex by infection, trauma, hemorrhage, or thrombosis. It may also follow surgery, anesthesia, or other acute stress in patients whose cortical reserve has already been diminished by disease, partial adrenalectomy, or previous treatment with corticoids or ACTH which suppresses endogenous corticotropin and causes secondary atrophy of the adrenal cortex.

Acute Adrenal Hemorrhage

This occasionally occurs in the newborn, most commonly following prolonged, difficult labor.

---

*Aldosterone, CLINICAL SYMPOSIA 15:23, 1963, Edward G. Biglieri, M.D.

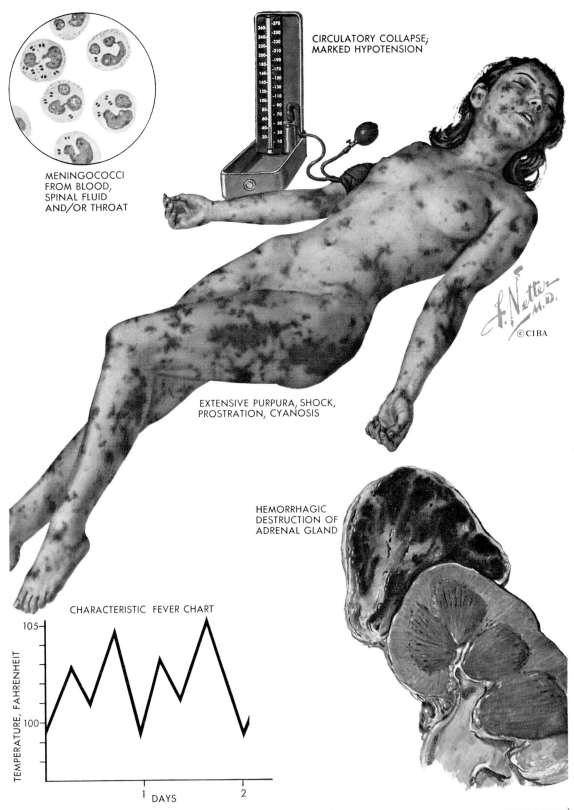

MENINGOCOCCI
FROM BLOOD,
SPINAL FLUID
AND/OR THROAT

CIRCULATORY COLLAPSE;
MARKED HYPOTENSION

EXTENSIVE PURPURA, SHOCK,
PROSTRATION, CYANOSIS

HEMORRHAGIC
DESTRUCTION OF
ADRENAL GLAND

CHARACTERISTIC FEVER CHART

TEMPERATURE, FAHRENHEIT

105

100

1 DAYS 2

PLATE I   ACUTE ADRENAL INSUFFICIENCY (WATERHOUSE-FRIDERICHSEN SYNDROME)

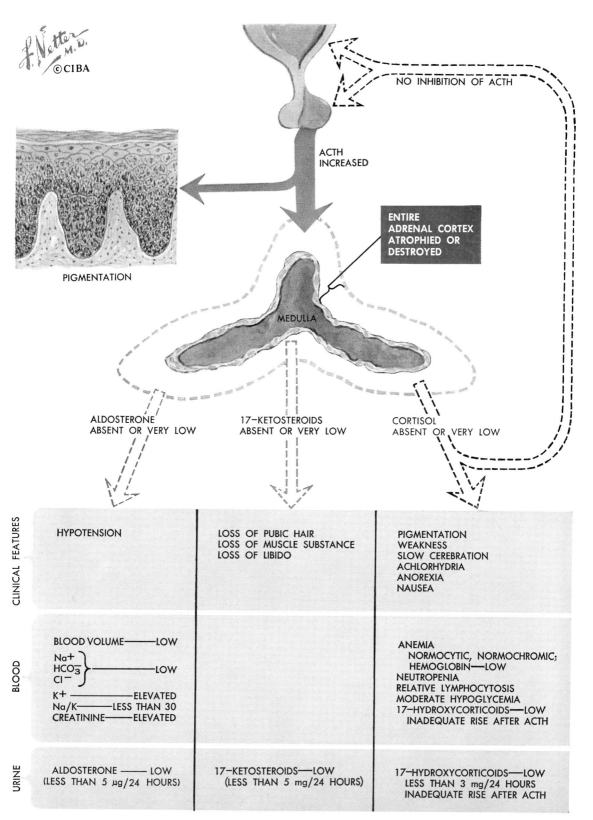

F. Netter
M.D.
©CIBA

NO INHIBITION OF ACTH

ACTH
INCREASED

PIGMENTATION

ENTIRE
ADRENAL CORTEX
ATROPHIED OR
DESTROYED

MEDULLA

ALDOSTERONE
ABSENT OR VERY LOW

17–KETOSTEROIDS
ABSENT OR VERY LOW

CORTISOL
ABSENT OR VERY LOW

CLINICAL FEATURES	HYPOTENSION	LOSS OF PUBIC HAIR LOSS OF MUSCLE SUBSTANCE LOSS OF LIBIDO	PIGMENTATION WEAKNESS SLOW CEREBRATION ACHLORHYDRIA ANOREXIA NAUSEA

BLOOD	BLOOD VOLUME——LOW
	Na+
	HCO₃⁻ } ——LOW
	Cl⁻
	K+ ——————ELEVATED
	Na/K————LESS THAN 30
	CREATININE———ELEVATED
			ANEMIA
			  NORMOCYTIC, NORMOCHROMIC;
			  HEMOGLOBIN——LOW
			NEUTROPENIA
			RELATIVE LYMPHOCYTOSIS
			MODERATE HYPOGLYCEMIA
			17–HYDROXYCORTICOIDS——LOW
			  INADEQUATE RISE AFTER ACTH

URINE	ALDOSTERONE ——— LOW (LESS THAN 5 µg/24 HOURS)	17–KETOSTEROIDS——LOW (LESS THAN 5 mg/24 HOURS)	17–HYDROXYCORTICOIDS——LOW LESS THAN 3 mg/24 HOURS INADEQUATE RISE AFTER ACTH

PLATE II

CAUSE AND RESULTS OF PRIMARY CHRONIC ADRENAL
INSUFFICIENCY (ADDISON'S DISEASE)

Waterhouse-Friderichsen Syndrome

An association of hemorrhage and infection (usually meningococcic septicemia) causes this syndrome (Plate I) seen predominantly in the younger age group. Here there is sudden hemorrhagic destruction of both adrenal glands with extensive purpuric manifestations, fever, cyanosis, circulatory collapse and death, usually within 48 hours. It has been suggested that the cause is the Shwartzman phenomenon, which can be produced experimentally in rabbits by injecting bacterial toxins intravenously at 6- to 32-hour intervals. The first injection "prepares" or "sensitizes" the vascular endothelium. The second injection given the rabbit during the critical 6- to 32-hour interval produces an accumulation of fibrinoid masses under the vascular endothelium with hemorrhagic infarcts in kidneys and adrenals.

Treatment: This consists in the administration of sulfadiazine, sulfisomidine, or other appropriate antibacterial compounds in large amounts to combat the meningococcemia. Every effort must be made to support the patient in profound shock, notably the infusion of 5 per cent dextrose in saline, albumin solutions and whole blood, the administration of 100 mg. of soluble cortisol or any of its modern equivalents, together with the judicious use of angiotensin amide.°

By energetically combining such supportive therapy, including relatively large amounts of hydrocortisone (50 mg. q 6 hours I.V., etc., see treatment, page 43) or one of its derivatives, survival has been made possible in a significant percentage of cases, whereas it was previously a universally fatal disease. Some presently feel that corticoids not only fail to contribute to therapy but actually lead to a more widespread septicemia. This opinion is held, however, by a very definite minority.

°Commercially available as Hypertensin-CIBA®.

Acute Adrenocortical Insufficiency Under Stress

Of greater importance because of its far greater frequency is adrenal crisis precipitated by stress. This condition occurs in those whose cortical reserve has been decreased by disease, previous partial adrenalectomy, or corticoid therapy. In such patients, it is precipitated by an operation, trauma, infection, or some other unusual stress.

After an insidious, prodromal period of 8 to 12 hours, weakness, hyperpyrexia, and vascular insufficiency with shock and loss of consciousness develop. Pigmentation, which may have been unrecognized, becomes obvious, being accentuated by the inadequate circulation. Or there may be no pigmentation because cortical insufficiency has been minimal or of too short duration.

Diagnosis: Determination of plasma levels of cortisol is too time-consuming. However, a *direct eosinophil* count may be helpful. In shock due to other cause, the count will be lower than 50 per cu. mm. In adrenal insufficiency it is usually, but not always, well above this level. The *potassium ratio* in the serum may show a downward shift from the normal of 30 toward 20.

Since there is no rapid, infallible laboratory test, treatment with cortisol must be started empirically, prophylactically, and immediately on suspicion, there being no real danger in its unnecessary administration for a short period of time.

Treatment: This includes the administration of adequate amounts of a soluble cortisol preparation such as cortisol hemisuccinate or phosphate 100 mg. intravenously, followed by 50 mg. at intervals of 6 hours. The dose is reduced to 25 mg. on the second day and to 10 mg. on the third day. Thereafter, it is given 3 times a day. Electrolyte solutions and whole blood must be given to combat dehydration and shock. Dextrose 1,000 ml. of 5 per cent solution in saline is given for hypoglycemia. If blood pressure does not respond, it may be necessary to give vasopressors such as angiotensin amide.*

Experimentally, aldosterone, as the sole agent in the therapy of adrenal crisis, has been most effective.

CHRONIC PRIMARY ADRENOCORTICAL INSUFFICIENCY (ADDISON'S DISEASE)

The normal adrenal cortex has an enormous reserve. Indeed, adrenocortical deficiency does not become clinically manifest until nine-tenths of the cortical tissue has been rendered unresponsive because of either tissue destruction, involution, or surgical removal.

Obviously, therefore, in a condition often so slowly progressive, the patient may live through a prolonged period of less apparent hormonal deficiency — a period during which secretion is adequate for everyday requirements, inadequate only when special stresses, such as operation, trauma, or infection, are encountered.

Fortunately, there are now available procedures which enable the physician to test the functional reserve of the gland without endangering the health and life of the patient. The widespread application of these screening tests and the use of *cortisol* in early therapy will undoubtedly prevent any sudden, unexpected deaths, and thus prolong the useful life of those with incipient deficiency.

Etiology

The most frequent cause of Addison's disease is *destructive atrophy*, which probably accounts for about 55 per cent of cases in the U.S.A. The reason for the atrophy is unknown, but toxic factors overwork atrophy, and more recently an auto-immune destructive process has been demonstrated.

Today, in the United States, probably about 40 per cent of cases are due to *tuberculosis*. Whether of the bovine or human strains, tubercular infection is almost always secondary to a focus elsewhere, usually in the lungs or genitourinary tract.

The remaining 5 per cent are accounted for by miscellaneous conditions such as hemorrhage due to trauma, metastatic carcinoma, histoplasmosis, amyloidosis, venous thrombosis, hemochromatosis, etc.

Incidence

Addison's disease is relatively rare in the United States, officially accounting for only 4 deaths per 1,000. However, the actual number is undoubtedly far higher, many unrecognized and incipient cases dying in crisis, the precipitating factor of which is given as the cause of death.

Signs and Symptoms

With atrophy or destruction of the adrenal cortex, all of the hormones there secreted become deficient with the signs and symptoms listed in Plate II and illustrated in Plate III.

Usually first noticed is *weakness and easy fatigability*. The patient looks tired and acts weary. Speaking even may be an effort. Mental weakness along with physical weakness increase as the day progresses, being least noticeable after a night's rest. The degree of muscle weakness depends not alone on the severity of the deficiency but also on the patient's muscular development prior to onset.

Acute prostration caused by a relatively minor infection or an unexplained long convalescence may be the first abnormality, suggesting that attention be given to the adrenal status. Since there is often increased nervousness and irritability with emotional instability and periods of depression, one may be tempted to brand the patient a neurasthenic or psychoneurotic unless functional tests are carried out.

Pigmentation is nearly always present in primary adrenal insufficiency. This

39

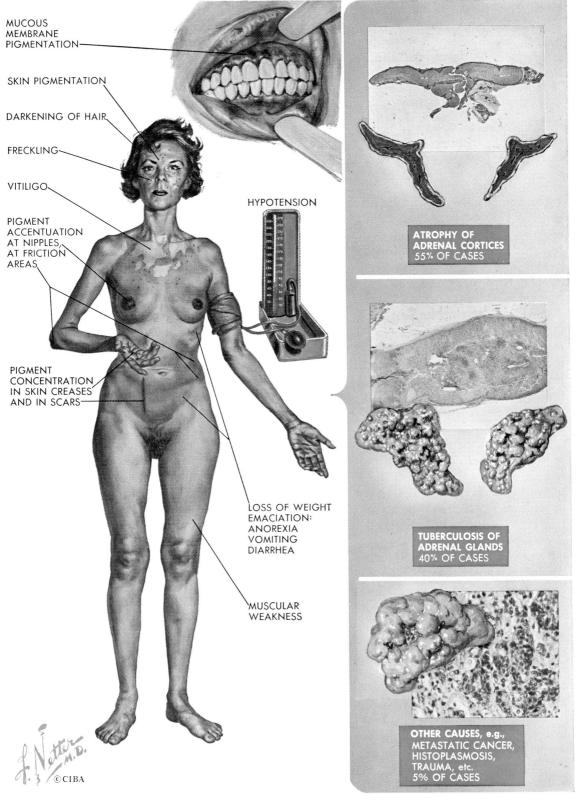

MUCOUS MEMBRANE PIGMENTATION

SKIN PIGMENTATION

DARKENING OF HAIR

FRECKLING

VITILIGO

PIGMENT ACCENTUATION AT NIPPLES, AT FRICTION AREAS

PIGMENT CONCENTRATION IN SKIN CREASES AND IN SCARS

HYPOTENSION

LOSS OF WEIGHT EMACIATION: ANOREXIA VOMITING DIARRHEA

MUSCULAR WEAKNESS

ATROPHY OF ADRENAL CORTICES 55% OF CASES

TUBERCULOSIS OF ADRENAL GLANDS 40% OF CASES

OTHER CAUSES, e.g., METASTATIC CANCER, HISTOPLASMOSIS, TRAUMA, etc. 5% OF CASES

PLATE III

CAUSES, SIGNS, AND SYMPTOMS OF PRIMARY CHRONIC ADRENAL INSUFFICIENCY (ADDISON'S DISEASE)

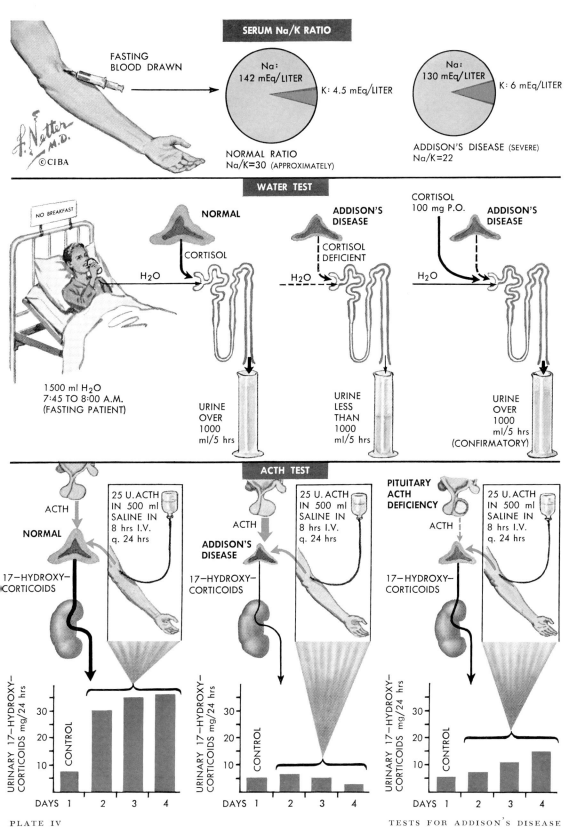

SERUM Na/K RATIO

FASTING BLOOD DRAWN

Na: 142 mEq/LITER   K: 4.5 mEq/LITER

NORMAL RATIO
Na/K=30 (APPROXIMATELY)

Na: 130 mEq/LITER   K: 6 mEq/LITER

ADDISON'S DISEASE (SEVERE)
Na/K=22

WATER TEST

NO BREAKFAST

NORMAL

CORTISOL

H_2O

1500 ml H_2O
7:45 TO 8:00 A.M.
(FASTING PATIENT)

URINE OVER 1000 ml/5 hrs

ADDISON'S DISEASE

CORTISOL DEFICIENT

H_2O

URINE LESS THAN 1000 ml/5 hrs

CORTISOL 100 mg P.O.   ADDISON'S DISEASE

H_2O

URINE OVER 1000 ml/5 hrs
(CONFIRMATORY)

ACTH TEST

ACTH

NORMAL

17—HYDROXY—CORTICOIDS

25 U. ACTH IN 500 ml SALINE IN 8 hrs I.V. q. 24 hrs

ACTH

ADDISON'S DISEASE

17—HYDROXY—CORTICOIDS

25 U. ACTH IN 500 ml SALINE IN 8 hrs I.V. q. 24 hrs

PITUITARY ACTH DEFICIENCY

ACTH

17—HYDROXY—CORTICOIDS

25 U. ACTH IN 500 ml SALINE IN 8 hrs I.V. q. 24 hrs

URINARY 17—HYDROXY—CORTICOIDS mg/24 hrs

CONTROL

DAYS 1 2 3 4

URINARY 17—HYDROXY—CORTICOIDS mg/24 hrs

CONTROL

DAYS 1 2 3 4

URINARY 17—HYDROXY—CORTICOIDS mg/24 hrs

CONTROL

DAYS 1 2 3 4

PLATE IV

TESTS FOR ADDISON'S DISEASE

pigmentation may serve to differentiate primary from secondary adrenocortical deficiency due to pituitary corticotropin deficiency, being absent nearly always in the latter condition. Assessment of pigmentation requires careful questioning as to the time of its development, previous exposure to sunlight, and racial characteristics of forebears back as far as three generations.

Weight Loss and Dehydration: Not all patients are emaciated but *all* will have suffered loss of weight in the recent past.

Hypotension and Small Heart Size: All patients have a reduction in pressure. However, those with previous hypertension may be found with pressure within the normal range, despite other signs of advanced adrenal disease.

Dizziness and syncopal attacks are caused by postural hypotension secondary to the dehydration, decreased plasma volume, hypotension, and muscle weakness.

Hypoglycemic Manifestations: Patients may have symptoms with relatively small reductions in blood sugar. These may consist of hunger, headache, weakness, sweating, trembling, blurring of vision, diplopia, disorientation, or even unconsciousness. Attacks are more likely in the early morning hours or several hours after a meal rich in carbohydrate — a reactive hypoglycemia.

Gonadal Function and Secondary Sex Characteristics: Growth of body hair is decreased in both sexes, more strikingly so in females who may show complete absence of axillary hair. Otherwise, secondary sex characteristics being maintained by ovarian or testicular secretions are little affected, unless the patient is very emaciated when amenorrhea and loss of potency are the rule.

Mental Depression: This varies from slight inability to concentrate to severe depression and schizoid behavior, all of which are rapidly abolished by cortisol treatment.

Diagnosis

Because of the rather nonspecific symptoms, it is most important to establish the diagnosis beyond reasonable doubt by appropriate laboratory measures. Otherwise the patient may carry the label of neurotic to an early death from a relatively minor accident, infection, or operation.

Moreover, the diagnosis should be established *before* treatment is commenced. Otherwise it may be impossible for many months to rule out the possibility of a secondary deficiency due to lack of pituitary corticotropin.

Sodium-Potassium Ratio in Plasma (Plate IV): In Addison's disease, deficiency of aldosterone causes a decrease in serum sodium with an increase in potassium. A determination of sodium alone might be misleading because of the concomitant dehydration. However, a calculation of the ratio between the two ions in effect cancels out the hemoconcentration factor and thus is far more reliable. Normally the ratio is 30:1. Anything significantly below this strongly suggests Addison's disease. In practice, this is really all that is necessary for determining a deficiency in salt regulation and, by inference, aldosterone.

Effect of ACTH on Direct Eosinophil Count: This relatively simple office procedure, which in an all-or-none test for cortical reserve, will exclude significant adrenocortical insufficiency but will *not* prove the diagnosis. *Procedure:* After a direct eosinophil count has been obtained from the patient, 25 units of lyophilized ACTH is injected intramuscularly (a meal can be given right after the blood sample). After 4 hours, blood is obtained for a second direct eosinophil count, after which the patient may have his next meal.

A decrease in circulating eosinophils of about 20 per cent normally occurs because of the diurnal rhythm of cortisol secretion.

However, a fall of 50 per cent or more definitely *excludes* adrenocortical insufficiency. Absence of such a fall is found in Addison's disease. However, it may be caused by an allergic eosinophilia or inactivation of the ACTH in sensitized individuals. In this case, therefore, additional tests must be carried out.

Water Diuresis: This test, which is based on the stimulating effect of cortisol on glomerular filtration, is probably the simplest and most widely used screening test for adrenocortical insufficiency. *Procedure:* The fasting patient, after urinating, drinks 1,500 ml. of water between 7:45 and 8:00 a.m. (Plate IV). He remains in bed for five hours, collecting all urine passed. If the five-hour specimen is above 1,000 ml. in volume, Addison's disease may be excluded. However, if much below, the diagnosis is likely. The procedure can then be repeated on the following day two hours after a dose of 100 mg. of cortisol by mouth. If this time the five-hour output is above 1,000 ml., the diagnosis is definite, and such conditions as heart failure and renal disease have been excluded.

Effect of ACTH on Urinary 17-Hydroxy-corticoids: This is the most sensitive and specific test of all. It estimates the actual functional cortisol reserve quantitatively and when repeated on successive days measures the potential functional reserve or the maximal production of corticoid. Thus it may reveal potential Addison's disease in patients whose basal output is still normal. *Procedure:* 25 units of ACTH in 500 ml. saline are given intravenously in *exactly* eight hours. A 24-hour urine specimen is taken on the day before the test and on each day the test is repeated.

As indicated in Plate IV, normally there is a three- to five-fold increase in urinary 17-hydroxycorticoids on the first day of the test, with further increases on successive days. In contrast, patients with Addison's disease show no increase or even a slight fall in urinary hydroxycorticoids.

This test also serves to differentiate patients with Addison's disease from those having pituitary deficiency. Patients whose corticoid deficiency is secondary to a lack of corticotropin show a gradual, slight, but sustained increase on successive days. As a rule, a definite diagnosis is possible after only one or two days on ACTH, as can be seen from Plate IV.

Patients undergoing this test should be closely observed because on rare occasions anaphylactic shock may occur due to pig or sheep proteins contained in the ACTH solution. This is easily controlled by stopping the infusion and giving epinephrine and hydrocortisone. However, the possibility of its occurrence rules against the use of depot ACTH given intramuscularly, absorption of which cannot be quickly terminated.

Fortunately, ACTH has now been synthesized. It works well and is free of the risk of reactions due to foreign proteins.

In order to prevent these frightening though rare reactions, administration of 1 mg. of dexamethasone* just before starting the test has been recommended. This will not materially affect results.

A number of tests formerly used have been abandoned because of the potential hazards and lack of specificity involved. These include salt withdrawal, potassium loading, and insulin tolerance.

Treatment

The availability of both glucocorticoids and mineralocorticoids for substitution therapy has rendered the treatment of Addison's disease relatively simple and has prolonged the lifespan of patients toward normal. However, a crisis complicating acute infection, trauma, or stress may still jeopardize life. Treatment of such episodes has been mentioned on page 38.

For maintenance a total of 15 to 30 mg. a day of cortisol should be given in three

---

*Dexamethasone is available as Gammacorten®.

43

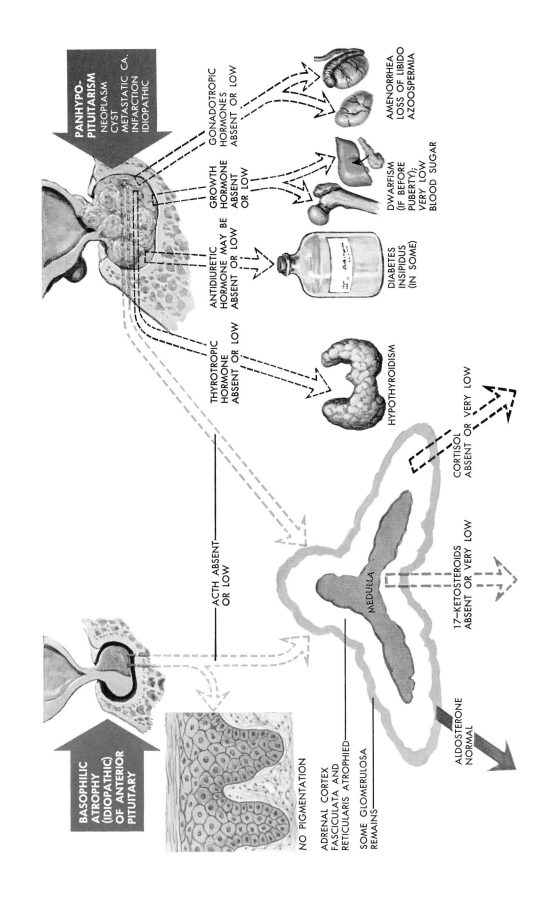

PANHYPO-PITUITARISM
NEOPLASM
CYST
METASTATIC CA.
INFARCTION
IDIOPATHIC

GONADOTROPIC HORMONES ABSENT OR LOW

AMENORRHEA
LOSS OF LIBIDO
AZOOSPERMIA

GROWTH HORMONE ABSENT OR LOW

DWARFISM (IF BEFORE PUBERTY); VERY LOW BLOOD SUGAR

ANTIDIURETIC HORMONE MAY BE ABSENT OR LOW

DIABETES INSIPIDUS (IN SOME)

THYROTROPIC HORMONE ABSENT OR LOW

HYPOTHYROIDISM

ACTH ABSENT OR LOW

CORTISOL ABSENT OR VERY LOW

MEDULLA

17-KETOSTEROIDS ABSENT OR VERY LOW

BASOPHILIC ATROPHY (IDIOPATHIC) OF ANTERIOR PITUITARY

NO PIGMENTATION

ADRENAL CORTEX FASCICULATA AND RETICULARIS ATROPHIED

SOME GLOMERULOSA REMAINS

ALDOSTERONE NORMAL

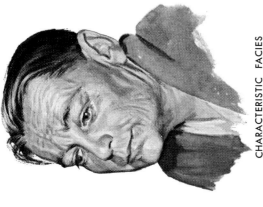

CHARACTERISTIC FACIES
IN PANHYPOPITUITARISM:
"FAWN" COLOR, "CROW'S
FEET"

CLINICAL FEATURES		
WEAKNESS SLOW CEREBRATION ACHLORHYDRIA MILD HYPOTENSION	LOSS OF SEX HAIR LOSS OF MUSCLE	NO DEHYDRATION

BLOOD		
ANEMIA NORMOCYTIC, NORMOCHROMIC HEMOGLOBIN——LOW NEUTROPENIA RELATIVE LYMPHOCYTOSIS BLOOD SUGAR——LOW 17-HYDROXYCORTICOIDS——LOW (SOME RISE AFTER ACTH)		Na+——NORMAL HCO₃——NORMAL Cl⁻——NORMAL K+——NORMAL Na/K——30 OR MORE CREATININE——NORMAL

URINE		
17-HYDROXYCORTICOIDS——LOW (SOME RISE AFTER ACTH)	17-KETOSTEROIDS——LOW (LESS THAN 5 mg/24 HOURS)	ALDOSTERONE——NORMAL TO LOW (RANGE 2 TO 20 µg/24 HOURS)

SECONDARY CHRONIC ADRENAL INSUFFICIENCY (PANHYPOPITUITARISM)

PLATE V

equal doses, preferably during meals to minimize gastric irritation. Sodium chloride intake should be increased to 10 Gm. per day. This can be accomplished by advising the patient to use plenty of salt and also take three or four 1-Gm. tablets of sodium chloride daily.

About 70 per cent of patients will require, in addition, a sodium-retaining hormone to maintain stable blood pressure. For this purpose 9-alpha-fluorohydrocortisone may be given in dosage of 0.1 mg. daily with breakfast. On rare occasions 0.2 mg. may be required. If edema develops the dose should be reduced to 0.05 mg. Dosage of this hormone is largely determined by the pre-breakfast weight of the patient.

Another sodium-retaining hormone has the advantage of bringing the patient back to the physician for repeated check-up and is indicated particularly in unreliable patients. This is desoxycorticosterone trimethylacetate,* a long-acting parenteral preparation, administered 25 mg. intramuscularly every three or four weeks. Occasionally there is somewhat excessive sodium retention with weight gain during the first week, with weight loss after the third week as the depot injection becomes exhausted.

SECONDARY ADRENOCORTICAL INSUFFICIENCY

This is one of the effects of panhypopituitarism in which there is usually also a deficiency of thyrotropic hormone and other hormones produced by the anterior pituitary (Plate V). Very rarely is there an isolated deficiency of corticotropin secretion.

Etiology

Atrophy or destruction of anterior pituitary tissue may be idiopathic or iatrogenic, total hypophysectomy being carried out for metastatic breast cancer with increasing frequency.

Several specific causes of pituitary destruction have been described. These include: *Postpartum pituitary necrosis (Sheehan's syndrome)*, developing late in pregnancy or during delivery, with shock and vaginal bleeding. Septic infarction of the pituitary due to puerperal infection (Simmonds' disease) is rare. This syndrome is characterized by relatively minor derangements of salt and water but severe asthenia and highly labile levels of blood sugar.

Prolonged corticoid therapy can cause pituitary corticotropin deficiency with adrenocortical atrophy. Therefore, any patient receiving prolonged corticoid (or corticotropin) therapy must be considered to have potential adrenocortical deficiency whenever intercurrent stress, such as a surgical operation, is encountered.

Signs and Symptoms

Because ACTH levels are low rather than increased as they are in Addison's disease, hyperpigmentation is nearly always absent.

Since aldosterone secretion is regulated only secondarily by corticotropin, levels of aldosterone in this type of adrenocortical insufficiency are essentially normal. Therefore, electrolyte disturbances and hypotension are much less severe than in Addison's disease and indeed are comparatively rare. However, on occasion, acute adrenal insufficiency with vascular collapse has been known to occur as a response to stress.

The effect of loss of pituitary hormones on the various glands of internal secretion is illustrated in Plate V.

Deficiency of gonadotropins causes amenorrhea or azoospermia with loss of libido and pubic hair. Growth hormone deficiency causes dwarfism if before puberty and is partially responsible for

---

*This is available as Percorten® trimethylacetate.

very low blood sugar. In some instances, antidiuretic hormone may be deficient with development of diabetes insipidus. Hypothyroidism results from deficiency of thyrotropic hormone. The skin takes on a fawn color and has a tendency to be dry and wrinkled. Deficiency of cortisol, 17-ketosteroids, and other cortical hormones (except aldosterone) produces the signs and symptoms listed in Plate V.

Diagnosis

The eight-hour ACTH test on two or three successive days, which differentiates Addison's disease from pituitary deficiency, has already been described (page 43) and illustrated (Plate IV).

The Metopirone test (Plate VI) is a shorter, more decisive test for deficiency and functional reserve of the anterior pituitary. This test depends upon the unique ability of Metopirone® (metyrapone) to block the action of 11-beta-hydroxylase, thus preventing the conversion of 11-desoxycortisol (Compound S) to cortisol in the adrenal cortex. As shown in Plate VI, cortisol normally inhibits production of pituitary corticotropin; thus, the more cortisol, the less ACTH (corticotropin) and vice versa.

With blockage of the action of 11-beta-hydroxylase, less cortisol is formed, inhibition to ACTH production is removed, and secretion of this pituitary stimulant to the adrenal cortex greatly increases. The result is a great (double or more) increase in 11-desoxycortisol and other cortisol precursors contributing to the 17-hydroxycorticoids found in plasma or urine by the Porter-Silber method.

However, in pituitary deficiency, removal of cortisol inhibition brings no response. There is *no* increase in ACTH production, and 17-hydroxycorticoids are only slightly increased or not increased at all.

Procedure: Levels of 17-hydroxycorticoids in a 24-hour urine specimen are measured before the test. Next, 30 mg./kg. of Metopirone (metyrapone) in 500 ml. of saline is infused intravenously over a four-hour period. A second 24-hour urine collection, begun when the infusion is started, is examined for 17-hydroxycorticoid content. Normally the second specimen will contain about double the 17-hydroxycorticoid content of the control specimen. If a deficiency of pituitary corticotropin exists, the rise will be minimal or absent, the degree of rise being proportionate to the pituitary corticotropin reserve. If the response is normal, *both* pituitary *and* primary adrenocortical deficiency are ruled out.

Treatment

These patients usually require less cortisol than addisonian patients. Therefore, cortisol 5 mg. after breakfast, lunch, and dinner should be sufficient for maintenance after controlling any initial crisis with parenteral therapy. Twenty-five mg. per day should be about the maximum, depending on body weight. Since there is usually no electrolyte defect, mineralocorticoids are rarely required, and if given should be kept to a minimum.

Other target gland deficiencies should also be treated, but not until after cortisol has been given for at least two days. After this, thyroid extract (30 to 120 mg. per day) may be administered without danger of crisis. Patients should also receive an anabolic agent such as methandrostenolone (Dianabol®).

An anabolic effect also can be obtained, together with sexual changes that might be desired, depending on the sex and age of the patient. To males, androgens can be given by injection of one of the long-acting esters, such as testosterone phenylacetate (100 mg. every three or four weeks). If oral therapy is preferred, methyltestosterone tablets can be given, or sublingual methyltestosterone can be prescribed in dosage of one 10-mg. Linguet

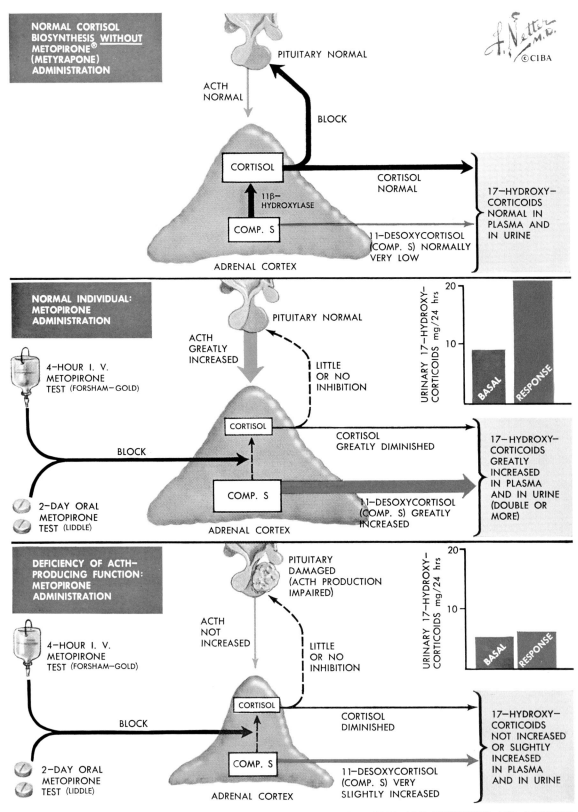

NORMAL CORTISOL BIOSYNTHESIS WITHOUT METOPIRONE® (METYRAPONE) ADMINISTRATION

PITUITARY NORMAL

ACTH NORMAL

BLOCK

CORTISOL

11β-HYDROXYLASE

CORTISOL NORMAL

COMP. S

11-DESOXYCORTISOL (COMP. S) NORMALLY VERY LOW

ADRENAL CORTEX

17-HYDROXY-CORTICOIDS NORMAL IN PLASMA AND IN URINE

NORMAL INDIVIDUAL: METOPIRONE ADMINISTRATION

4-HOUR I. V. METOPIRONE TEST (FORSHAM—GOLD)

2-DAY ORAL METOPIRONE TEST (LIDDLE)

PITUITARY NORMAL

ACTH GREATLY INCREASED

LITTLE OR NO INHIBITION

BLOCK

CORTISOL

CORTISOL GREATLY DIMINISHED

COMP. S

11-DESOXYCORTISOL (COMP. S) GREATLY INCREASED

ADRENAL CORTEX

17-HYDROXY-CORTICOIDS GREATLY INCREASED IN PLASMA AND IN URINE (DOUBLE OR MORE)

URINARY 17-HYDROXY-CORTICOIDS mg/24 hrs

20

10

BASAL RESPONSE

DEFICIENCY OF ACTH-PRODUCING FUNCTION: METOPIRONE ADMINISTRATION

4-HOUR I. V. METOPIRONE TEST (FORSHAM—GOLD)

2-DAY ORAL METOPIRONE TEST (LIDDLE)

PITUITARY DAMAGED (ACTH PRODUCTION IMPAIRED)

ACTH NOT INCREASED

LITTLE OR NO INHIBITION

BLOCK

CORTISOL

CORTISOL DIMINISHED

COMP. S

11-DESOXYCORTISOL (COMP. S) VERY SLIGHTLY INCREASED

ADRENAL CORTEX

17-HYDROXY-CORTICOIDS NOT INCREASED OR SLIGHTLY INCREASED IN PLASMA AND IN URINE

URINARY 17-HYDROXY-CORTICOIDS mg/24 hrs

20

10

BASAL RESPONSE

PLATE VI

METOPIRONE TEST FOR PITUITARY FUNCTION AND RESERVE

once or twice a day. Androgen therapy, in addition to its anabolic effect, has the advantage that it will promote growth of pubic hair and increase the libido in both sexes. However, because of the possible virilizing effect of androgens, women should be given estrogens. In women of child-bearing age, estrogens promote breast development, and if given cyclically (three weeks out of four) the menstrual cycle can be simulated usually without bleeding. After the menopausal age, sex steroid therapy, possibly using a combination androgen-estrogen mixture or anabolic therapy with Dianabol (methandrostenolone), decreases the tendency to osteoporosis.

CUSHING'S SYNDROME

This syndrome bears the name of the neurosurgeon, Harvey Cushing, who first described the signs and symptoms produced by a basophilic adenoma of the pituitary. Therefore, one is tempted to think first of a pituitary tumor when this syndrome is encountered. However, as indicated in Plate VII, identical symptoms may arise from a number of other causes.

Incidence

Cushing's syndrome is a relatively rare condition, found about once in a thousand autopsies. It occurs far more frequently (four to one) in females than in males. Highest incidence is in the third and fourth decades, particularly following pregnancy, suggesting that pituitary overactivity during gestation may be predisposing.

Pathogenesis (Plate VII)

Normally there is an inverse relationship between levels of ACTH and cortisol. Due to the inhibiting "feed-back mechanism" of cortisol, the higher the level of cortisol, the lower the level of ACTH and vice versa.

However, under certain conditions this inhibitory action of cortisol on the production of ACTH is ineffective. Despite excessive levels of cortisol, the pituitary continues to secrete ACTH in abnormally large amounts. These conditions include:

Pituitary Basophilic Adenomas: Even though small in size, these tumors secrete abnormal amounts of ACTH, regardless of the high levels of cortisol secreted by the secondary bilateral adrenocortical hyperplasia which they stimulate. However, ACTH levels are not sufficiently high to cause hyperpigmentation.

Pituitary Chromophobe Adenomas: These are usually much larger tumors, tending to erode the sella turcica and even affect vision by pressing on the optic chiasm. Moreover, the more massive amounts of ACTH produced by chromophobe tumors often cause hyperpigmentation, as well as a secondary adrenocortical hyperplasia, with a resulting excess of cortisol.

Functional Pituitary Overactivity: Presumably due to excessive hypothalamic stimulation, the pituitary gland, even though histologically normal in appearance, may produce corticotropin (ACTH) in excessive amounts, despite abnormally high levels of cortisol.

Thus, all of these pituitary abnormalities produce bilateral hyperplasia of the adrenal cortex, with the increase in cortisol production responsible for the symptoms so characteristic of Cushing's syndrome. However, practically identical symptoms can be produced by tumors of the adrenal gland itself. In these cases the overproduction of cortisol suppresses ACTH secretion. This leads to atrophy of the ipsilateral adrenal cortex. Adrenal tumors producing Cushing's syndrome may be either of two varieties:

Adrenocortical Adenomas: These tumors are usually found in the zona fasciculata, and in rare cases they are multiple. Cells of the adenoma are quite

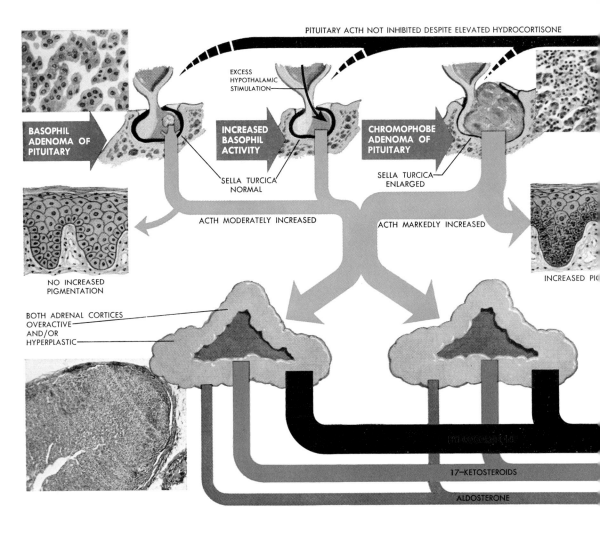

PITUITARY ACTH NOT INHIBITED DESPITE ELEVATED HYDROCORTISONE

EXCESS
HYPOTHALAMIC
STIMULATION

BASOPHIL
ADENOMA OF
PITUITARY

INCREASED
BASOPHIL
ACTIVITY

CHROMOPHOBE
ADENOMA OF
PITUITARY

SELLA TURCICA
NORMAL

SELLA TURCICA
ENLARGED

ACTH MODERATELY INCREASED

ACTH MARKEDLY INCREASED

NO INCREASED
PIGMENTATION

INCREASED PIG

BOTH ADRENAL CORTICES
OVERACTIVE
AND/OR
HYPERPLASTIC

HYDROCORTISONE

17-KETOSTEROIDS

ALDOSTERONE

PLATE VII

PATHOLOGY, SIGNS, AND SYMPTOMS OF CUSHING'S SYNDROME

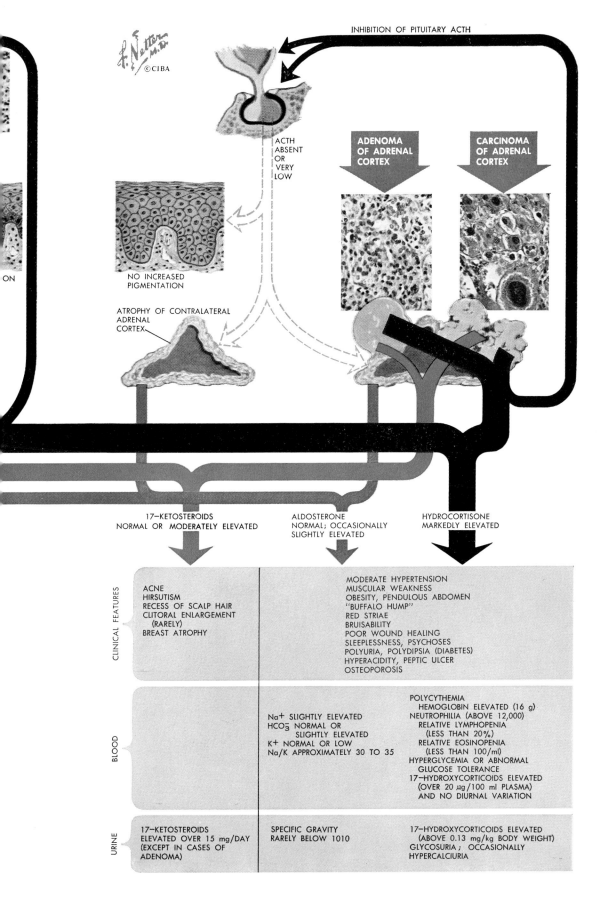

INHIBITION OF PITUITARY ACTH

ACTH ABSENT OR VERY LOW

ADENOMA OF ADRENAL CORTEX

CARCINOMA OF ADRENAL CORTEX

NO INCREASED PIGMENTATION

ATROPHY OF CONTRALATERAL ADRENAL CORTEX

17–KETOSTEROIDS NORMAL OR MODERATELY ELEVATED

ALDOSTERONE NORMAL; OCCASIONALLY SLIGHTLY ELEVATED

HYDROCORTISONE MARKEDLY ELEVATED

CLINICAL FEATURES	ACNE HIRSUTISM RECESS OF SCALP HAIR CLITORAL ENLARGEMENT (RARELY) BREAST ATROPHY		MODERATE HYPERTENSION MUSCULAR WEAKNESS OBESITY, PENDULOUS ABDOMEN "BUFFALO HUMP" RED STRIAE BRUISABILITY POOR WOUND HEALING SLEEPLESSNESS, PSYCHOSES POLYURIA, POLYDIPSIA (DIABETES) HYPERACIDITY, PEPTIC ULCER OSTEOPOROSIS

BLOOD		Na^+ SLIGHTLY ELEVATED
		HCO_3^- NORMAL OR
		    SLIGHTLY ELEVATED
		K^+ NORMAL OR LOW
		Na/K APPROXIMATELY 30 TO 35
			POLYCYTHEMIA
			  HEMOGLOBIN ELEVATED (16 g)
			NEUTROPHILIA (ABOVE 12,000)
			  RELATIVE LYMPHOPENIA
			  (LESS THAN 20%)
			  RELATIVE EOSINOPENIA
			  (LESS THAN 100/ml)
			HYPERGLYCEMIA OR ABNORMAL
			  GLUCOSE TOLERANCE
			17–HYDROXYCORTICOIDS ELEVATED
			  (OVER 20 μg/100 ml PLASMA)
			  AND NO DIURNAL VARIATION

URINE	17–KETOSTEROIDS ELEVATED OVER 15 mg/DAY (EXCEPT IN CASES OF ADENOMA)	SPECIFIC GRAVITY RARELY BELOW 1010	17–HYDROXYCORTICOIDS ELEVATED (ABOVE 0.13 mg/kg BODY WEIGHT) GLYCOSURIA ; OCCASIONALLY HYPERCALCIURIA

uniform in type, in spite of overcrowding. The tumor is usually surrounded by a narrow rim of atrophic cortical tissue, forming a pseudocapsule.

Carcinoma of the Adrenal Cortex: In these tumors the typical cellular zoning is lost. Pleomorphism is marked. In early stages the tumor may not be invasive and may not metastasize. However, once the cells invade the adrenal vein, metastases to liver and lungs occur. In these new locations the cells continue their hyperfunction and may be responsible for persistence of symptoms after surgical removal of the primary tumor.

In all of the conditions that have been mentioned, the secretion of cortisol predominates over other cortical steroids. Usually aldosterone is normal, although very rarely it may be slightly increased. In conditions other than cortical carcinoma, 17-ketosteroids are normal or only moderately elevated. However, in this latter condition these adrenal androgens may be markedly elevated.

Pathologic changes in other organs may include atherosclerosis of larger vessels, nephrosclerosis, and sometimes calcinosis of the kidney, gonadal atrophy, pancreatic islet cell hyperplasia, and occasionally fatty necrosis of the pancreas.

Signs and Symptoms

As listed in Plate VII, there may be signs and symptoms of increased 17-ketosteroid secretion, particularly in the presence of adrenocortical carcinoma. In some cases there is hirsutism, acne, and other signs found more typically in the adrenogenital syndrome (see page 62). Also, even without elevation of aldosterone, a few abnormalities, including hypertension and hypokalemia, may simulate an excess of this hormone.

Most of the signs and symptoms listed in Plate VII and illustrated in Plate VIII are due to excess cortisol and are similar in nature to the side effects produced by corticosteroid therapy, given in large doses over rather prolonged periods. These include:

Abnormal Fat Distribution: This is due to the effect of cortisol on fat metabolism and may take place without marked gain in weight, since it is confined to the face and trunk. The face is rounded (moonface). There is a "buffalo hump" behind the shoulders, enlarged supraclavicular fat pads, and a pendulous abdomen. The uninvolved arms and legs look thin in contrast.

Skin is thin, almost paperlike. The transparency of facial skin produces an unnatural redness caused by underlying vasculature and a polycythemia. Disappearance of elastic fibers, coupled with stretching due to abnormal accumulations of fat, produces depressed *purple striae* over the abdomen, buttocks, upper thighs, breasts, and even upper arms.

Poor wound healing, with high susceptibility to infection, is characteristic, as is *easy bruisability,* ecchymoses being produced by the slightest blow or even an expert venipuncture.

The *catabolic effect* of excess cortisol, with protein loss, brings about *muscle wasting and weakness* and the early development of *osteoporosis.* This latter condition is responsible for *backache,* which may be severe. The loss of protein matrix of bone and bone calcium due to increased urinary loss may result frequently in *compression fractures of vertebrae, rib fractures,* and *dorsal kyphosis.* Often the skull is involved in osteoporosis, an involvement hardly ever found in postmenopausal or senile osteoporosis.

Due to the stimulatory effect of cortisol on gluconeogenesis, blood sugar tends to rise with ultimate exhaustion of the pancreatic islet cells. Therefore, in 80 per cent of cases there is *latent diabetes,* with *overt diabetes* in 25 per cent. *Arteriosclerosis* develops rapidly, with hypertension which is at first systolic but later diastolic.

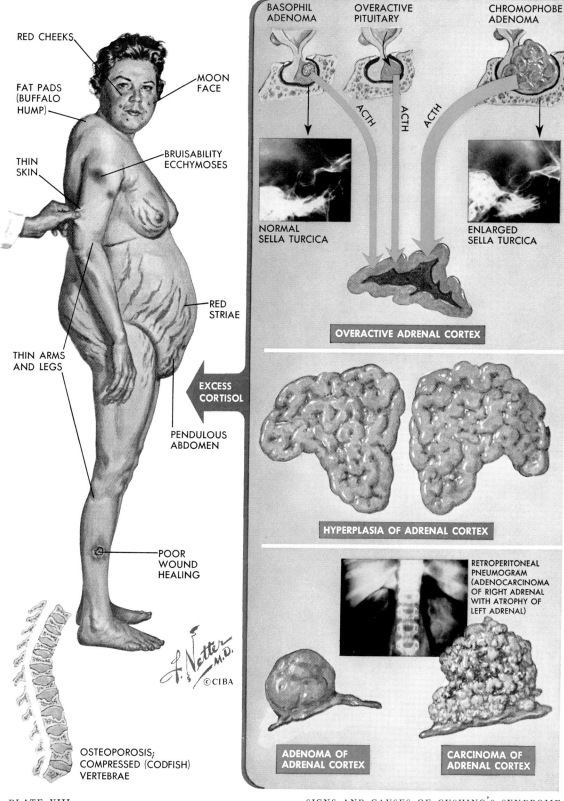

RED CHEEKS

FAT PADS (BUFFALO HUMP)

MOON FACE

THIN SKIN

BRUISABILITY ECCHYMOSES

RED STRIAE

THIN ARMS AND LEGS

EXCESS CORTISOL

PENDULOUS ABDOMEN

POOR WOUND HEALING

OSTEOPOROSIS; COMPRESSED (CODFISH) VERTEBRAE

BASOPHIL ADENOMA

OVERACTIVE PITUITARY

CHROMOPHOBE ADENOMA

ACTH

ACTH

ACTH

NORMAL SELLA TURCICA

ENLARGED SELLA TURCICA

OVERACTIVE ADRENAL CORTEX

HYPERPLASIA OF ADRENAL CORTEX

RETROPERITONEAL PNEUMOGRAM (ADENOCARCINOMA OF RIGHT ADRENAL WITH ATROPHY OF LEFT ADRENAL)

ADENOMA OF ADRENAL CORTEX

CARCINOMA OF ADRENAL CORTEX

PLATE VIII

SIGNS AND CAUSES OF CUSHING'S SYNDROME

Psychoses: There may be only a pronounced lability of mood. However, a definite psychosis may develop, ranging from depression to mania. Indeed, one of Harvey Cushing's first cases was found in an institution for the insane.

Course

The onset is usually insidious, changes being ascribed initially to increasing obesity. With transitory remissions and exacerbations, the disease progresses until the patient becomes bedridden because of muscle weakness and vertebral fractures. If untreated, death ensues, usually in about 5 years, from general debility, vascular accident, infection, or rarely diabetic coma.

Diagnosis

Finding three or more of the following signs, one should strongly suspect Cushing's syndrome: (1) muscle weakness and muscle wasting, (2) obesity, sparing the extremities, (3) red and depressed striae, (4) ecchymoses with a normal platelet count, (5) osteoporosis, (6) diabetes mellitus or abnormal glucose tolerance, and (7) hypertension. On rare occasions only one of these signs is present initially. A recent, rather sudden onset of any of these suggests adenoma or adenocarcinoma rather than hyperplasia.

Laboratory Findings (Plate VII): Suggestive laboratory findings include: (1) a low relative lymphocyte count (less than 15 per cent of total leukocytes), (2) a neutrophilia of 10,000 to 20,000 which may be increased to 30,000 or 40,000 in the presence of infection, (3) polycythemia with packed red cells of 50 per cent or more, (4) during more acute phases a direct eosinophil count of 50 or less (normal 100 to 300), (5) diabetic glucose tolerance curve (present in 80 per cent), and (6) hypokalemic alkalosis occurring in 15 per cent.

Definitive laboratory procedures require estimation of 17-hydroxycorticoids in plasma or urine. These tests are illustrated in Plate IX.

Normally there is a definite *diurnal variation* in plasma hydroxycorticoids, as shown in the upper figure, Plate IX. The minimum level occurs soon after midnight, followed by a sudden rise to a maximum between 6 and 8 a.m. Then there is a gradual decline throughout the day.

In Cushing's syndrome, whether from bilateral hyperplasia or tumor, the diurnal variation is practically absent. Therefore, if almost identical levels of plasma hydroxycorticoids are found at 8 a.m. and at 4 p.m., Cushing's syndrome is strongly suspected.

Unfortunately, false positives occur. If the patient becomes upset emotionally, the level may remain elevated in the absence of Cushing's syndrome, as it may with a central nervous system lesion and occasionally for no demonstrable reason whatever. Also, on rare occasions a false negative may result, a Cushing patient having diurnal rhythm. Therefore, additional tests should be carried out. Easiest is giving of 1 mg. dexamethasone* by mouth about 10 p.m. If the plasma level is found unchanged at 8 a.m., the patient is presumed to have Cushing's syndrome. Normally, this medication will greatly reduce morning hydroxycorticoids because of its inhibition of corticotropin formation (Plate IX, upper right).

Urinary Unconjugated Cortisol: Normally, about 10 per cent of biologically active cortisol exists in the plasma in the unconjugated and unreduced form, the remainder being bound to transcortin and to a lesser extent and more weakly to albumin. However, as the titer of plasma cortisol rises, the percentage of the free, active form increases rapidly. This free form spills over into the urine in increas-

---

*Dexamethasone is available as Gammacorten®.

54

ing amounts. Indeed, the free cortisol in the urine rises much more rapidly than does the free form in the plasma (Plate IX). In Cushing's syndrome, urinary free cortisol is usually much higher than the upper limit of normal of 200 micrograms in 24 hours.

Unfortunately, this determination involves repeated chromatographies and a double-isotope technique. Therefore, a somewhat less accurate method which can be carried out in many laboratories may be substituted. This determines the methylene chloride-extractable urinary unconjugated 17-hydroxycorticoids by the Porter-Silber color reaction. Any values in excess of 500 micrograms in terms of cortisol per day are diagnostic of Cushing's syndrome.

Thirty per cent of the cortisol and related glucocorticoids secreted by the adrenals are rapidly reduced to biologically inactive di- and tetrahydrocortisol by only one passage through the liver. Thus at any one time in the blood approximately one-half the total 17-hydroxycorticoids (Porter-Silber chromogens) is in the reduced and inactive form; the other one-half in the form of active unaltered hormone, 10 per cent of which is in the free state. The reduced material is rapidly conjugated with glucuronic acid in the liver, and the glucuronides are excreted by the kidney, making up 95 per cent of the so-called urinary 17-hydroxycorticoids of Porter-Silber chromogens. The diagnosis of Cushing's syndrome is strongly implied by *total* urinary 17-hydroxycorticoids (conjugated and unconjugated) much above 10 mg. per day, provided obesity is corrected for on the basis of 0.13 mg./kg. of body weight.

The diagnosis having been made, it remains to be determined whether the syndrome is caused by hyperplasia, an adenoma, or an adenocarcinoma.

The *differentiation between hyperplasia and tumor* can be made by the dexa-

methasone suppression test. A 24-hour control urine is obtained for 17-hydroxycorticoid determination. Then the patient is placed on 0.5 mg. dexamethasone by mouth every 6 hours for two days, and 2 mg. given at the same intervals for two more days. Urines are collected on the second and fourth days of dexamethasone administration. On the lower dose the patients without adrenal abnormality have a 50 per cent or better suppression of 17-hydroxycorticoids, whereas patients with Cushing's syndrome, regardless of cause, do not.

On the higher dose of dexamethasone, patients with normal adrenals show still greater suppression. More important, patients with hyperplasia have a 50 per cent or better suppression; those with tumor are unaffected. This, whether the tumor is an adenoma or an adenocarcinoma.

The *differentiation between hyperplasia and tumor* can also be made by the Metopirone test, which has the advantage that it is less time-consuming. This compound selectively blocks 11-beta-hydroxylation and, therefore, prevents the formation of cortisol (and also of aldosterone). The inhibition of cortisol on the pituitary having been removed by this blockade, increased amounts of ACTH (corticotropin) are formed with increase in the amounts of cortisol precursors still measured as 17-hydroxycorticoids in the urine. After a 24-hour control urine is obtained, 30 mg./kg. of Metopirone (metyrapone) are given by intravenous infusion over a period of 4 hours. Then a second 24-hour urine specimen is obtained. Patients with normal adrenals and those with hyperplasia will about double their 17-hydroxycorticoid output as a result of the infusion. However, in patients with tumor there will be no change, since the self-sufficient, cortisol-producing tumor has long since maximally reduced pituitary ACTH reserve and production.

The *differentiation between adenoma*

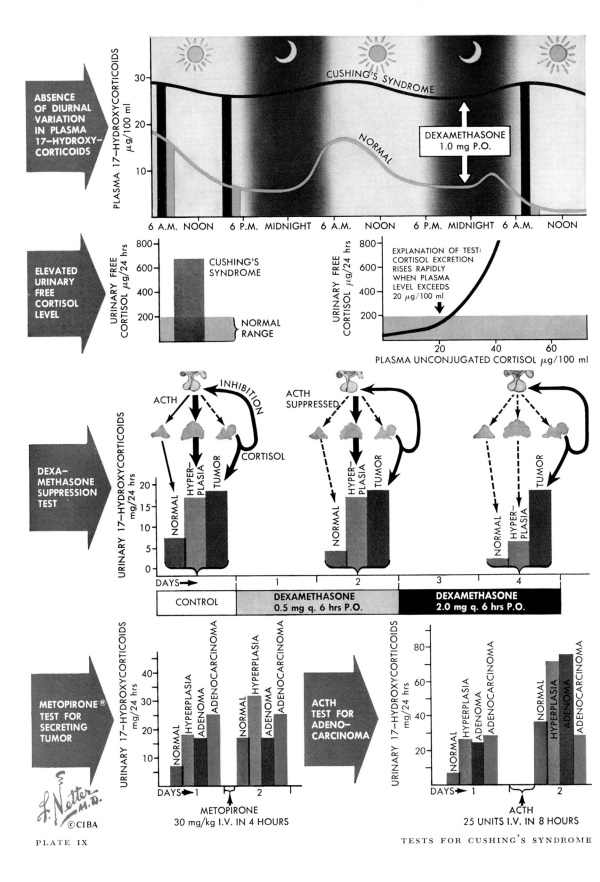

ABSENCE OF DIURNAL VARIATION IN PLASMA 17–HYDROXY–CORTICOIDS

ELEVATED URINARY FREE CORTISOL LEVEL

DEXA–METHASONE SUPPRESSION TEST

METOPIRONE® TEST FOR SECRETING TUMOR

ACTH TEST FOR ADENO–CARCINOMA

PLASMA 17–HYDROXYCORTICOIDS μg/100 ml

CUSHING'S SYNDROME

NORMAL

DEXAMETHASONE 1.0 mg P.O.

6 A.M. NOON   6 P.M. MIDNIGHT   6 A.M.   NOON   6 P.M. MIDNIGHT   6 A.M.   NOON

URINARY FREE CORTISOL μg/24 hrs

CUSHING'S SYNDROME

NORMAL RANGE

EXPLANATION OF TEST: CORTISOL EXCRETION RISES RAPIDLY WHEN PLASMA LEVEL EXCEEDS 20 μg/100 ml

PLASMA UNCONJUGATED CORTISOL μg/100 ml

ACTH   INHIBITION   ACTH SUPPRESSED   CORTISOL

URINARY 17–HYDROXYCORTICOIDS mg/24 hrs

NORMAL   HYPER–PLASIA   TUMOR

DAYS→   1   2   3   4

CONTROL   DEXAMETHASONE 0.5 mg q. 6 hrs P.O.   DEXAMETHASONE 2.0 mg q. 6 hrs P.O.

URINARY 17–HYDROXYCORTICOIDS mg/24 hrs

NORMAL   HYPERPLASIA   ADENOMA   ADENOCARCINOMA

DAYS→   1   2

METOPIRONE 30 mg/kg I.V. IN 4 HOURS

URINARY 17–HYDROXYCORTICOIDS mg/24 hrs

NORMAL   HYPERPLASIA   ADENOMA   ADENOCARCINOMA

DAYS→   1   2

ACTH 25 UNITS I.V. IN 8 HOURS

PLATE IX

TESTS FOR CUSHING'S SYNDROME

and adenocarcinoma can often, though not invariably, be made by an 8-hour intravenous ACTH test. Again a 24-hour control specimen of urine is obtained, after which 25 international units of ACTH are given intravenously in 500 ml. of saline over a period of 8 hours.

With hyperplasia, a second 24-hour urine specimen will show a three- to five-fold rise of 17-hydroxycorticoid excretion. There may be an equal rise in adenoma, but no rise with an adenocarcinoma which behaves as a totally independent structure. An adenocarcinoma usually produces excessive urinary levels of estrogen, dehydroepiandrosterone, and 11-desoxycortisol to name a few.

By a judicious selection of these modern tests, the nature of the pathology leading to Cushing's syndrome may be determined with a 90 per cent degree of accuracy. In the case of tumor there remains the need to localize it. This can be done usually by a careful tomogram of the adrenal region. Rarely, one requires a retroperitoneal pneumogram or CO_2 gram.

Treatment

The treatment of an adrenal cortical tumor is obviously extirpation. With regard to bilateral hyperplasia, there is some controversy at the present time. Everyone now agrees that bilateral hyperplasia is caused by a slight to considerable elevation of pituitary ACTH secretion. Since this is often due to increased hypothalamic stimulation of what on section appears to be a normal pituitary gland, one might wish to attack first the hypothalamus by administering various tranquilizers. This has met only with partial success.

The next approach might be removal of the anterior pituitary. This has been tried on a few occasions. However, such a radical approach is unwarranted, except when there is clear-cut indication (see below). With total removal of the pituitary by surgery or, to a much lesser extent,

various radio-destructive processes, the patient loses not only ACTH but also some thyrotropin, gonadotropins, and perhaps some antidiuretic hormone of the posterior pituitary as well. Therefore, one might try the administration of x-ray to the pituitary in *less* than a totally destructive dose. When 4500 r was given in the past as the exclusive treatment, the number of remissions was certainly less than 30 per cent. When this same procedure was used following removal of one adrenal as practiced by Soffer and his colleagues, remissions as high as 70 per cent were obtained. These results appear excellent but require further confirmation. However, one unquestioned advantage of this procedure lies in the complete verification of the original diagnosis by a meticulous, histological examination of the removed adrenal.

Irradiation of the pituitary at lower than totally destructive dosage, by the use of the proton beam or the implantation of yttrium pellets without removal of any adrenal tissue, is presently a promising experimental procedure, but cannot be recommended as yet for general use.

One is therefore left very largely with the choice of bilateral adrenalectomy, a procedure that becomes mandatory in the presence of psychoses, multiple fractures, or uncontrollable, debilitating diabetes, or subtotal adrenalectomy.

Admittedly, total adrenalectomy converts Cushing's syndrome to Addison's disease. Nevertheless, substitution therapy now available for Addison's disease enables the patient to live in comparative normalcy and for a normal lifespan.

Certainly total adrenalectomy is preferable to subtotal procedures, which may leave the patient teetering between Addison's disease and Cushing's syndrome, depending upon the regenerative potency of the remaining adrenal tissue on the one hand and the perennial problem that the remaining tissue has no further reserve of cortisol available when the patient is exposed to stress.

The one clear-cut indication for *partial hypophysectomy* is in cases of chromophobe adenoma of the pituitary interfering with the optic chiasm. This is found in about ten per cent of cases of Cushing's syndrome with bilateral adrenal hyperplasia. As a rule, it is accompanied by melanin hyperpigmentation. The diagnosis is confirmed by x-ray of the sella turcica, revealing enlargement. And if visual fields show increased bilateral hemianopsia, hypophysectomy becomes mandatory.

It is interesting to note that such tumors have been described as occurring more frequently to date after bilateral adrenalectomy. The exact reason for this has not been elucidated. However, the higher incidence of such tumors after pregnancy suggests that hyperactivity due to reduction of preoperative cortisol inhibition may be the stimulant.

Preoperatively, potassium chloride (4 to 12 Gm. daily by mouth) should be given for at least a week, and testosterone propionate 50 mg. daily should be given intramuscularly for a similar period for its anabolic effect in patients with chronic protein and potassium depletion. A soluble preparation of cortisol (100 mg.) should be given just after the incision is made, and 50 mg. given at six-hour intervals thereafter during the day of surgery. Succeeding therapy and course we have outlined elsewhere.*

ADRENOGENITAL SYNDROMES

The adrenal cortex normally secretes a number of androgenic (masculinizing) compounds. As shown in Figure 1 (page 60), these include the 17-ketosteroids, dehydroepiandrosterone, etiocholanolone, androsterone, and 11-oxy derivatives thereof, all of which are weakly andro-

---

*Textbook of Endocrinology, Third Edition, page 357. (W. B. Saunders Company.)

genic and excreted as sulfates and glucuronides. Total 17-ketosteroids amount to 5 to 15 mg. daily in the urine. In addition, the adrenal cortex is capable of synthesizing testosterone which has some 40 to 60 times the androgenic activity as any of the 17-ketosteroids.

The bulk of testosterone, of course, arises from the male testicle and to a smaller extent from the ovary in females. But in both sexes, the normal adrenal cortex makes a significant contribution of androgenic hormones. It is not surprising, therefore, that these adrenal androgens, when secreted in excess, will produce changes in sex characteristics.

The clinical findings and anatomic abnormalities will depend not only upon the nature of the adrenal disturbance, but also upon the age of the patient and the state of his or her development when abnormalities of steroid secretion first begin.

Action of Adrenal Androgens

The action of these androgens may be divided into their anabolic effect on the synthesis of protein and their effect on secondary sex characteristics.

Anabolic Effects: These are largely dependent on the ability of androgen to increase the synthesis of protein from amino acids. This leads to greater muscle strength and development. Since protein is a vital constituent of bone matrix, the androgens improve bone development and increase the utilization of calcium, while reducing its loss in the urine. Epiphysial closure, however, is wholly dependent upon:

Androgenic Effects: Stimulation of male sex characteristics and inhibition of female sex characteristics include: atrophy of müllerian duct structure in utero in the female, development of phallus and prostate, deepening of voice, and growth of sexual hair in the male, with shrinkage of breasts and uterus, hirsutism, amenorrhea,

58

enlargement of the clitoris, deepening of the voice, and acne in the female. Closure of epiphysis is hastened in both sexes.

Pathogenesis of Adrenal Androgen Excess

Starting with cholesterol, a great many chemical modifications are required of the adrenal cortex in order to produce the final biologically active steroids. Each of these steps in biosynthesis requires the action of a specific enzyme, capable of introducing a chemical group at a specific location in the cyclopentanophenanthrene ring. Each of the adrenogenital syndromes is produced by inhibition or blockade of one of these enzymes (Plate XI and Figure 1). The congenital androgenic states have in common a deficiency of cortisol (and therefore an excess of ACTH) and some change in sex characteristics.

Prenatal Adrenogenital Syndromes

Lipoid Hyperplasia: The first of the blocks in chemical modification occurs in the transformation of cholesterol to pregnenolone (Figure 1 and Plate XI). Formation of all steroid hormones ceases, and the adrenal cortex becomes overfilled with lipid material (Plate XI). The ovaries or the testes are also involved in the lipoid hyperplasia. When this enzymatic block occurs during fetal life, the intra-uterine müllerian duct system of the female type is preserved indefinitely, even in genotypic males, because of the loss of the normal influence of androgens on urogenital development. Therefore, such an infant has female external genitalia and is in fact a male pseudohermaphrodite.

Fortunately, this is a rare condition. Infants have rarely survived their severe total adrenal insufficiency. With earlier recognition and adequate substitution therapy, more may survive in the future.

Salt-Losing Syndromes: These syndromes may be caused by an enzymatic block in one of two locations. When block

occurs of the dehydrogenase and isomerase, responsible for transformation of pregnenolone to progesterone (Figure 1 and Plate XI), all adrenal steroids, with the exception of androgens (with their masculinizing effect), are lacking or deficient. The typically high titers of pregnanetriol found in the other types of androgenic adrenal hyperplasia are not found in this variant. There is profound adrenocortical insufficiency, with sodium loss, circulatory collapse, and early death. Fortunately this is also a rare condition.

The most common type of prenatal adrenogenital syndrome is produced by a block at C-21, preventing normal formation of 11-desoxycortisol and hence cortisol from 17-alpha-hydroxyprogesterone and of desoxycorticosterone from progesterone (with deficiency of aldosterone, Figure 1). This block is only a partial one in two-thirds of the cases, so that enough aldosterone is produced to minimize sodium loss, and enough cortisol is produced to prevent serious signs of adrenal insufficiency. However, the unblocked production of excess 17-ketosteroids, stimulated by abnormally high levels of ACTH, and a shift in the direction of 17-ketosteroid production, produce masculinization with great enlargement of the phallus in males and pseudohermaphroditism in females. Most of these patients are hyperpigmented due to the excess of ACTH.

As a result of the excess corticotropin, overproduction of progesteroids occurs. Typically, pregnanetriol rises above the upper limits of normal of 2 mg. per day in the urine. This may occur even when 17-ketosteroids are only showing a borderline elevation. In about one-third of these cases, titers of both cortisol and aldosterone are quite low. The excess progesteroids compete with reduced amounts of aldosterone in the renal tubules, producing a salt-losing syndrome of sufficient severity to cause vascular collapse and early death, unless vigorously treated with

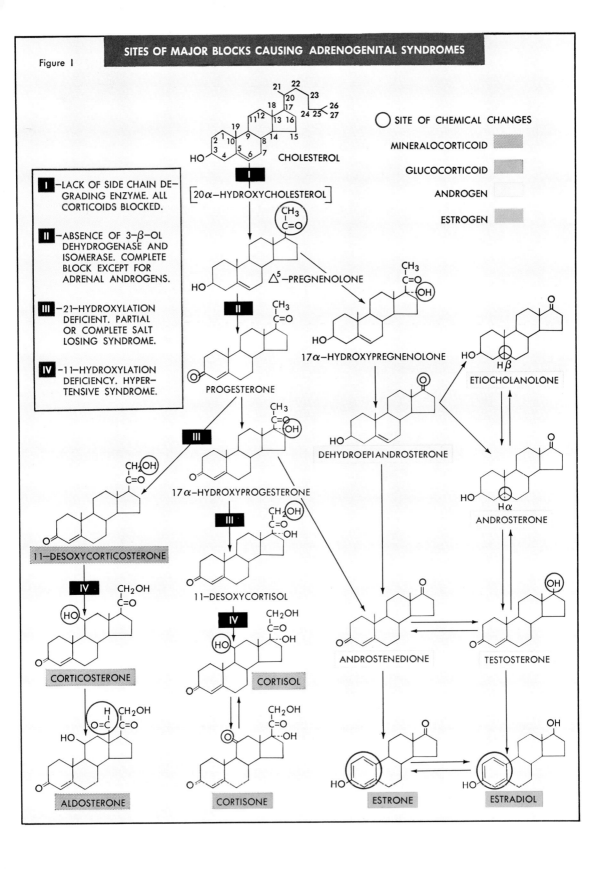

Figure I

SITES OF MAJOR BLOCKS CAUSING ADRENOGENITAL SYNDROMES

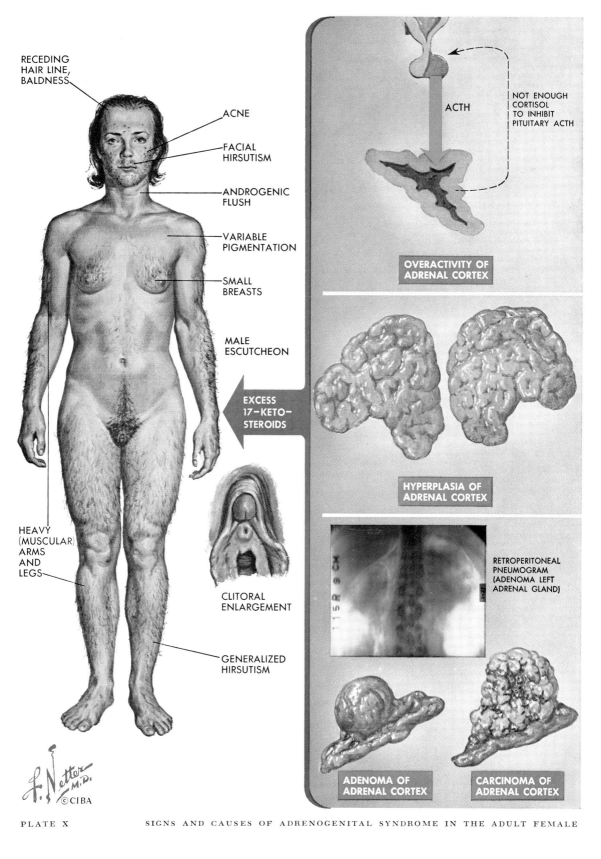

RECEDING
HAIR LINE,
BALDNESS

ACNE

FACIAL
HIRSUTISM

ANDROGENIC
FLUSH

VARIABLE
PIGMENTATION

SMALL
BREASTS

MALE
ESCUTCHEON

EXCESS
17–KETO–
STEROIDS

HEAVY
(MUSCULAR)
ARMS
AND
LEGS

CLITORAL
ENLARGEMENT

GENERALIZED
HIRSUTISM

ACTH

NOT ENOUGH
CORTISOL
TO INHIBIT
PITUITARY ACTH

OVERACTIVITY OF
ADRENAL CORTEX

HYPERPLASIA OF
ADRENAL CORTEX

RETROPERITONEAL
PNEUMOGRAM
(ADENOMA LEFT
ADRENAL GLAND)

ADENOMA OF
ADRENAL CORTEX

CARCINOMA OF
ADRENAL CORTEX

PLATE X   SIGNS AND CAUSES OF ADRENOGENITAL SYNDROME IN THE ADULT FEMALE

relatively large doses of mineralocorticoids, such as 9-alpha-fluorohydrocortisone or desoxycorticosterone acetate, as well as cortisol.

Hypertensive Syndrome: A block of hydroxylase at C-11 prevents production of cortisol and of aldosterone (Figure 1 and Plate XI). As in other cases there is an abundance of unblocked 17-ketosteroids and of the precursors of the blocked hormones. In this case one of the precursors is 11-desoxycorticosterone, itself a potent salt-retaining hormone, capable in excess of causing hypertension. In this instance, therefore, male macrogenitosomia and female pseudohermaphroditism are complicated by hypertension.

Postnatal Adrenogenital Syndrome

This is quite rare. In an overwhelming majority, symptoms are caused by a tumor and most frequently by an adenocarcinoma.

Signs and symptoms caused by an excess of 17-ketosteroids are similar to those found in the adult, except that androgenic changes are exaggerated. In the male the phallus assumes adult proportions, while the testicles remain small. Rarely the presence of adrenal rests in the testicles causes enlargement. In any case, there is absence of sperm in the ejaculate, differentiating the condition from precocious puberty. In the female the clitoris is enlarged, and there is male distribution of hair.

Diagnosis of the syndrome before maturity rests on the finding of elevated 17-ketosteroids or pregnanetriol in the urine.

Treatment consists of the administration of cortisol or one of its modern derivatives (see Table 1) in physiologic amounts but enough to suppress the excess of ACTH which becomes manifest by a sharp reduction in 17-ketosteroid output. This usually requires between 15 and 20 mg. of cortisol or between 0.5 and 0.75 mg. of dexamethasone daily per square meter of surface area. It is of inter-est that a more sensitive indicator of the effectiveness of suppressive therapy than 17-ketosteroid excretion is the daily urinary output of pregnanetriol, which normally does not exceed 2 to 3 mg. in children close to puberty.

In children who have the salt-losing syndrome, one would have to add a mineralocorticoid, such as small amounts (0.05 to 0.2 mg.) per day of fluorohydrocortisone or Percorten (desoxycorticosterone trimethylacetate) 10 to 25 mg. by injection every 3 to 4 weeks.

Adrenogenital Syndrome in the Adult
(Plate X)

The female develops a more masculine habitus, with receding hairline, hirsutism of body and face, atrophy of breasts and uterus, a male escutcheon, and enlargement of the clitoris. The latter, together with an excess of androgen, is probably responsible for the frequent increase in heterosexual sex drive. Deepening of the voice, whether induced by the adrenogenital syndrome or androgen therapy, is always irreversible. Menstruation usually ceases as does ovulation. Feminine distribution of fat disappears, to be replaced by heavier masculine musculature. The skin, in contrast to that of Cushing's syndrome which is thin and almost paperlike, becomes thick and resilient, reflecting the anabolic effect of the excess androgens.

This fully developed picture is relatively rare and must be differentiated from *benign androgenic adrenal hyperactivity* which is seen far more frequently. In this latter condition, women are somewhat obese, have quite a feminine habitus, the only abnormality being increasing hirsutism and sometimes an amenorrhea.

Among patients with benign androgenic adrenal hyperplasia with at most a slight bilateral enlargement of the adrenal cortices, one occasionally finds cases which have the same biochemical blocks found in the prenatal varieties. This is charac-

TABLE 1.

RELATIVE ANTI-INFLAMMATORY POTENCY AND SODIUM-RETAINING EFFECT OF VARIOUS CORTICOIDS USED IN THERAPY

COMPOUND	RELATIVE POTENCY COMPARED TO CORTISOL	RELATIVE SODIUM-RETAINING ACTIVITY
Cortisol	1	+ +
Cortisone Acetate	0.8	+ +
Prednisolone	4	+
Prednisone	3.5	+
Triamcinolone	5	0
6-Methylprednisolone	5	0
Haldranolone	10	0
Betamethasone	25	0
Dexamethasone*	30	0
9-α-fluorohydrocortisone	15	+ + + + +

*Available commercially as Gammacorten®.

terized by a partial block of cortisol synthesis, an accumulation of pregnanetriol which is diagnostically elevated above the upper normal limit of 2 mg./day in the urine, and the overproduction of 17-ketosteroids leading to rises up to 20 to 40 mg. in the urine in 24 hours. Such rare instances of the "prenatal syndrome" in adults are treated just as other androgenic hyperplasias or overactivities of the adrenal cortex — suppression with cortisol or one of its modern derivatives.

Course: In the adult, unless caused by rapidly growing adenoma or adenocarcinoma, the course is usually benign, although psychologically and socially traumatizing.

Diagnosis: This depends on laboratory determination of urinary 17-ketosteroids, which are usually only moderately elevated in hyperplasia (15 to 20 mg. per day), but quite high (30 to 150 mg. per day) in adenoma or adenocarcinoma. In the benign syndrome, 17-ketosteroids may be in the upper range of normal, remain-

ing constant from day to day even prior to ovulation instead of rising as they do normally.

Any elevation in 17-ketosteroid excretion above 20 mg. per day points to the adrenal as the source of excess androgen. In the absence of a 17-ketosteroid elevation, one is probably dealing with an ovarian androgenic tumor, such as an arrhenoblastoma, which tends to have normal or only slightly elevated 17-ketosteroid levels which are not suppressed by dexamethasone. Where abnormal amounts of androgen are being secreted by an ovarian or testicular tumor, 2,000 units of chorionic gonadotropin given intramuscularly on arising will cause a three- to five-fold increase in testosterone excretion in the urine specimen obtained during the next 24 hours. Where androgens are of adrenal origin, no such increase will be produced.

The differentiation between hyperplasia and tumor is made by the dexamethasone suppression test described on page

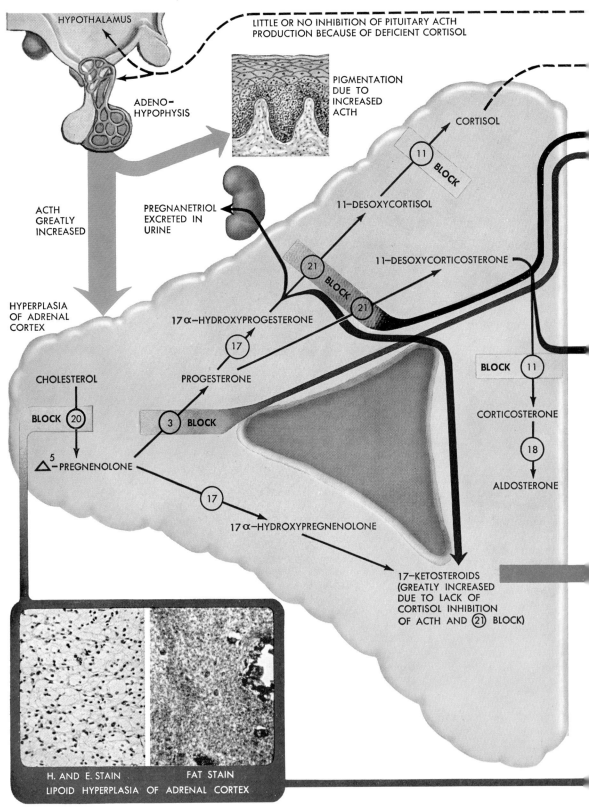

HYPOTHALAMUS

LITTLE OR NO INHIBITION OF PITUITARY ACTH
PRODUCTION BECAUSE OF DEFICIENT CORTISOL

ADENO-
HYPOPHYSIS

PIGMENTATION
DUE TO
INCREASED
ACTH

CORTISOL

11 BLOCK

11-DESOXYCORTISOL

ACTH
GREATLY
INCREASED

PREGNANETRIOL
EXCRETED IN
URINE

21 BLOCK

21

11-DESOXYCORTICOSTERONE

17α-HYDROXYPROGESTERONE

17

HYPERPLASIA
OF ADRENAL
CORTEX

PROGESTERONE

CHOLESTEROL

BLOCK 11

BLOCK 20

3 BLOCK

CORTICOSTERONE

$\triangle^5$-PREGNENOLONE

18

17

ALDOSTERONE

17α-HYDROXYPREGNENOLONE

17-KETOSTEROIDS
(GREATLY INCREASED
DUE TO LACK OF
CORTISOL INHIBITION
OF ACTH AND 21 BLOCK)

H. AND E. STAIN   FAT STAIN
LIPOID HYPERPLASIA OF ADRENAL CORTEX

PLATE XI

ADRENOGENITAL SYNDROMES PRODUCED BY BLOCK

- - - → CORTISOL DEFICIENT OR ABSENT

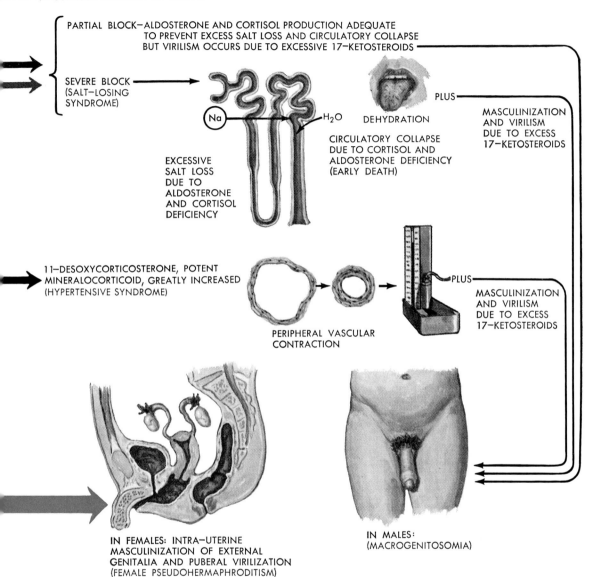

PARTIAL BLOCK—ALDOSTERONE AND CORTISOL PRODUCTION ADEQUATE TO PREVENT EXCESS SALT LOSS AND CIRCULATORY COLLAPSE BUT VIRILISM OCCURS DUE TO EXCESSIVE 17—KETOSTEROIDS

SEVERE BLOCK (SALT—LOSING SYNDROME)

Na → H_2O

DEHYDRATION

PLUS

MASCULINIZATION AND VIRILISM DUE TO EXCESS 17—KETOSTEROIDS

CIRCULATORY COLLAPSE DUE TO CORTISOL AND ALDOSTERONE DEFICIENCY (EARLY DEATH)

EXCESSIVE SALT LOSS DUE TO ALDOSTERONE AND CORTISOL DEFICIENCY

11—DESOXYCORTICOSTERONE, POTENT MINERALOCORTICOID, GREATLY INCREASED (HYPERTENSIVE SYNDROME)

PERIPHERAL VASCULAR CONTRACTION

PLUS

MASCULINIZATION AND VIRILISM DUE TO EXCESS 17—KETOSTEROIDS

IN FEMALES: INTRA—UTERINE MASCULINIZATION OF EXTERNAL GENITALIA AND PUBERAL VIRILIZATION (FEMALE PSEUDOHERMAPHRODITISM)

IN MALES: (MACROGENITOSOMIA)

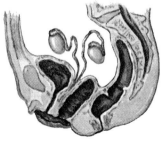

COMPLETE DEFICIENCY OF STEROID HORMONES, INCLUDING 17—KETOSTEROIDS: TESTICULAR ANDROGEN PRODUCTION ALSO IMPAIRED (LIPOID HYPERPLASIA)

GENOTYPIC MALE DEVELOPS FEMALE EXTERNAL GENITALIA DUE TO ABSENCE OF MASCULINIZING INFLUENCE OF ANDROGENS IN UTERO

54 and Plate IX. At 2 mg. per day, with tumors there is no suppression of 17-keto-steroids. In hyperplasia they are reduced 50 per cent or more. Unfortunately, differentiation between adenoma and adenocarcinoma by the 8-hour intravenous ACTH test utilized in Cushing's syndrome (page 57 and Plate IX) is not reliable in the adrenogenital syndrome.

Treatment

In the benign form, suppression with cortisol or one of its derivatives, such as dexamethasone which is nonsalt-retaining, is carried out. The equivalent of 10 mg. of cortisol is given by mouth on arising, at 3 p.m., and as late in the evening as compatible with sleep in order to suppress the maximal ACTH secretion occurring, as a rule, from 2 a.m. to 6 a.m. After suppression has been achieved for a matter of months, dosages may sometimes be reduced without recrudescence. The supplementary administration of small dosage of estrogens has been advocated to reduce hirsutism.

In the presence of adenoma or adenocarcinoma, extirpation is required. The pre- and postoperative therapy required in Cushing's syndrome is not usually nec-essary since, in the absence of an excess of cortisol, ACTH and the contralateral adrenal gland are not suppressed and the patient can stand the stress of operation well. Wound healing is exceptionally good.

SUMMARY

Within the relatively few years that have passed since the synthesis of 11-des-oxycorticosterone by Reichstein in 1939, truly stupendous progress has been made in the field of adrenal pathophysiology.

Relatively simple tests have been evolved, and laboratory methods for determining hormone levels have become generally available. Moreover, hormones have been synthesized so that complete and adequate substitution therapy is easily achieved.

Thus the definitive medical management, as well as the surgical correction of nearly all adrenal diseases, is now well worked out.

It is hoped that this brief and somewhat oversimplified discussion will be found both stimulating and helpful to my colleagues in their handling of these admittedly complex conditions.

ACKNOWLEDGMENTS

We are indebted to Professor A. Prader, Head, Pediatric Clinic, Zurich University, and Dr. R. E. Seibenmann, Pathological Institute, Zurich University, Switzerland, for kindly providing the photomicrographs from their cases, used in Plate XI, pages 64-65.

Plate VI, which appears on page 48, was developed in collaboration with Calvin Ezrin, M.D., F.R.C.P., Toronto General Hospital, Associate, Department of Medicine, Research Associate, Department of Pathology, Division of Neuropathology, University of Toronto, Canada.